Physical Therapy for Horses

An Illustrated Guide to Anatomy, Biomechanics, Massage, Stretching, and Rehabilitation

Helle Katrine Kleven

Translated by Karen M. Brittle and Anja Cain

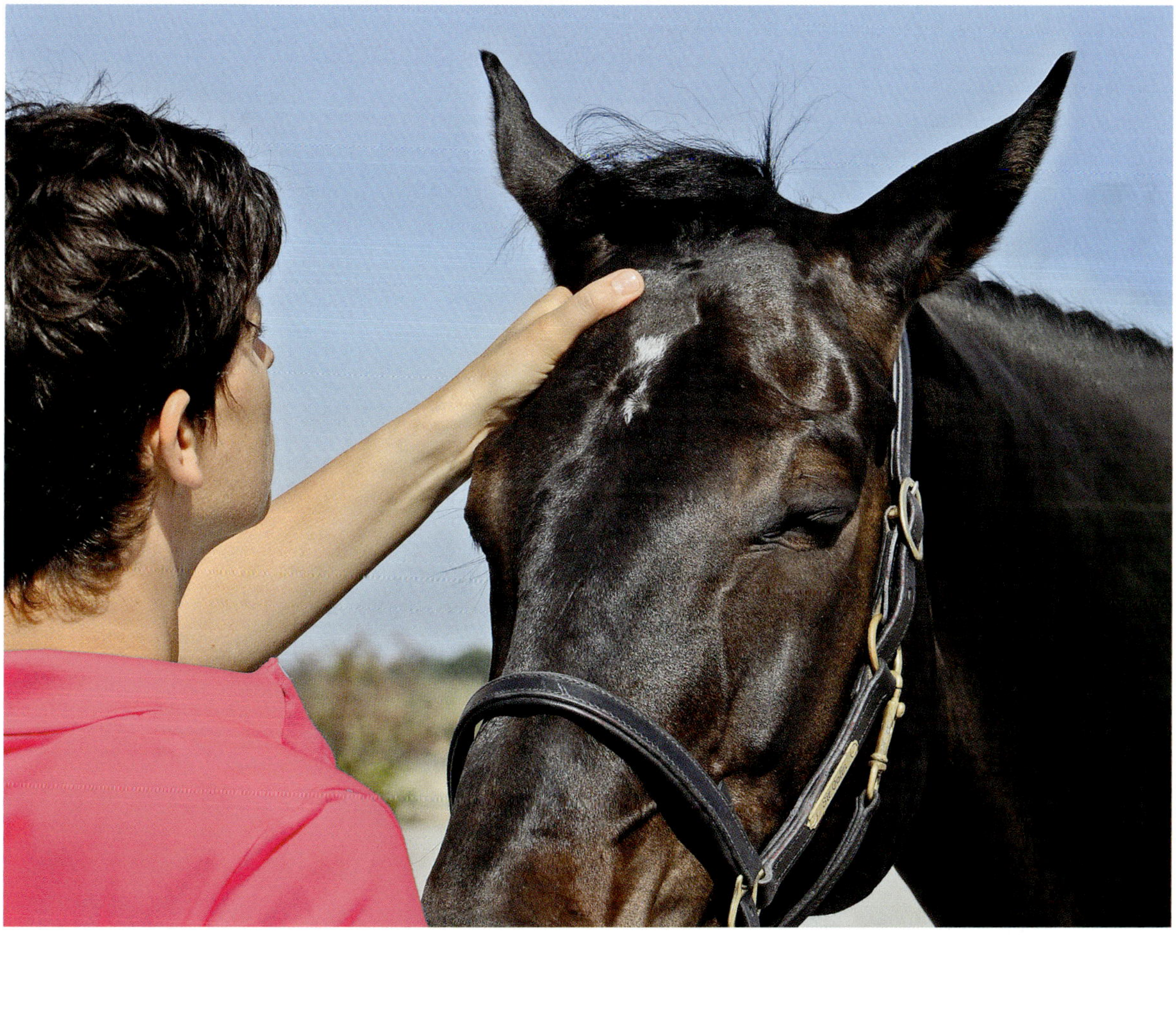

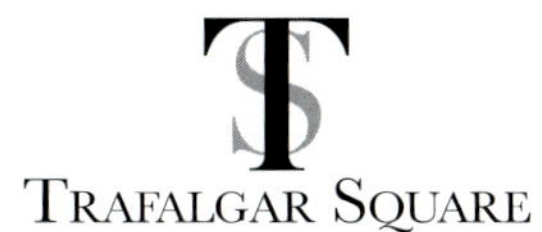

Trafalgar Square

First published in the English language in 2019 by
Trafalgar Square Books
an imprint of the Stable Book Group
32 Court Street, Suite 2109
Brooklyn, NY 11201
www.trafalgarbooks.com

Originally published in the German language as *Biomechanik und Physiotherapie für Pferde* by FNverlag
der Deutschen Reiterlichen Verienigung GmbH, Warendorf

ISBN: 978 1 57076 938 2
Library of Congress Control Number: 2019937923

All photographs by Maximilian Schreiner, except: p. 67 *left* (Arnd Bronkhorst from *FEI World Equestrian
Games Aachen 2006*); pp. 133 *left*, 138 *right*, 151 *left*, 158 *right*, 200, 203 *right* (Petra Huml); pp. 60 *top*, 199
(Fotohaus Kiepker from *Ausbildung junger Pferde*); pp. 3, 4, 6, 9, 16, 27 *left top*; 32, 35, 57 *right*, 60 *bottom*,
69, 83, 85, 92, 93, 96, 98, 99, 100, 102, 119, 139, 168 *right bottom*, 169, 171 *left*, 185 *bottom*, 189, 203 left,
213, 230 (Helle Katrine Kleven); p. 91 (Ulrich Neddens & Sabine Kämper GbR—Tierfotografie from *Siege
warden im Stall errungen*); pp. 13, 81 (Peter Prohn from *Gesunde Hufe—kein Zufall* and *FN-Handbuch
Pferdewirt*); p. ix (Julia Rau); pp. 171 *right*, 177, 179, 181 *right*, 185 *top*, 187, 201 (Norbert Schamper from
Physiotherapie für Pferde); pp. 34, 47 *right*, 215 (Rika Schneider); pp. 110, 111, 195 (Barbara Schnell from
Ausbildung junger Pferde); p. 27 *left top* (Jacques Toffi from *Physiotherapie für Pferde*); pp. 71 *left*, 123,
196, 197, 198 (Julia Kathmann).

Design by Ute Schmoll, Captain Pixel, Brad Schwalbach
Cover design by RM Didier
Index by Andrea M. Jones (www.jonesliteraryservices.com)
Typefaces: DIN

Printed in China

10 9 8 7 6

Many thanks to my family, especially my daughters,
Kristin and Malin. I want to dedicate this book to you.
When "Mama" needed to work on this book, your
understanding and support was fantastic. I promise
you now that it is finished, we'll catch up on everything.
The first thing we're going to do: travel to Rome!

TRANSLATORS' NOTE

*The concepts of muscular engagement, tone, and tension are vital components of Helle Kleven's philosophy and work. It seems important to note that these words have the same root in German—*Spannung*—and therefore, are also used somewhat interchangeably. For the purpose of the English text, we translated *Spannung* as "engagement" (positive connotation) or "tone" (neutral implication); and *Verspannung* as "tension" or "accumulated tension" (negative connotation).

Karen M. Brittle and Anja Cain

Contents

Contents

Contents

Foreword by Bettina Hoy

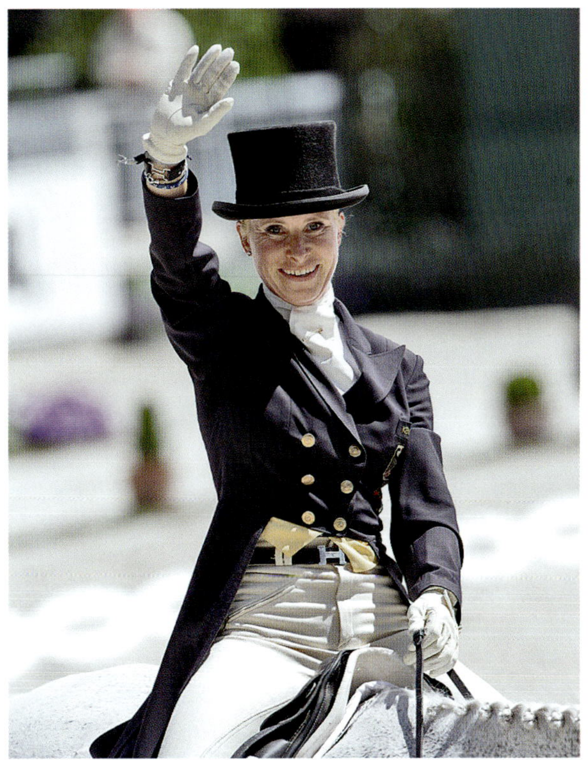

Some years have passed since the publication of Helle Kleven's first book, for which I also had the pleasure of writing the Foreword. During this time, the use of physical therapy for both competitive sport horses and pleasure horses has become firmly established. The inclusion of physical therapy practices in equestrian sport marked a milestone for the prevention and treatment of soft tissue injuries, and as such, for the optimization of horse care.

I remember well, back in 1996, when I got to know Helle Kleven during the preparatory courses for the Olympic Games. I was so excited. It was easy to recognize how important—and how helpful—the practical exercises such as massage and stretching were. I noticed what positive effects these techniques had when regularly applied.

Later, in England, I also worked regularly with horse physical therapists: when training to avoid certain problems, but also at competitions. I determined that through this work, my horses were both more ready to work and more relaxed. This prevented and reduced musculoskeletal injuries. If a horse had to break from training due to an injury, physical therapy provided excellent support to the rehabilitation process. In the meantime, it's now become commonplace for every serious team, including most of today's internationally competitive riders, to include a physical therapist as part of the medical care team.

This book elaborates on an extremely important area of biomechanics, the functional ability of the musculoskeletal system. For human athletes, biomechanics is now an established component of sports science—above all, helping to improve movement patterns. I'm so pleased that such knowledge will now be available for equestrian sports.

With knowledge about the correct movement patterns, riders and trainers will be able to recognize how to support the developmental success and physical resilience of the horse, and can adjust their conditioning and training plan accordingly. This applies to all branches of equestrian sport, from amateur riders to pleasure riders to top professionals.

Bettina Hoy
German Olympic Event Rider

Foreword by Victoria Max-Theurer

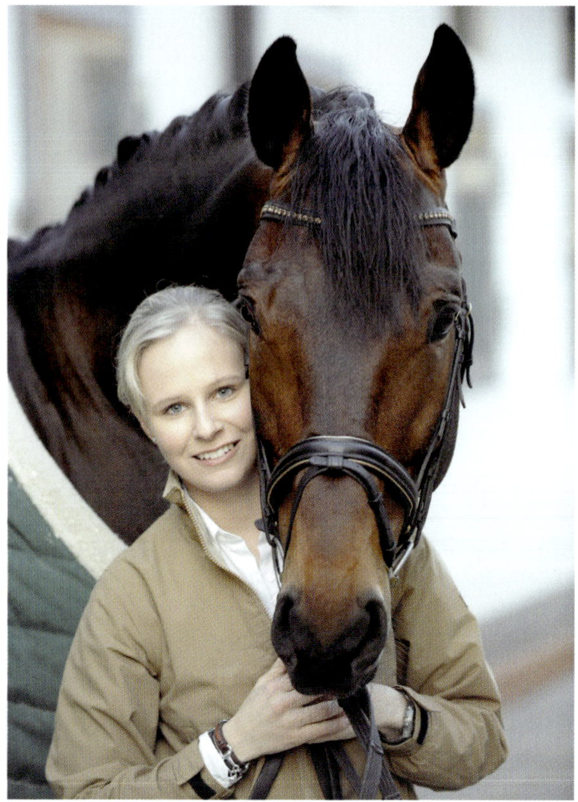

For a long time now, top human athletes have recognized the application of physical therapy as a training measure. In equestrian sport, too, recent years have brought more and more recognition of its value. My family and I have had our horses treated by a physical therapist for many years now and have had very positive experiences. Today, we consider this essential. Helle Kleven has treated our horses regularly since 2010. She comes to us in Austria every other week and has accompanied us to all major competitions, including the Rio Olympics in 2016.

I especially value that Helle can easily adjust her techniques to meet the needs of each individual horse, whether a stallion or a sensitive mare, and how she genuinely takes an interest in the horse and his development. To me, it's so important that she does not simply treat them and then leave, but rather regularly observes the horses go under saddle. In this way, we can both describe what we're seeing and seek solutions. This makes for a solid and trustful partnership.

Our continuous collaboration offers the advantage that we do not have to work wonders in a short amount of time, which most often only leads to short-term success anyway. Problems, such as a muscular issue, can be identified and treated much more effectively over time. This applies not only to horses that are already in training but even during the early conditioning phases or when they are getting started with more intense work. Physical therapy at these times prepares horses for more intense work and helps to avoid strain.

The possibilities that physical therapy offers are multifaceted. Helle is proficient in and uses a broad spectrum of techniques and is, therefore, very flexible and versatile in how she approaches her work. New developments are happening all the time in this area. New scientific findings and treatment possibilities should be used in order to achieve optimal well-being for the horse and, thereby, also improve his performance. Therefore, I see it as extremely positive that Helle continues to educate herself further. She shares so much of her extensive knowledge in this book. All riders who care about their horse's health will benefit from this, as well as the many practical tips offered.

Victoria Max-Theurer
Austrian Olympic Dressage Rider

Preface

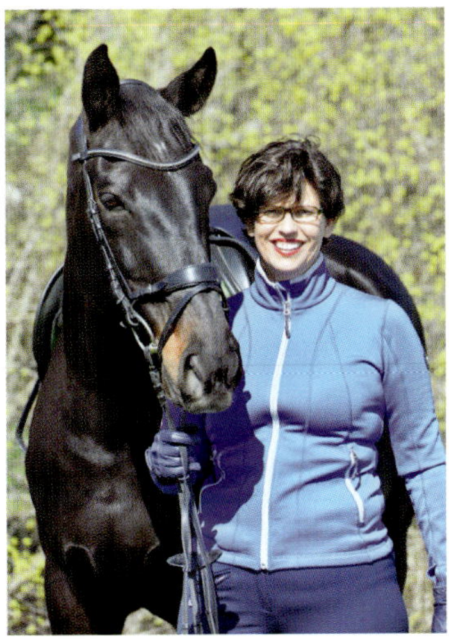

So much has happened in the field of physical therapy since the publication of my first book, which was published in German in 2000. It has been wonderful to experience how this form of therapy has become an important part of health management for horses. This motivated me anew to write this, my second book, which was originally published in German in 2009, and which I have now expanded even further, including newly acquired knowledge in the field of physical therapy.

Because we influence the movement patterns of our horse on a daily basis, it is my wish that all riders, horse owners, and trainers become familiar with their horse's movement patterns. With this in mind, I've written this book in such a way that prior medical knowledge is not needed to understand it. In the sections on biomechanics (see p. 34), I describe the movement patterns of the horse. What movements take place and where? What can your horse do? What can't he? How can you recognize when "blockages" are present? How can you tell whether your horse has the physical stability for the task at hand? Seeing that we train our horse every day with the goal of strengthening his musculoskeletal system and achieving suppleness, basic knowledge of anatomy and biomechanics is a "must," regardless of your riding level or discipline. Within my description of biomechanics, you'll find many practical examples.

After explaining the theory, I want to educate your eye and "feel," so that you can see and palpate when something isn't right. You'll find guidelines for massage and stretching. You can apply these techniques both preventively and as a supplement to therapy. In addition I've written about therapies that incorporate ice, water, heat, Matrix Rhythm therapy, TENS, and laser and magnetic therapy. I discuss kinesiology tape and the Equicore System, both of which are important techniques for rehabilitation. These therapies are especially suited for minimizing the extent of an injury as much as possible, for supporting the affected structures during rehabilitation, and for promoting quick and successful healing.

In addition, active rehabilitation presents possibilities for reestablishing the physical condition that existed before an injury or drop in performance. With the help of a rehabilitation plan, the body can be built back up again, physically and/or mentally.

Last, I'll introduce preventive measures, which can be employed to avoid musculoskeletal injuries and accumulated tension.

I am thoroughly convinced that the better a rider or horse owner understands the horse's anatomy and biomechanics, the better she can develop the horse's natural movement under saddle and avoid tension, injury, and "wear and tear." In this sense, I hope that you will find the science around the horse's musculoskeletal system just as interesting and fascinating as I do. You will certainly find it automatically slips into your daily work with your horse. Now, I wish you lots of fun reading and practicing!

Helle Kleven

Introduction to Physical Therapy for Horses

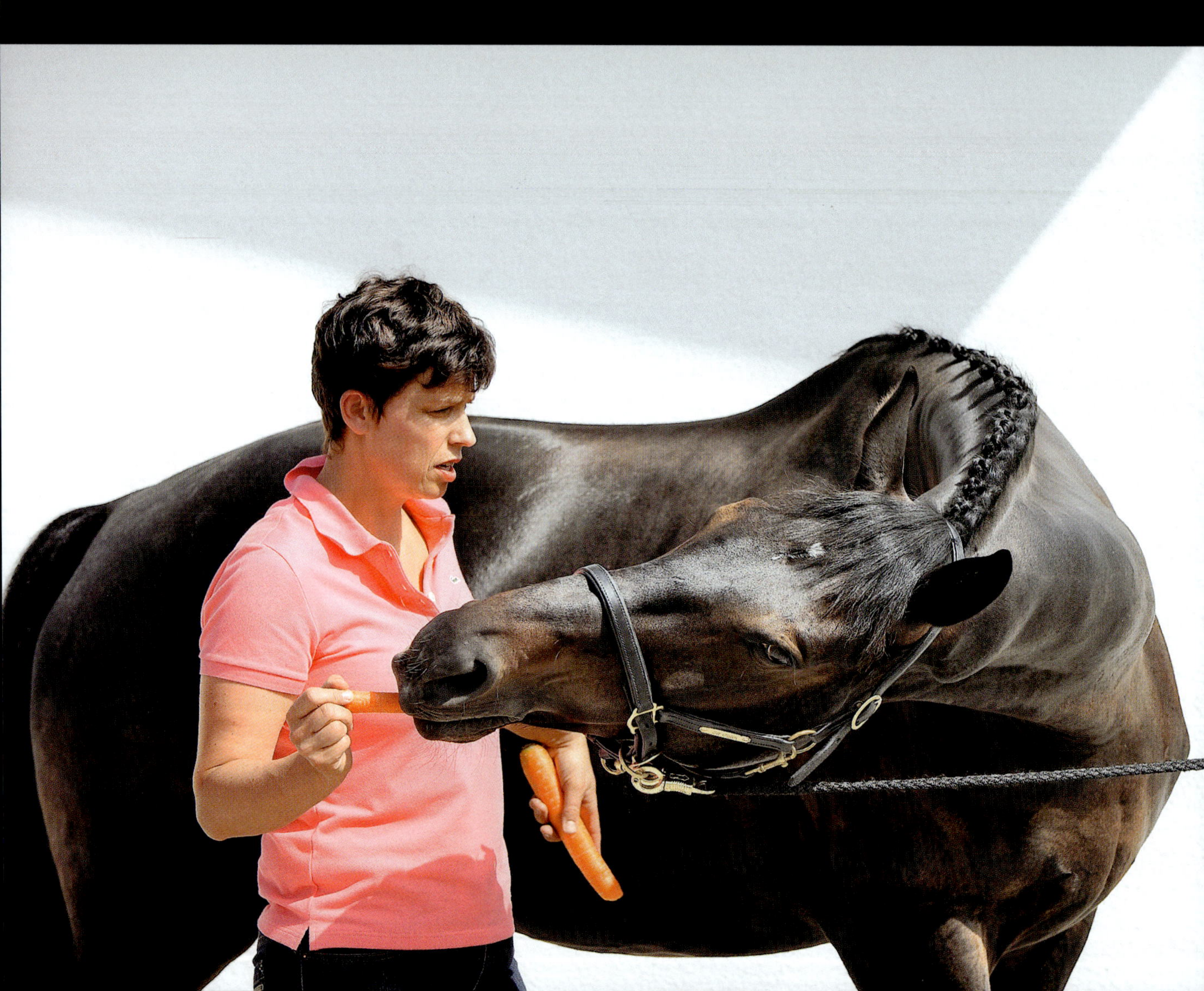

You've likely already benefited from physical therapy treatment at some point in your life due to injury. With our way of living today, we use our musculoskeletal system in a one-sided way, and therefore, develop problems over the course of our lifetime, whether through work, trauma, or our hobby—riding! Pleasure riders and competitive riders are equally affected.

In human medicine, physical therapy is already an important component of medical training and has essential significance for the care and treatment of many complaints. Everyone can benefit—from newborn babies to seniors of advanced age. Moreover, physical therapy has also come to play an important role in an athlete's success. When we think about major events, such as the European or World Championships or the Olympic Games, we see physical therapy in application across all kinds of sports. In the meantime, professional teams have hired specialists who work daily with their athletes, checking in on their musculoskeletal system and directly influencing them. Even in the amateur realm, there are hardly any athletes who haven't had a physical therapy treatment at least once if not on a regular basis.

It's become quite similar in equestrian sports. In the past few years, this form of therapy has won increasing importance here, too. Most professional riders have already seen its advantage for human athletes. So, they arrange for their "investment"—their horse—to be checked and treated regularly. However, a treatment can also work wonders for the pleasure horse. Every rider knows the feeling: "something's not right with my horse." Exercises aren't working anymore, the horse isn't supple, he's stiff on one side, he's falling out with his back, looks unwell, and more. For most of us, sooner or later, it becomes impossible to ignore these changes in performance.

In recent years, larger equine veterinary clinics have begun employing physical therapists to supervise physical therapy and rehabilitation for their patients. But, there's a long way ahead of us and the future is exciting. There's hope that veterinarians and animal physical therapists will work together even more closely, in order to successfully treat horses and restore their good health.

The three foundational components of equine physical therapy are the clinical diagnosis, treatment (evidence based), and supervised rehabilitation. Our treatment area primarily encompasses the musculoskeletal system, including back problems, muscular problems, "blockages," and instabilities, to mention a few, all of which can lead to compromised performance. To successfully treat these ailments, you need expert knowledge about the function of muscles and their relationship to the joints and about the movement patterns in the body (functional biomechanics). A physical therapist must be able to assess the horse's nutritional state, overall condition, farrier work and equipment (saddle, girth, reins, cavesson, auxiliary reins, for example). In addition, she must be able to evaluate the dynamics between rider and horse. As you can see, a good physical therapist demonstrates diverse and vast competency around horses.

Why the Current Trend Toward Physical Therapy?

The developments in horse breeding go hand in hand with what riders are looking for. No matter what element of riding you engage in at home, whether jumping, dressage, Western, or endurance riding, you want a horse that is best suited to your purpose. It's even noticeably easier to train a horse that is already "heading in the right direction" because of his innate ability to move well than it is to train a horse that has to work against his natural tendencies. Breeders want to make things easier for you. Horses are being bred with lots of capability for movement and they are also very sensitive and responsive to your body language. This makes it easier for you and, at the same time, more difficult. In contrast to the highly specialized horses of today,

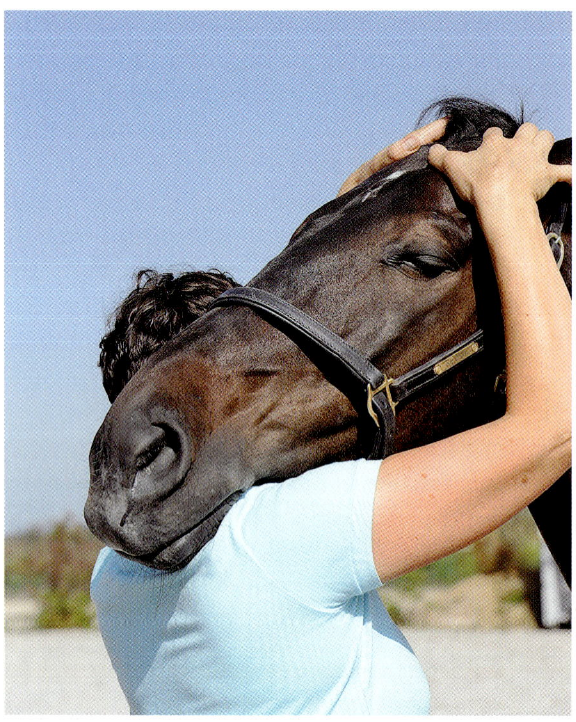

During a massage, the horse can truly relax. This fosters trust between horse and human.

humans have generally lost some of the body awareness they had in earlier times. From the time they are children in school, through college and the workplace, they spend most of their time sitting. Therefore, humans often noticeably lack mobility, stability, and coordination. You can certainly imagine that this leads to communication problems between horse and rider, through which horses often feel the stress the most.

In this, physical therapy for horses can be a true help and can bring relief. Experience has shown that horses benefit and enjoy it when they are "loosened up" and "blockages" are resolved through physical therapy treatments. This is also true with just massage and stretching, which the "layperson" can do. You will notice that your horse can become wonderfully relaxed from this. The practice of massaging and stretching the horse can also lead to improved trust. Even after a short time, you'll see that your horse enjoys the unusual way of

interacting with you, and you will soon notice a positive change when riding. In addition, physical therapy offers the possibility to keep your horse fit if he has to take time off due to injury, is being rehabbed, or is lacking in positive tone throughout his body.

When and Where Can Physical Therapy Be Applied?

Physical therapy can be successfully applied for many health problems. I'd like to give you a few hints about the sources of problems, how they come to pass, and how you can recognize the symptoms. You'll then find treatment tips and methods in the following chapters.

Back and Neck Problems

There's nothing better than when a horse engages his back and you have the wonderful feeling of being carried along with his movement. For this to happen, your horse needs a healthy, mobile, and strong neck and back, not to mention a well-balanced rider! But how can you recognize that all is well with your horse's spinal column?

When your horse will quietly stand with his weight evenly distributed on all four feet, his musculature will give you your first hint about the status of his spinal column. In the neck, his topline must be more pronounced than the underside of the neck, and the neck should be filled out evenly—with no dips in front of the shoulder blade. From withers to tail, you should see a round, fleshy, evenly pronounced musculature.[1] When grooming, you can press firmly, without causing the horse to "fall out" through his back.

When riding, a sign of an engaged back is that the horse is comfortable with sitting trot, for example. When observing a horse at walk or trot, you should

---

[1] These body conditions cannot be expected in a young or untrained horse. Here, I'm describing an adult horse that is in regular training.

Physical Therapy for Horses

see an alternating contraction and relaxation of the muscles on the right and left side of the back behind the saddle area. The relaxed tail swings gently left and right, except for specific breeds that carry their tail to one side as a breed characteristic. (In chapter 5, "Observation," I explore this subject more closely.)

Initial signs that the horse is unwell can be noticed during grooming. It's likely the horse will behave restlessly, "moving about," or he'll move away from touch with his back or neck. Perhaps you've already noticed one that demonstrates tension and resistance when being saddled. Your horse might also arch his back when you go to mount, hollow his back or, in extreme cases, even go down on his knees. Have you ever ridden a horse that takes a really long time to get "through"? Is one side noticeably stiffer than the other? A horse with neck or back problems may also have problems with his rhythm or appear lame. This horse can no longer take weight onto his hindquarters. He travels more on the forehand and "leans" on the reins. When the normal movement of the back is restricted, it will also affect the length of stride. The horse will take shorter steps. Even just the presence of a single one of these symptoms will show you—as an observant rider—that there's a problem in the spinal region. This can lead to a performance injury or even a refusal to work.

Unfortunately, the spinal column is often affected by various other malfunctions in the body. Pain in this area can be a primary or secondary complaint. This means the source of a problem may be in the spinal column for degenerative ailments (I'm sure you've heard of "kissing spine" often enough), but it could lie in an acute or chronic blockage. The problem could, in fact, have its source in a completely different location in the body, such as in the extremities. For example, an underlying lameness could cause back pain because it alters the movement pattern, and the symptoms of back pain may overshadow the lameness. New studies have proven that when there's a lameness in a limb, it only takes a few days for that to lead to a change in muscle

tone. A decrease in strength in the deep, stabilizing musculature will result.

In addition, organ dysfunction, such as an ailment of the liver or lungs, can have a secondary effect on the back.

Unnatural Head and Tail Carriage

An unnatural head and tail carriage is a sign that the spine is not how it should be. This can indicate limitations in movement and/or that the spinal column is so positioned to avoid pain.

The more relaxed a horse can stand, the less muscular power he needs to use. A sign of a functional disorder in the poll can already be observed when the horse is standing still. You can recognize that the horse is not carrying his neck in a relaxed position. The head is either stretched out or bent too tightly. When riding, you'll notice that your horse will not allow himself to be bent to one side when positioned, and gets crooked at the poll or won't move toward the bit.

During movement, the tail should hang in a relaxed manner and swing loosely back and forth. If the horse

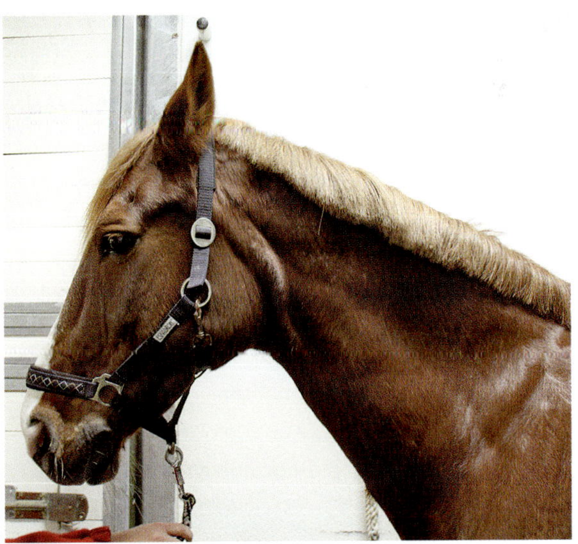

With this 19-year-old horse, you can see that the underside of the neck is overly pronounced and his head and neck carriage is not relaxed.

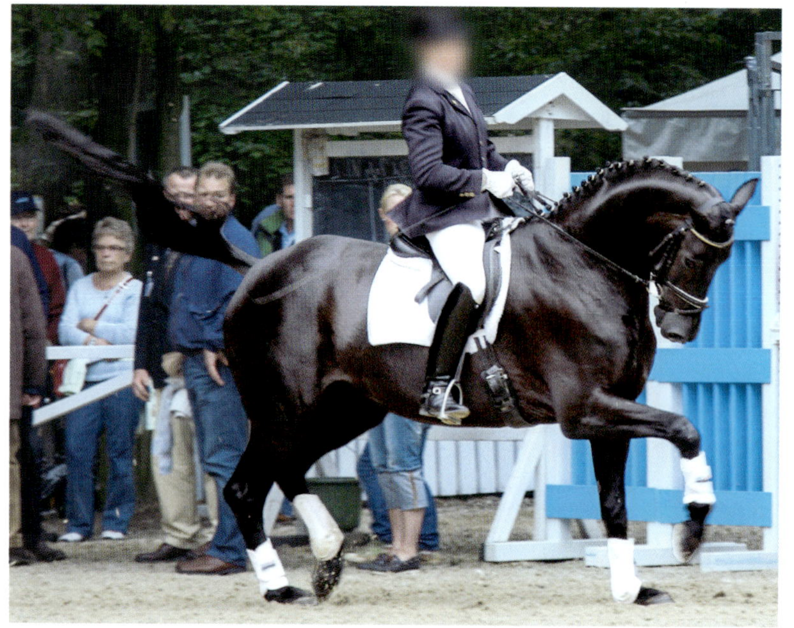

Pay attention to tail carriage. Because of the hyper-flexion (overstretch) of the neck, the tension goes all the way to the tail. At the same time, this horse is physically unstable. Although he appears muscular, he has no stability in his body. This is recognizable through the weak pastern and sagging of the trunk.

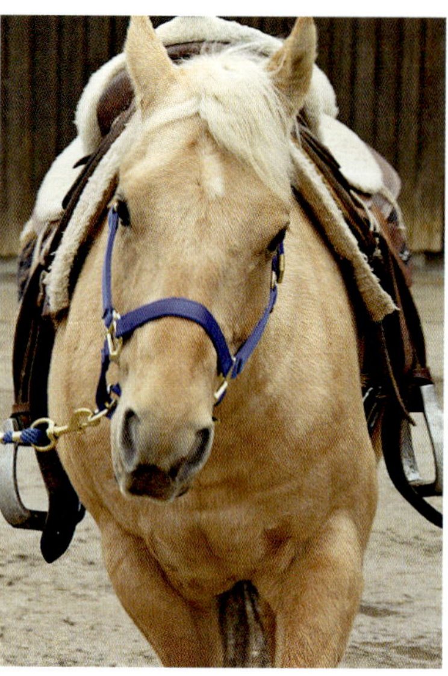

A horse with a crooked head carriage. The source can be a blockage in the poll.

doesn't carry his tail in the middle, it can be a sign that the muscles in the back are short on one side. The tail will travel toward the side where the muscles are shortened. Caused by the shortened musculature on one side, the horse may have trouble bending the other way and getting the necessary longitudinal bend. Another way of saying this: when the horse carries his tail off to the left, you'll likely have problems getting longitudinal bend tracking right. The symptom of a tail that's carried off to one side can even be an indication of limited movement in the neck. In this case, the source of the problem and the symptom are found far apart from one another.

There are exceptions: Arabian horses often carry their tails off to the left but without being limited in the bend to the right.

Another possibility is that this dysfunction is caused by the stretch of the sacrum against the iliac bone or heightened tension in the large pelvic ligaments. These horses either hold their tails too high, clamp them down, and/or carry them off to one side. In these cases, horses often also have problems shifting weight onto the hindquarters. They may demonstrate an uneven rhythm or regularly switch leads behind when cantering (cross-cantering).

A little observation: horses have no problem reaching their back with their teeth. That's an indication of a good moving neck according to many horse owners. But horses are "movement artists," with a repertoire of trick movements. These "abilities" are also a problem when you ride. A simple example: you're riding a volte, during which you want to see the horse's inside eye and nostril. That's how you'll know your horse is positioned correctly. Let's imagine the horse has a blockage in his poll. What does he do? He turns his head instead of positioning it. You definitely can see his inside eye, but not the inside nostril. Yes, it's possible to ride a ring figure that looks like a volte, but it won't be correct. The horse cannot bend around your inside leg optimally and you must do too much with your hand.

Physical Therapy for Horses

Stiff or Blocked Joints

Has one of your riding friends ever determined that your or her horse has a "popped-out vertebra?" In your mind, you see before you a vertebra that's clearly positioned to the side of the spinal column. But luckily, that's only your imagination.

More accurately, it looks like this: when a horse is worked incorrectly over a long period of time or, for example, he makes a sudden movement that's too much for the joint, the soft tissue that surrounds the joint will be overburdened or overstretched. The musculature that lies around the joint is also rich in nerves and receptors, which measure the length of the muscles. This means the musculature shortens to protect the affected joint. This can only occur for a short period of time or else, worst case, the musculature will remain in this contracted state. This, in turn, leads to a blockage.

You've almost certainly experienced this yourself; for example, when you wake up in the morning and have a stiff neck, and can neither turn your head nor stretch. That's a blockage in the neck and the pain that you feel is a tensing of the muscles—it's not the joint. The joint experiences a movement limitation. (Unfortunately, as I mentioned above, people often describe this as a "popped-out vertebra," which I don't like to hear.) This blockage can affect both sides or just one side. Apply this to a horse, and it could mean that you ride to the right without any problem, but tracking left, it feels as if you're riding a completely different horse.

Where does the description "popped out a vertebra" even come from? This term unfortunately became common after years of use by the medical layperson, perhaps because it's easier to picture and it's a catchier phrase.

In fact, the individual vertebrae of the spinal column link together in such a way that a major shift of a vertebra would only be possible with enormous strength applied from the outside. If this should happen, the damage to the spinal cord would

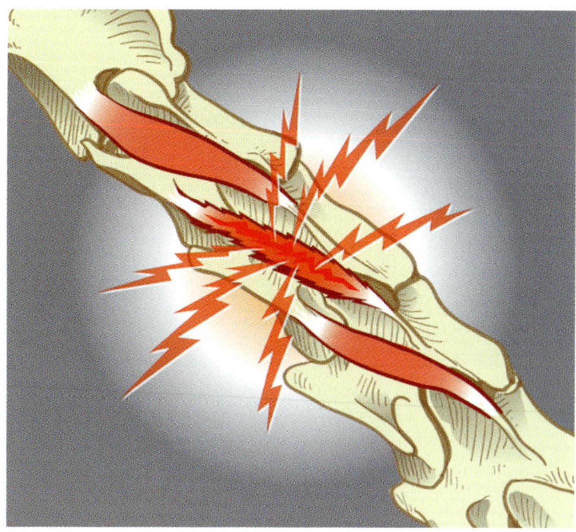

Ligaments, joint capsules, menisci of the neck vertebrae and musculature, which lie near to joints, can cause a blockage like we see here in a neck vertebra. The affected deep muscles tense up and cause immobility of the joint.

unfortunately be so significant that the horse would not survive this accident. The true source of blockages, which is what we're talking about here, is the braced/tensed soft tissue, which can develop so much strength that it causes a vertebra to rotate or can even deform one. This disorder can be perceived both through touch and visually. You can feel the muscular tension and/or see a sideways tilted spinous process in the thoracic or lumbar vertebra compared to other spinal processes, which are aligned. When you look down on the horse from above, it will be evident that the line of the spinal column includes small curves. Even the large pelvic bone can get pulled out of line by a tight muscle, resulting in a so-called misaligned pelvis. With such an example, it will become very clear how much strength the muscles can apply.

Fact: The bones of the small joints in the neck vertebrae do not fit together exactly. Small discs made of cartilage even out this imprecision. It is believed that if something causes them to shrink or "get caught" during movement (for example, a trauma such as a fall, hit, or bump), they become inflamed, which can also trigger an acute blockage.

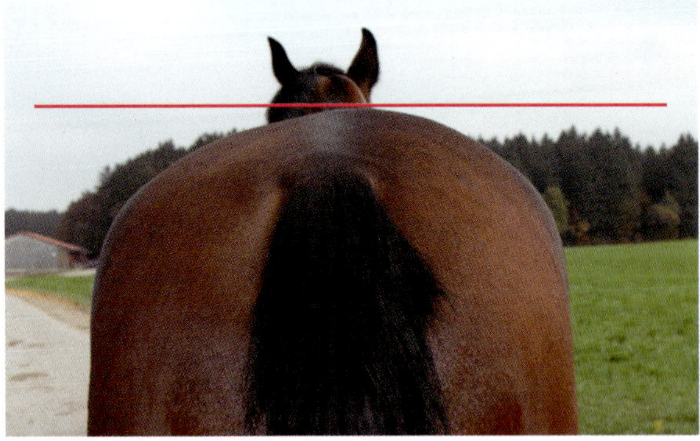

A misaligned pelvis can originate from blockages in the spinal column or trauma.

When the blockage is in the region of the spinal area, the connection between body and brain is interrupted. The reason is because the nerve must pass through a tight canal between two vertebrae before leaving the spinal column. Through the blockages in the vertebrae, the soft tissue swells around the column, which leads to pressure on the nerve. This, in turn, causes problems with coordination such as stumbling and uneven rhythm, lost strength, muscular tension, circulatory and metabolic disorders, and even lamenesses because the compressed nerve signals pain. As with people who have problems with their sciatic nerve, the pain may not show up in the back. These patients feel pain in the area of the hip joint, upper thigh, knee joint, or even ankle joint. In horses, unnatural sweat patterns (round, wet spots) can also be a hint about blockages in the spinal region, which demonstrates how the symptom can be located far from the source of the problem!

In an acute state, this muscular tension/blockage is very painful, as the circulation to the muscle is no longer good and it can very quickly become acidic. When the blockage exists over a long period of time, the affected soft tissue begins to change. The muscles "go to sleep" and, in the short term, they begin to work like a corset surrounding the joint. The blocked joint can no longer move optimally. In this condition, the joint itself is not the source of any pain, but for the musculoskeletal system it's a major strain, which can quickly lead to secondary tension and injury. Somehow, the body must balance out the limitations on movement. So, the other areas must move more strongly, even "over moving," which once again can lead to overstressing those joints and, therefore, creating even further injury. It starts a vicious circle, which over time can lead to more secondary blocks or cause more injury—all originating from the primary blockage.

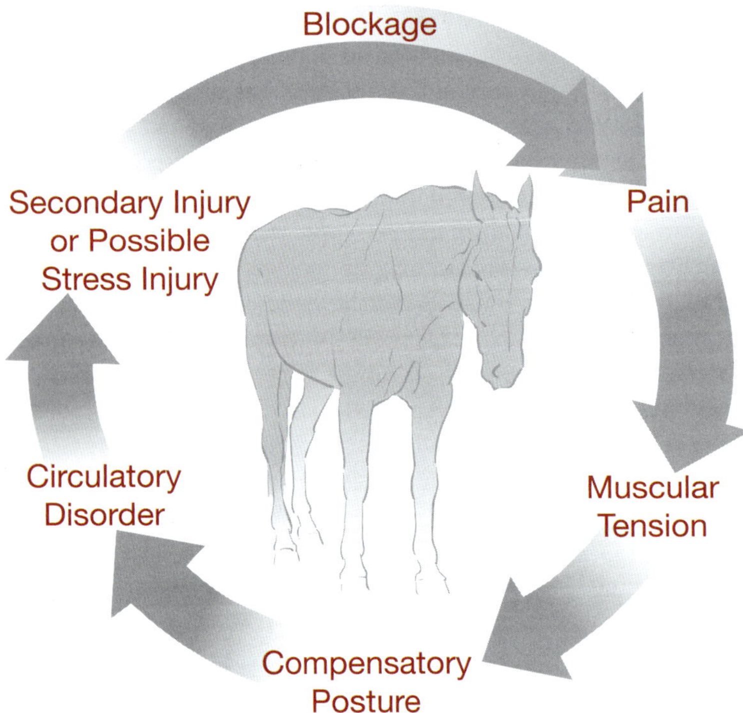

An acute blockage is always painful. This pain automatically triggers muscular tension and the horse attempts to relieve pain by adopting an "avoiding" posture. All of the factors lead to a circulatory disorder and secondary blockages. Injury and overstressing a body part are hardly avoidable. Over time, more and more body parts will continue to be pulled into this vicious circle. The intensity and number of problems will increase for the horse.

Physical Therapy for Horses

Normally, acute blocks that originate from a trauma or out-of-control movement go away by themselves in one to three days. If they stay or if they're caused by ill use, they will be difficult to "release" through riding. It's highly recommended that you allow them to be released by treatment from a physical therapist or osteopath.

During this treatment, you'll now and then hear a noise like a joint cracking. The customer then thinks that the joint has now been brought back to the right position and the vertebra has been "shoved back into place." But one cannot shove something back into place that was never "popped out of place" to begin with! This crackling noise is instead caused by a vacuum in the joint (see "Clicking Joints," p. 20).

A blockage can also originate in the limbs. For all joints in these areas of the body, bending and stretching are the major movements. In addition, almost all joints in the limbs can, to a lesser extent, turn sideways and to the inside and outside. These small movements are important in order for full range of motion to be possible. This means that if these small movements are blocked, the horse is not in the position to stretch or bend to the max with the affected joint. These small movements are not only significant to the limbs, they are essential to all joints in the body.

Instability in the Body

Blockages aren't the only problem that your horse faces. The opposite, meaning too much mobility (also referred to as instability/hypermobility) is just as problematic for the horse's performance as are mobility limitations. In my more than 20 years of professional experience, I had to realize that horses can also tend toward instability/hypermobility. There are many reasons for this, such as a trauma or training methods. So, too, horses that have been bred for big movement can tend toward instability/ hypermobility.

Actually, horses have little mobility in their back. The thoracic and lumbar vertebrae are relatively immobile when compared to those of dogs, cats, and cheetahs. This condition offers horses the enormous advantage that they can travel a long distance at a fast pace with relatively little output of energy. In contrast, the "hunters" have a very flexible spine, but they require a lot more energy for muscular activity.

If you observe the movement of dressage horses over the last 30 years, you can see a clear change. Horses now have more impulsion and overall spectacular movement. This way of going is only possible because of a breeding trend for more mobility in the back. The danger is that consequently we're also reducing the horse's stability through the back. The result is a higher risk of musculoskeletal injury.

For this reason, too, it's important to build up the horse's training systematically: namely by deliberately strengthening the deep, stabilizing muscles (see chapter 9, "Stabilization/Strengthening," p. 166), as well as the abdominal muscles and the hip flexors (trunk stabilization). When that doesn't happen, movements will be executed incorrectly over time, predestining the horse for injury and tension in the musculoskeletal system.

The following is an example of how instability can appear in your horse: when being ridden, he won't allow himself to be positioned and bent to the inside. The horse holds himself tightly, as if he has a blockage in his spine. However, the movement

Fact: A joint that's blocked will unfortunately also be less adequately supplied with nutrients and minerals. This causes a deficit. No new nutrients and minerals are being supplied, so what's there will become depleted. Without important building blocks, the cartilage degrades. As a result of a longstanding blockage, joint arthrosis can begin. This causes musculature to not get used and it loses its strength and elasticity. The degrading of muscle mass happens really quickly. In three days, it will already be recognizable on an ultrasound.

test with the carrot stretches (see p. 152) demonstrates that the horse can actually bend just fine in all directions. In this example, the source of the problem with positioning to the inside could be that the horse can't stabilize his outside. You'll find more about stability in chapter 9 (p. 166).

Tendon, Ligament, and Muscle Injuries

A variety of studies has shown that exposing the tendons, ligaments, and muscular tissue to movement stimuli has the exact same effect as it does on bone tissue. This means that tissue responds by getting stronger with use and weaker when underused.

Irritation and injury to these structures are often the result of wrong movement patterns or too much stress stimuli. The latter refers to exercise and movement that either lasts too long, is one-sided, or too hard. When such symptoms present themselves, you really should ask yourself if any of these circumstances could be the cause. But, of course, it's also possible that injury, a misalignment of the limbs (either from conformation or developed from use), instability, tension, and blockages in the neck, back, or upper limbs could lead to the development of these problems.

You can recognize these injuries through a daily inspection of your horse's musculoskeletal system. Look for swelling and determine if there's heat anywhere in the horse's body. These signs mean that something isn't right and inflammation is brewing. In order to avoid worsening the injury or irritation, I'd advise you to contact your vet. Always remember that a horse may not necessarily appear lame because of something like a swollen deep flexor tendon. But if the horse continues to work, this can quickly lead to a serious injury that requires months of rehabilitation.

Unfortunately, tendons and ligaments are just by nature going to receive less blood supply than muscle tissue. That's why, after a soft tissue injury, optimal circulation is just so crucial to foster a good healing state. The delivery of the blood determines the repair of the injury site. Just imagine a giant construction zone. The road must be clear for all the delivery trucks to get through with the necessary building material. The empty trucks then drive away with the waste and any damaged building material. But, if the road is blocked—for example, by a swelling—then one truck can't drive away and all repair work stops.

Back to the horse. It's crucial that after an injury you prevent swelling as much as possible, which stops the inflammatory reaction in the body. Swelling compromises the tissue and, thereby, also the blood vessels. As a result, circulation is restricted. It's helpful when the damaged tissue (such as with a hematoma) can be transported away from the injury site as quickly as possible.

Here, physical therapy offers many possibilities to support the healing of tendon, ligament, and muscle injuries (see chapter 10, "Physical Therapy," p. 176).

Muscular Atrophy and Hypertrophy

Simply put, muscular atrophy refers to a lessening of the muscle mass; muscular hypertrophy refers to too much muscular bulk. Both are problematic and hint at discord in the body. Often, these symptoms present together; for example, when a muscle no longer functions correctly, another muscle takes over to compensate for the lack of function and, therefore, begins to bulk up.

Another source can be the rider's attempt to achieve collection with a young, not very developed horse through the hand. This young horse can develop a disharmonious muscular structure because of too much physical strain, too soon.

Of course, imbalances can also develop from a trauma, for example, a nerve injury. The related muscle can no longer be cared for properly by the body. The result is a decrease in muscle mass. This often happens in jumping when the horse hits a

Physical Therapy for Horses

> **Example:** The way the muscles are built up allows you to recognize when the horse is compensating at work. You observe your horse from the side. In the poll area, there are pronounced muscles, but lower in the neck there's a dip just before the shoulder blade. The muscles around the withers and in the saddle area are also reduced. Farther back behind the saddle area, there's a "good" pronounced muscle in the lumbar region (also the kidney area). The muscles of the croup ascend and descend like a rollercoaster. The gluteal muscles are too small, but at the top of the tail, the hamstring muscles are too strongly pronounced. Most of the time, the abdominal muscles also hang down as if asleep, but they may also be pulled up tightly.

pole with his shoulder. The nerve that runs there is injured, and the horse can no longer move his front leg correctly.

The muscular pattern described in this example is almost a catastrophe for the horse. This will quickly lead to overstressing of the weaker places. And the impulse to move, which is developed from the hindquarters, can't travel over the horse's back to the forehand. It is already "broken" in the back, because

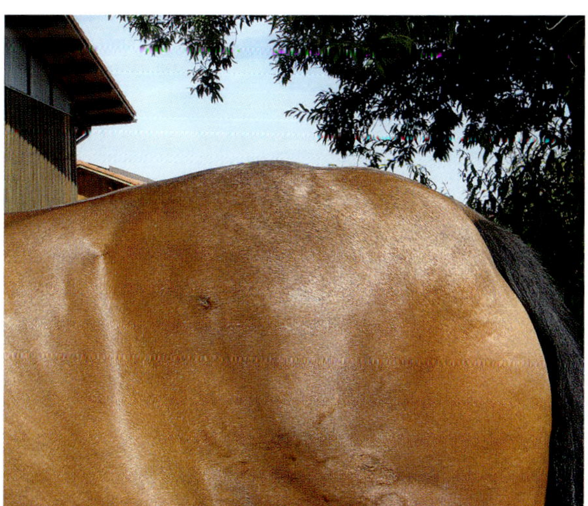

With this horse, all muscles of the hindquarters are hardened, tensed up, and unevenly developed. On one side, he presents with too much muscle; on the other side, not enough. This is a clear sign that this horse has been compensating at work for a long time.

the back is not relaxed. Therefore, the energy never reaches its goal: over the forehand to the rider's hand.

Organ Dysfunction

An illness in the digestive tract can also lead to tightening in the back. The reason is that the organs are supplied by nerves and these nerves exit along the spinal canal. For example, liver problems can lead to blockages around the 14th thoracic vertebra. Because there's a connection between the liver and the 14th thoracic vertebra, either can affect the other. When there's a blockage at the 14th thoracic vertebra (for example, due to an ill-fitting saddle), this can also lead to reduction of function in the liver as the muscular tension can cause the nerve to become constricted.

Teeth Problems

A perfect jaw and teeth connection is imperative for the overall balance and performance ability of the horse. The formation of hooks can lead to painful injuries to the gums, bad mouth hygiene, and a misaligned jaw. All these problems can have an immense impact on the rider.

For example, a misalignment causes constant tension in the jaw and prevents movement of the hyoid (tongue) bone. This results in tension in the connecting muscles and fascia of the second and third vertebrae. The gears don't work anymore. When you're riding, you notice this horse no longer allows himself to be positioned through the neck and poll. Over time, the problem will travel farther back and become noticeable, for example, in the reduced extension of the front limbs.

> **My Tip**
>
> **In order to avoid unnecessary stress on the musculoskeletal system, it's best to have an equine dentist/veterinarian check your horse's teeth at least once a year.**

The musculoskeletal system functions like the inner workings of a clock—all gears affect the others when they move. This is what makes optimal movement patterns possible. When a "gear" stops moving, it has an effect on the entire body.

rehabilitation and, thereby, avoid secondary injuries. However, you must realize that when lameness occurs, the back will almost always be affected. Therefore, it's important that after veterinary treatment, the back is given therapy in order to support overall healing.

If the veterinary exam is negative, it means the vet hasn't found the source of the problem. It follows that you must search further. In my experience, the two professional groups see problems from different vantage points and work with different examining practices. When seeking a diagnosis, this can be a great advantage.

Wound and Scar Tissue

Often, systemic disorders associated with wound healing occur after a major injury. Because of open wounds or surgical incisions, widespread tissue changes occur. If the wound healing proceeds too slowly, more and more scar tissue will build, which can later have a negative effect on freedom of movement. Scar tissue, in general, is less elastic and allows less blood circulation. In rare cases, a scar in the neck or abdominal region can even lead to a shoulder injury, for example, because freedom of movement has been so reduced due to the constriction of the tissue.

Example: The following example is to provide better understanding of the cause of an unclear but oft-encountered lameness. In your mind, picture the musculoskeletal system as the inner workings of a clock. Many gear wheels hold one another. When one gear wheel no longer turns, the others won't work optimally and can even come to a standstill.

For example, the molars can develop so-called "hooks." This means, the teeth are not even and constantly rub. Unevenness builds and it begins to hurt the horse when he chews food. The horse will move his jaw differently to avoid the pain. This incorrect use causes a reduction in movement of the poll, which perhaps limits forward movement of the forelimbs. This can lead to incorrect use and alignment of the vertebrae in the thoracic and lumbar regions and further to lameness of the hindquarters—a small problem has major effects!

"Mystery" Lameness

When a lameness presents itself, a vet must be called first. If the exam goes well and the vet finds the source of the problem, it will be treated. The physical therapist will subsequently work in collaboration with the veterinarian to support the

General Difficulties Under Saddle

Here, you'll find a list of symptoms that you may have already encountered in the course of your "riding life," followed by suggested solutions, which are then elaborated on later in the book.

Long-Term Stiffness

Just like people, every horse has a good and bad side. In daily work, it should, therefore, become the goal to gymnasticize the horse evenly, allowing him to become more supple and stronger and preparing him for more advanced movements.

Sometimes it just doesn't work this way, no matter how much you wish it did.

Example: The horse develops fantastically on one side. When you change direction, it's as if you're sitting on a different horse. Unfortunately, there are still riders who don't heed this alarm and simply "ride away" at this point. Many riders still have the idea that they can accomplish a lot with force.

BUT: Horses are "movement artists." They will evade and bend themselves somehow in order to satisfy the rider. In any case, this is not a foundation from which you can build. What follows these thoughtless proceedings causes harm to the horse in the form of lameness, back pain, uneven movement, deterioration in performance, resistance, to name a few issues.

Resistance

Most horses enjoy working with you. But when they're in pain or the performance expectations are too difficult, they may also respond with resistance. Bucking and rearing are the most common defense mechanisms. If your horse demonstrates these behaviors, please don't punish him, but rather apply critical thinking and begin searching for a possible cause. Few horses are "buckers"; they're just misunderstood by their rider.

Decline in Performance

Example: During jumping training, your horse suddenly begins to make mistakes with his hind legs. Or, in dressage, the flying change from left to right no longer works the way it has in the past. As described in "Mystery Lameness" (p. 10), the musculoskeletal system functions like the gears of a clock. If one of the gears gets caught, the rest of the body will be

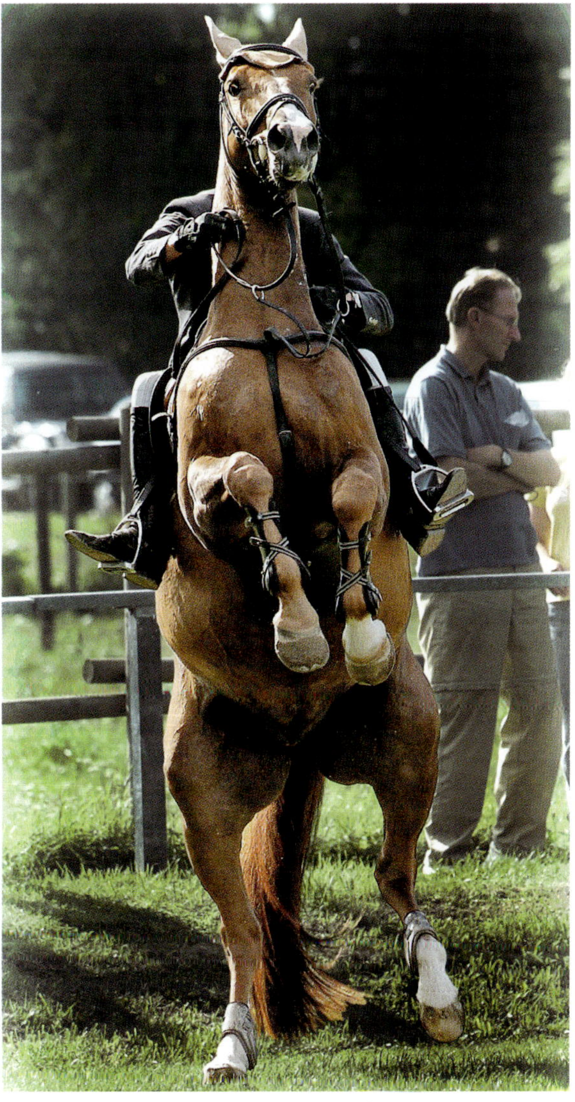

When in pain or under psychological pressure, resistance can be the horse's cry for help, like the rearing pictured here.

affected by the problem. A decline in performance signals a disorder. In this case, your alarm bells should be going off!

Headshaking

The horse constantly nods or shakes his head. There can be many causes of this behavior. A common cause is a neurological disorder, such as hypersensitivity to light, environmental influences, vaccines, flies, or pollen. Headshaking can definitely also be triggered by tension in the neck and/or back region. A poorly fitted saddle could be the problem, or so could limited mobility of the spine overall.

Playing with the Tongue and Grinding the Teeth

When a horse moves around his tongue and sticks it out while being ridden, he's said to be "playing with the tongue." The behavior is a sign something is not right and, as with headshaking, can originate from tension. Playing with the tongue can also occur when the rider applies too much pressure and the horse is being overwhelmed in terms of his performance ability. Obviously, playing with the tongue can also be a sign of a bit that doesn't fit well, a blockage in the tongue bone/hyoid bone or pain in the mouth area. With this problem, you often lose *losgelassenheit* (most commonly translated as relaxation, supple relaxation, or "looseness").

When horses are regularly worked at the limit of their ability or develop inner tension due to pain, they also tense their jaw muscles and begin to grind their teeth. A little later in this book (see chapter 3, "Biomechanics," p. 34), I'll explain how the jaw joint connects in a specific way to the rest of the musculoskeletal system and how pain and unwellness in the jaw joint immediately spreads.

It's important that teeth grinding isn't mistaken for teeth "chattering." "Chattering" is a sign of *losgelassenheit* and very welcome by us riders! It's not only a sign of a well horse, in higher collected work, the horse must, in fact, be able to move along with his jaw in order to execute a perfect piaffe and passage. Therefore, I request that you don't make the noseband too tight because doing so blocks your horse's freedom of movement.

Uneven Rhythm

There's a difference between lameness and uneven rhythm. In contrast to most lameness, uneven rhythm has no clinical explanation! It only happens

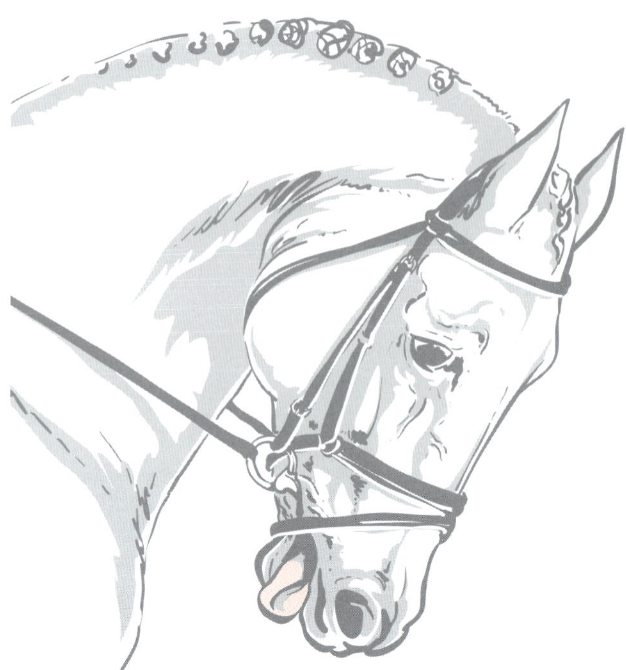

This horse is uncomfortable, which you can recognize because his tongue is hanging out. Because of the forced frame, he can't see well and his topline and neck muscles are under excessive stress.

under saddle and is sometimes called "rein-lame." It doesn't appear in the beginning when the horse is being led and isn't always present in all gaits. Unevenness is a clear sign that something is wrong with the flow of movement in the body. You can trace this back to a muscular imbalance and to tension in the spine. Typically, uneven rhythm has a rider error as part of the background; for example, too tight hands or an un-elastic seat. If the rein-lameness is not corrected, it can become a true lameness, which you will then certainly see when the horse is being led in hand.

What Causes Injury and Tension?

With horses, there are many reasons for tension and injury to the musculoskeletal system. In order to best avoid them, you should know in advance about the potential threats.

Trauma

Accidents happen! Horses spend most of their time in a stall or pasture. Often, no one even knows that the horse has slipped and fallen while running around the pasture or become temporarily cast in his stall. When you arrive at the barn for a ride, you often don't even recognize that anything out of ordinary has happened. Unfortunately, it's also true that the resulting injury won't necessarily be noticeable at first but it becomes more obvious over time. The source of the injury can then be difficult to diagnose.

Hoof Conformation and Shoeing

The horse's trim and shoeing have an enormous influence over his musculoskeletal system. When the horse's hoof falls are incorrect or uneven, it can lead to a biomechanical imbalance within the limbs. Unequivocally, this leads to unhealthy compression of the joints. What follows can result in overstressing and/or permanent damage to the musculoskeletal system, which moves up to influence the back and neck areas. So too, the incorrect shoe size or weight can have a negative effect on the musculoskeletal system. In addition, you see toes that are far too long, which lead to the horse's inability to roll over his toe quickly enough so that the standing phase is extended. In this case, the pull on the flexor tendons and suspensory ligaments gets more intense and the horse must dig in more with the shoulder and neck muscles in order to strike off and bring his limbs forward.

With tendon and ligament injuries of the lower extremities, you often see a raised heel position. This is the most commonly utilized solution to relieve the injured area. However, you should definitely not forget that this can be at the expense of other structures. For example, when you want to relieve the flexor tendon, you can put too much stress on the suspensory ligament. In this adjustment phase, you should watch the horse really carefully and not overdo it.

In addition, you often see orthopedic fittings used during rehabilitation as a short-term solution. For

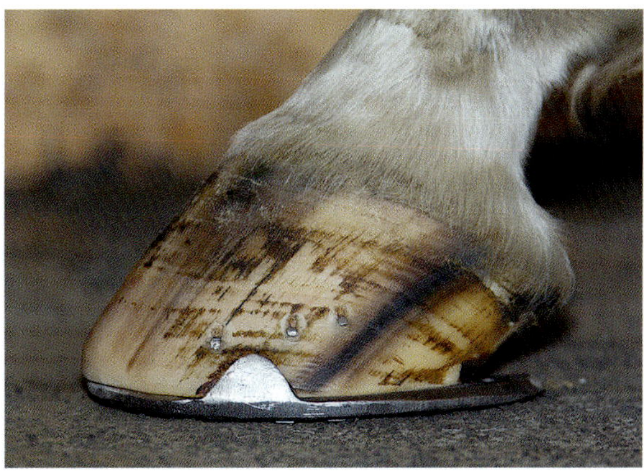

Shoeing has enormous influence on the musculoskeletal system. In this picture, you can see a correctly shod horse; the shoe is large enough.

example, when the horse is prescribed an egg-bar shoe, this should not be a long-term solution but rather only used for as long as the tissue needs to heal. These special shoes can also have negative effects on other structures.

My Tip

Immediately inform your farrier and/or veterinarian when you notice a worsening condition due to new corrective shoes.

Tack and Equipment

Another common reason for injury and tension is equipment that fits poorly. Attention is often only given to ensure a good saddle fit, and the condition of the rest of the equipment is overlooked. But there's more to consider: your complete equipment! Other essential elements include a well-fitting bridle cavesson, the right bit, correctly applied polo wraps, boots that fit, the right girth and so forth. Very often, you can solve riding problems just by correcting the fit of various equipment. And these mistakes are so easy to avoid. In chapter 12 of this book (p. 200), I'll describe how you can self-check your equipment to make sure it fits.

Overstressing

Stress injuries can develop through work that incorporates little variety. Continually riding dressage movements or always galloping a racehorse are good examples. Also, always riding on the same type of footing can cause stress injuries.

Unfortunately, this mistake often begins with young horses. Frequently, young dressage horses are only ridden in dressage, never getting out for a hack, and absolutely never turned out in a paddock. Here's the reason: they might get injured. Obviously, there's a risk of injury associated with turnout, but if you take away the horse's ability to move freely and only do one type of training, you're absolutely guaranteeing that he'll have health issues. Therefore, under no circumstances should you neglect the horse's intrinsic needs.

In order to bring a horse along so that he's sure-footed, strong, and coordinated, the musculoskeletal system requires a variety of stimuli. Being worked on different footing/ground is extremely important, as opposed to only riding in the indoor and outdoor arenas at home. A horse—even a dressage horse—can and should jump small jumps and cavalletti, and he should be able to gallop out in the open without "falling on his nose." This rich variety and diverse training leads to a balanced, positive use of all structures in the musculoskeletal system, which leads to even muscular development and muscular coordination.

When a horse hasn't been exposed to this type of work and comes upon an unfamiliar surface, he'll feel insecure, tense up, shorten his stride, and lose his *losgelassenheit*.

Stabling Conditions

In nature, horses are always in movement and, therefore, always producing more synovial (joint) fluid. They maintain an intact musculoskeletal system and flexibility. In addition, their metabolism stays turned on and their muscles are stretched and developed.

Today, because horses are often kept in a box stall, which for many horses means 23 hours a day, horses lose their natural mobility and suppleness. This type of horse-keeping also has implications beyond the musculoskeletal system. We shouldn't overlook the effects on mental health, which again has a close relationship with the musculoskeletal system. This psychological stress is heightened in stables that are very loud or when the horse doesn't get along well with his neighbors but hardly ever gets away from them.

Let's not forget horses are herd animals and need contact with members of their own species. They love to play, scratch one another, and require a herd hierarchy to orient themselves. When we take these possibilities away , we can cause psychological damage and, thereby, higher levels of tension in the body.

Inadequate Warm-Up and Cool-Down

When a training session begins, the rider must take enough time to warm up the horse's musculoskeletal system and, of course, her own as well, in order to prepare for the planned work under saddle.

Much too often you see a horse at the barn being brought directly from the box stall to the arena. The horse is mounted and, if he's lucky, walked around for a lap or two. This is not adequate as in this little time, the musculoskeletal system does not have the opportunity to prepare well enough for work. The synovial fluid is not flowing enough to protect the cartilage in the joints; the ligaments and tendons are not supple enough, and the muscles are not yet receiving enough blood supply. All of these structures require at least 15 minutes of warm-up in order to be ready for optimal use.

The same goes for the end of the training session. Now, the horse's body should be given the opportunity to come back to normal (breathing, pulse, temperature). An old rule that many riders go by is that you should ride the horse until he's dry. But many horses don't sweat that much! This definitely does not mean that they don't need a cool-down phase.

The heightened metabolic processes of the body are still flowing. This includes the muscles, which have been highly engaged, oxygen, and nutrients. Waste products also are contained in the muscles, which the system needs to transport out. Until this process is over, the horse will continue to have an elevated pulse and respiration. But he won't necessarily be sweating. Regardless of how hard the horse has worked, the cool-down phase should last approximately 10 to 15 minutes.

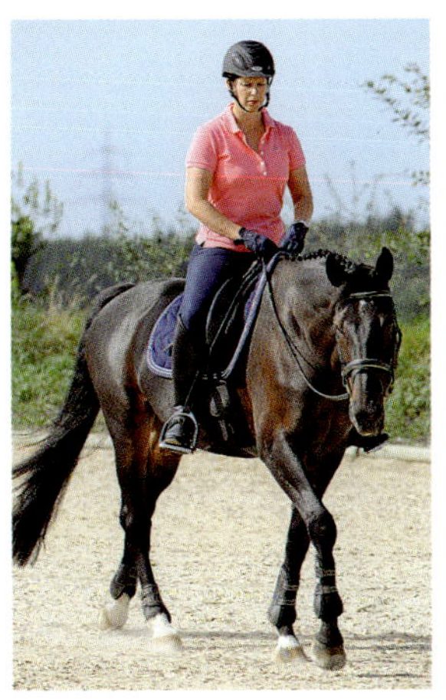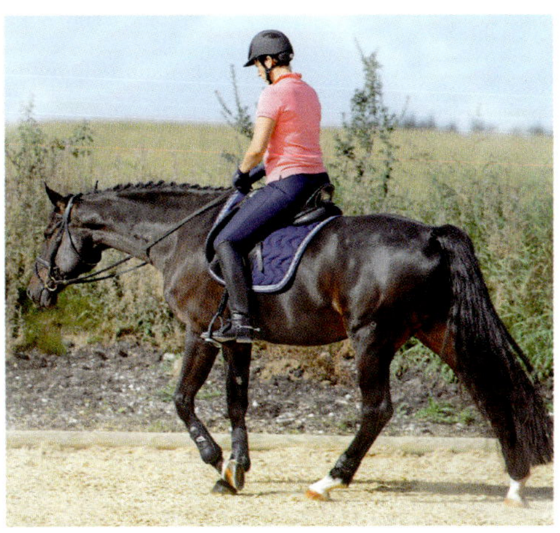

Approximately 15 minutes of walking at the start of your ride and 10 minutes at the end are indispensable to maintaining your horse's health.

Incorrect Riding

We've all heard this saying, "Most riding problems are not caused by the horse." This saying should make us feel good (and be seen by us riders as a stroke of luck!) as this means we can improve the situation. Let's take the rider's seat. The rider's seat is the "be all and end all" in riding. Without a good seat, you'll quickly encounter misunderstandings in the communication and harmony between rider and horse, and the desired *losgelassenheit* will be lost for both. An example, it's enough for a rider to have poor hand position, such as riding with a clenched fist. This mistake initiates a chain reaction in her body. The result is blocked shoulders and hips. The horse immediately senses this loss of movement and must take countermeasures, often with loss of rhythm and his supple relaxation. In this case, using draw reins, special bits or other tools will be totally counterproductive!

In addition, the correct stirrup length has a big effect on the rider's seat and, therefore, on the horse. When they're too long, the rider's hip joint is overstretched and locked. Because of this, the pelvis will be unable to swing with the horse's movement and the weight and leg aids will be impeded. If the hip joint is locked, the shoulder won't be free. This leads to the rider's hand, which is in direct connection with the horse's mouth, becoming tight. With these conditions, can you be at all surprised when the horse loses his suppleness and relaxation? Therefore, you must always be ready to work on yourself, too. And be honest—that's also the whole point of riding, right?

Many riders sit asymmetrically on the horse without realizing it. However, the horse feels this precisely. It impedes him from balancing himself, just as when a person carries a backpack that's clearly heavier on one side or the other. The muscles on the opposite side tense up automatically in order to balance out the heavier weight. If the asymmetry continues over a long period of time, it will lead to permanent tension and pain in the horse's back.

My Tip

Have a riding instructor with a good eye help you. She can precisely analyze and correct your seat. Even professional riders get help from the ground. Or, have someone film you so that you can recognize problems with your seat. The visual perception is invaluable.

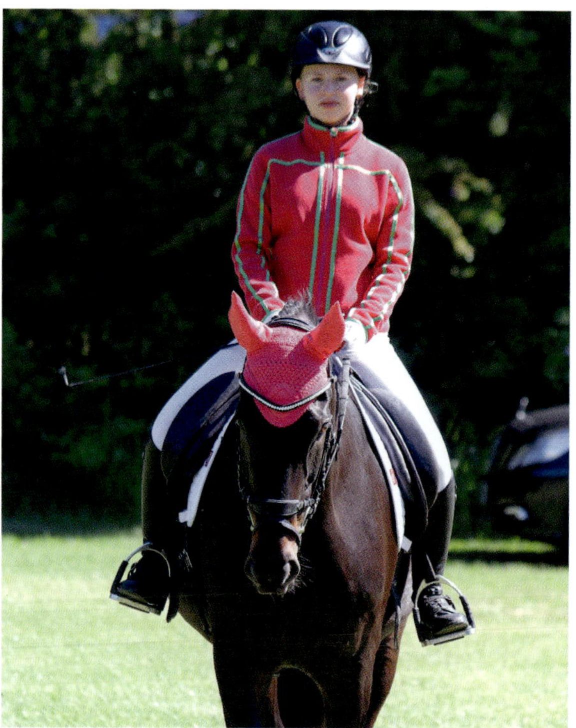

Visual aids are always a big help in riding: for example, a jacket with a painted-on stripe. With its help, you can see for yourself if you're sitting in the middle or not. This rider's whole axis is off-center.

The Goal of Physical Therapy—What Can Physical Therapy Accomplish?

Much can be accomplished through a physical therapy treatment. An animal physical therapist has the same goal as a human physical therapist: based on her knowledge, she wants to recognize the animal's ailments and determine the source of his health problems. It's about making a functional diagnosis, which means she is examining the body for existing or possibly developing physical impairments but in addition, she must also look for clues in the horse's environment such as stabling, feed, and equipment. She's looking to integrate the case history and the treatment. This is the only way that a treatment will be successful long-term. With a physical therapy treatment, it's about relieving neurological and movement disorders in order to restore functional patterns of movement and stabilize the body.

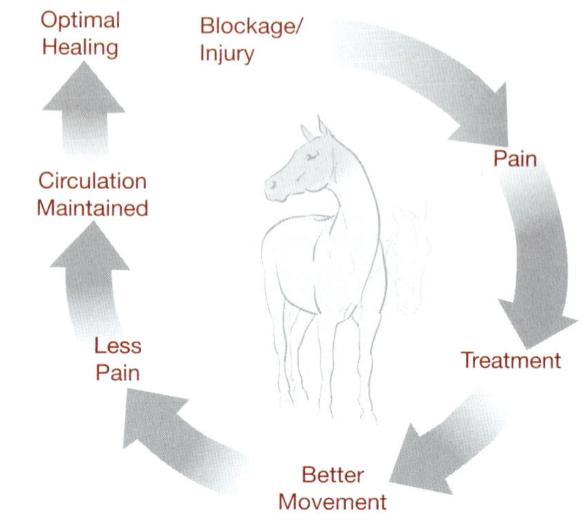

Every injury or blockage is accompanied by pain. Through a timely treatment, you can avoid muscular tension and pain. Blood flow and movement remain stable and the result is reduced muscular tension/pain. Thereby, the recovery time can go smoothly.

Improving Circulation and Metabolism

Imagine a muscle as a sponge. Blood flow is promoted in the sponge through various physiotherapeutic techniques such as massage, stretching, electrotherapy, and others. With blood, nutrients are transported to the muscle. At the same time, waste products are transported out. Only then can the new nutrients once again be delivered to the muscles. After this cleanup, there is better blood flow and, thereby, also more optimal metabolic status.

Avoiding/Releasing Adhesions

When tissue is damaged because of an injury, the body transports building blocks to this area in order to rebuild and repair. If circulation is disrupted, the by-products and the affected area remain immobile, unable to stretch or contract. A new injury in the surrounding tissue is predestined.

Promoting Relaxation

Horses enjoy it so much when you spend quiet time with them without being in a hurry. By sensitively laying your hands on the horse for a massage, the horse notices quickly that it doesn't hurt and he'll enjoy the contact. Massages bring both physical and mental relaxation.

Relieving Pain

Pain can be caused by poor blood flow to the muscles. The acid levels in the muscles will become too high and that is a source of pain. In physical therapy, we use various measures such as massage to release hormones and endorphins and relieve pain. You'll recognize it from your own reactions. When you bump into something, you automatically stroke the spot you hit—and the pain disappears faster!

Restoring Mobility

When a blockage is limiting the movement of a joint, the cartilage will be stressed unevenly, and the joint will tend more quickly toward joint disease and, eventually, inflammation. By relieving tension and blockages, the joints become more mobile again and a wider area will be impacted. A joint that is fully mobile will also stay healthy longer.

Restoring Performance Capability

Through all of these measures, the horse's musculoskeletal system will (again) become reliable. With the right kind of—and regularly given—support, the horse learns how to move optimally once again, correctly engaging his muscles and joints. He avoids injury. You can find tips about optimal rehabilitation in the forthcoming chapters.

Prevention

In chapters 7, 8, 9, and 12, I'll describe active manual techniques, such as massage techniques, stabilizing exercises and stretching exercises, and passive techniques, such as electrotherapy and

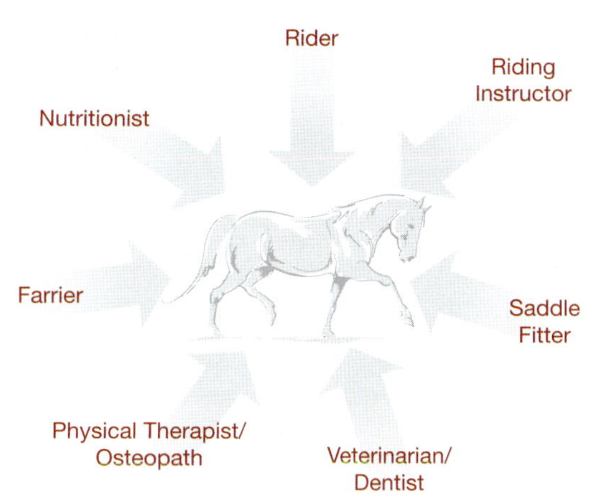

Physical therapy is a part of your horse's collaborative maintenance, care, and treatment. All the people involved should understand they're part of a team and work together. Only in this way is it possible to provide the horse with optimal care and keep him healthy.

water therapy, all of which can be executed by the layperson. It's an invitation to you to implement physical therapy as a preventive measure, to avoid injury and improve performance.

For injury and blockages/limited movement, there are also exercises that you should not execute yourself, such as specific mobilization and manipulation of the joints and soft tissue. This part of the treatment must be done by a veterinarian or qualified therapist! Information to help you recognize when you should definitely call an expert can be found in chapter 6, "Palpation," chapter 7, "Massage," chapter 8, "Mobilizing and Stretching," and chapter 9, "Stabilizing and Strengthening."

My Tip

Success lies in teamwork.

The Anatomy of the Musculoskeletal System

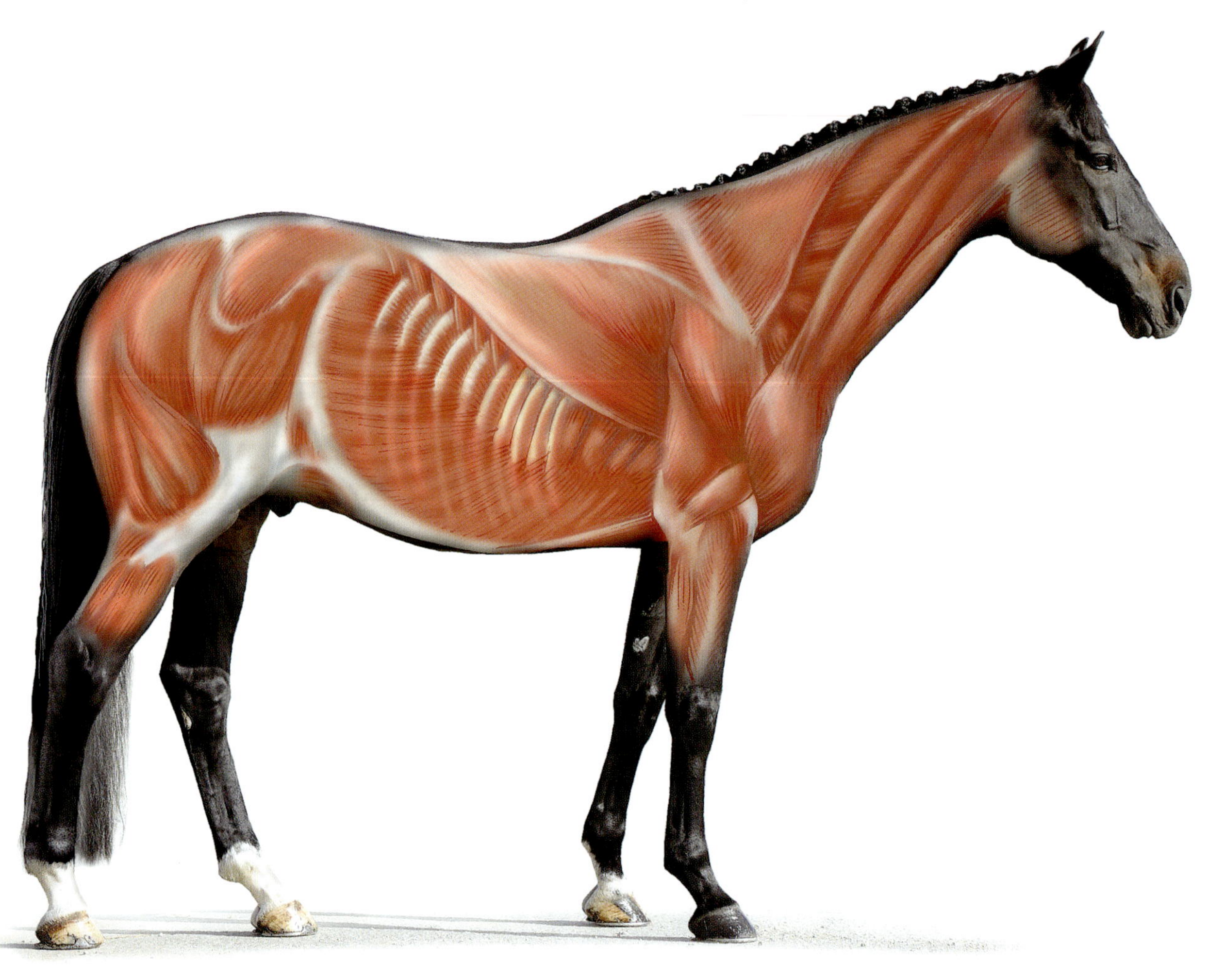

Why Is Understanding Anatomy Important?

We work with our horses every day with the goal of improving their strength and performance. To find the correct path to this goal, it helps to have general knowledge about the anatomy of the musculoskeletal system. Through knowledge of anatomy, you get a glimpse of what's going on inside the horse.

For a start, the musculoskeletal system can be divided into:

- **The "passive" musculoskeletal system.**
  The bony skeleton and the connective joints —static.
- **The "active" musculoskeletal system.**
  The skeletal muscles and ligament system —dynamic.

The "Passive" Musculoskeletal System

Bones

The bones have two important jobs: they provide support and elasticity. Contrary to popular belief that bones are just a rigid mass, they are actually a combination of organic substance, water, and minerals, which make it possible for them to be flexible but resilient at the same time.

The flexibility is important for the bones to absorb and distribute impact, stress, and vibrations. In this way, they're protected from fractures and other types of injury. The bones are regularly remodeled; this means the old bone tissue will be exchanged for new tissue. The two most important components for healthy building of bones are good nutrition and systematic training. The training should be designed specifically for the type of work. For example, a jumper must be trained so that his bone structure has elevated strength upon landing and for tight turns. A racehorse must be trained with the stress of galloping at a high tempo in mind. A dressage horse must strengthen the bones of his hindquarters in order to be able to carry a lot more weight during the collected movements.

Training heightens risk. Because of training-related stress, microtraumas occur over and over in the bony tissue. This means, you must also give the tissue time to heal. Otherwise, you'll quickly encounter macro-trauma, or even fractures in the worst case scenario! Ganglia on the cannon bone are an alarm bell as they result from the workload being elevated too quickly: the body is trying to stabilize the bones with inappropriate bone building using weak bone building materials.

Giving the bones time to recover doesn't mean that the horse has to have a day off. It much more implies that cross-training should be part of his routine. You shouldn't run a racehorse every single day, nor should you jump a jumper daily or constantly school collected movements with your dressage horse. Rather, you need to ensure your training is rich in diversity.

The bones allow the body to continue working. They carry calcium, magnesium, phosphorus, and produce red and white blood cells.

Every bone (and by the way, your horse has more than 200 bones) has its own special shape. Designed for its unique task, the bone inserts into the skeleton's structure. In every place where bones meet one another, there is a joint. The joints give the skeleton mobility, crucial for movement.

Joints

There are three types of joints: fibrous joints (like sutures, they are the seams between the cranial bones); cartilaginous joints (like the connective tissues between the vertebrae); and synovial joints. The latter are the most common joints of the body. In this category, there are many subcategories, such as ball joints and hinges, which allow mobility and range of movement because of the special shape of the joint surface. Likewise, movement is also fostered or limited through ligaments, muscles, and even bone structures.

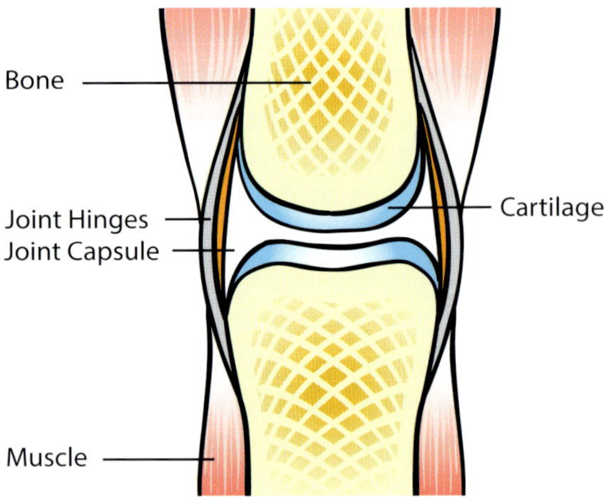

A schematic diagram of a joint.

Fact: The job of a joint is to permit movement and absorb impact and/or stress.

The end of the bones (on the joints) are covered in cartilage. The bone has a hard, elastic, and smooth surface. Its job is to facilitate smooth movement for the joint and to mute impact.

As joint cartilage doesn't possess blood vessels or nerves, it doesn't receive any blood flow. In the joint, metabolic processes occur like a sponge. Through work, the "junk" is pressed out of the joint and through relaxation, the nutrition is sucked in. The cartilage benefits especially from this metabolic process when there is regular movement. If horses don't move enough, the metabolic process is not

My Tip

Good nutrition and regular, moderate movement with lots of variety when the horse is still young brings great advantages for healthy and strong joint cartilage. In addition, it's advisable to work the horse on diverse surfaces such as hard asphalt and soft trail, grass, or sand footing.

achieved for the joint and that can have the effect that the cartilage gets stiff and thick.

Example: Horses that are only worked in the arena each day will eventually have weaker cartilage than horses who regularly train on diverse footing/surfaces.

Every joint is contained by a capsule. On the inside of this capsule, which is covered by synovium, synovial fluid is produced. Its job is to nourish the cartilage. In addition, the joint membranes collect waste products and transport them from the joint. On the outside of the joint capsule, you'll also find joint hinges, which give stability to the joint.

Think about it please: when your horse has been standing a long time, which includes overnight in his stall, the synovial fluid is significantly thicker. Therefore, it can't optimally serve the joint. The synovial fluid needs about 15 minutes to get flowing to be able to provide the joint with optimal protection. If the joint is stressed too much before this time has passed, the joint surfaces rub against one another, which can lead to irreparable damage to the joint.

In practice, you often see a horse come directly out of the stall, head to the arena and be allowed to run free. This includes fast turns, racing tempos, and abrupt stops in the corners. It is a real challenge for your horse's cartilage (as well as for the entire musculoskeletal system). Please avoid this form of movement at all costs.

Clicking Joints

One often hears the crack of a joint—your own or your horse's. Where does this noise come from and what does it mean?

Clicking joints are much less worrisome than is generally believed. You'll often hear this in the horse's joints at the beginning of your ride when the synovial fluid has not yet reached the right "working temperature."

Physical Therapy for Horses

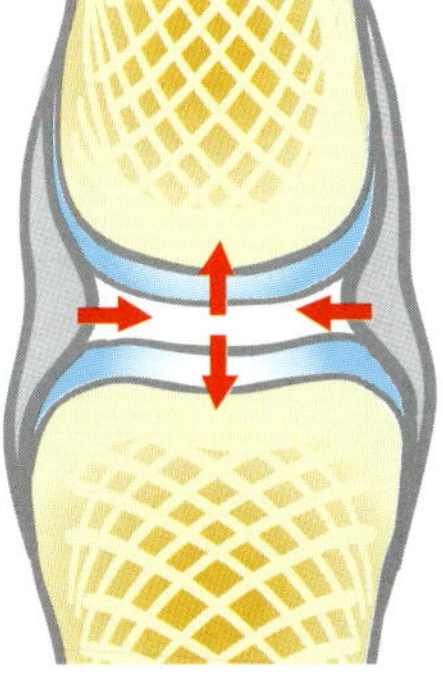
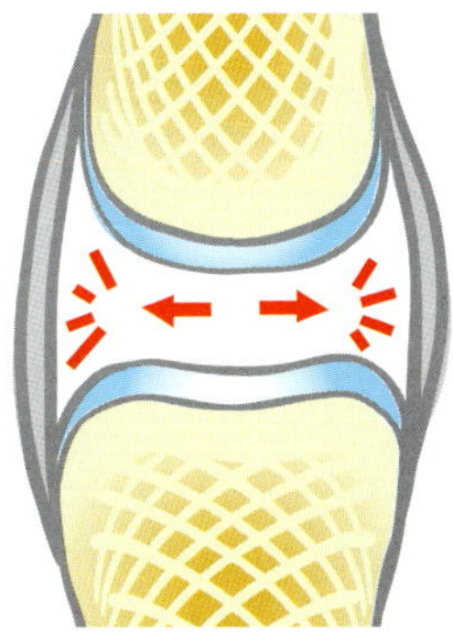

Clicking joints. First the joint surfaces meet each other; the joint capsule is pulled to the inside. Next, through a reaction in the joint, the joint capsule will be pushed outward again and that's when you hear the clicking.

The cracking actually comes from two noises, although you'll only hear one "crack." The noise occurs when the surfaces of two joints meet. When they part, there's a vacuum (negative pressure) created in the joint. In addition, the joint capsule is pulled a bit into the space between the joints. The separation of the joint surfaces is the source of the first crack. At the same time, a gas bubble forms in the joint. This gas bubble again enlarges the volume in the space between the joints. Thereby, the joint capsule gets pushed out again, very quickly. This snapping back of the joint hinges is the source of the second crack.

When a joint cracks, it is indicating energy being released in the joint's membranes, but it's definitely too little to hurt the joint. Certainly, if it always cracks, it eventually could lead to an unstable joint due to the repeated overstretching of the joint capsule and hinges. This could have negative consequences (premature wear). This is not common among horses, but much more among people who for example constantly pull on their fingers to crack their knuckles.

The Skeleton

All the bones combine to form the skeleton, which all vertebrate animals have. It's an important scaffolding that supports the musculoskeletal system. In other words, the skeleton cannot stand erect without the support of the soft tissues, and the soft tissues can't build up stabilizing (traction) power without the skeleton.

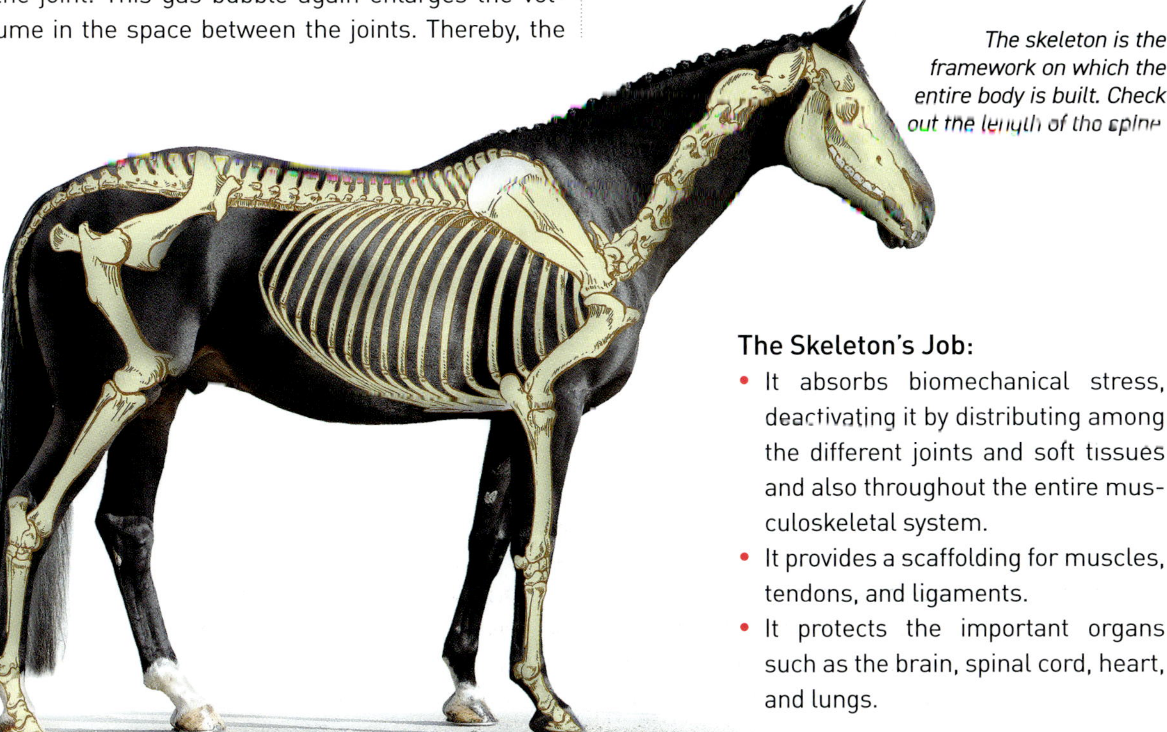

The skeleton is the framework on which the entire body is built. Check out the length of the spine

The Skeleton's Job:
- It absorbs biomechanical stress, deactivating it by distributing among the different joints and soft tissues and also throughout the entire musculoskeletal system.
- It provides a scaffolding for muscles, tendons, and ligaments.
- It protects the important organs such as the brain, spinal cord, heart, and lungs.

The "Active" Musculoskeletal System

The active musculoskeletal system consists of soft tissue, which executes, slows, and stabilizes movement.

Joint Capsules
The joint capsules enclose the two bone ends and "envelop" the joint. Inside the capsule, synovial fluid is produced, which fills up the capsule, protecting and nourishing the cartilage. On the outside, the joint capsule is strengthened by taut connective tissue, which gives the joint additional security (see "Structure of the Joints," p. 20).

Ligaments
Around every joint, there are multiple joint ligaments, whose job is to hold the joint together, support the muscle contractions, and stop the joint's movement when it reaches the physiological limits of its range of motion; in this way, they control and manage the joint. The hinges work closely with the surrounding muscles. For a long time, it was believed that the joint ligaments could only passively and powerlessly support the joint. With the advancement of scientific knowledge, we know that they actually also actively support the muscle contractions.

Because joint ligaments have hardly any blood flow, they heal poorly when injured. When these ligaments are badly overstretched, for example after a fall, there can be so much stress on the joint that the ligaments overstretch or even tear. When this occurs, the ligaments can lose their ability to support the joint forever, causing the affected joint to become unstable. The surrounding muscles must then take over this missing functionality. This means that they must become even stronger in order to stabilize the joint. Unfortunately, that's not always possible as, for example, with a cruciate ligament rupture in the stifle joint.

An example of muscular stability that actually functions well is that of loose stifle ligaments (though not the cruciate). Here, the stifle joint is unstable.

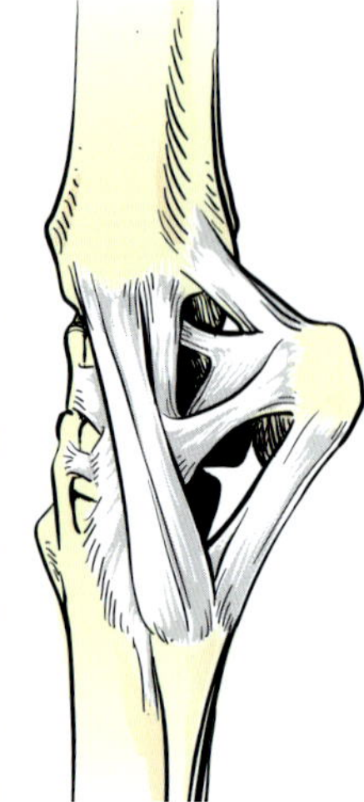

Here, you can clearly recognize the large number of joint ligaments, which hold the knee joint together and stabilize it.

Symptoms include the horse constantly "giving out" with his hindquarters, especially during transitions to the walk or on bending lines. This happens because the stifle ligaments are too loose and there's not enough basic engagement or strength in the muscles of the hindquarters. With young horses, you'll often see this during a growth spurt, but afterward the horse regains his stability.

With older horses, you'll often find a muscular imbalance accompanies loose joint ligaments in the stifle. In particular, the biceps and quadriceps of the thigh (see chapter 3, "Biomechanics," p. 34) are too weak when there's instability of the stifle joint. It's their job to ensure the engagement of the stifle joint ligaments. With the right training plan, you can possibly strengthen these muscles enough to support the stifle's stability. This plan might include lots of uphill work, jumping, or riding many transitions.

Muscles
In order to help you understand the largest component of the musculoskeletal system—namely, the muscles—the following will delve more deeply into the subject of "muscles and their function." The muscles are among the most important components of our body and our horses' body. Without them, the horse (like us) would be unable to move or to absorb and digest nutrients. As you'll soon read, there are different types of muscle work, but in essence, all muscles work alike—by contracting or expanding the muscle fibers. It's the tissue over which you'll later have great influence with massage and stretching exercises, as well as when you ride.

There are three groups of muscles: smooth, cardiac, and skeletal. The first two types work

Physical Therapy for Horses

involuntarily, without us initiating them. You'll find these involuntary muscles in the digestive tract, respiratory tract, and urogenital system. The cardiac muscles also belong in this category. In contrast, the skeletal muscles are voluntary and you can initiate them: your brain sends a signal to a muscle, telling it what you want it to do.

■ Muscle Development

Every muscle is comprised of fiber bundles, which themselves are composed of many millions of muscular fibers. Every fiber consists of many fibrils. They're the smallest building blocks of the muscles and are primarily made up of two types of protein: myosin and actin.

■ Muscles and Tendons

Striated muscles (skeletal muscles) are responsible for movement. Each individual striated muscle is divided into three parts: the muscle origin, the muscle belly, and the muscle insertion. The skeletal musculature is secured to the skeleton and fascia via its sinewy (connective tissue) attachments.

Every muscle is enveloped by connective tissue, which begins at the end of the muscle and is referred to as tendons. The tendons are composed of coarse connective tissue and make up the origin and the insertion of the muscle. They have different lengths and anchor the muscle to the skeleton and muscle fascia. They are less elastic than the belly of the muscle and have less blood flow. Contraction of the muscle takes place in its belly; therefore, it's highly elastic/flexible and is well-nourished with the help of much blood flow.

In anatomy books, muscles are represented schematically and distinguished clearly from one another. Their insertion and origin on the bones are listed schematically as well. Furthermore, the functions of each individual muscle are described as bending, stretching, turning, etc.

In reality, it looks a lot different. If you're dissecting a horse and, for example, you want to clearly separate the large-headed *brachiocephalicus* muscle, you'll realize that the muscular fibers and fascia from the *trapezius* muscles permeate the *brachiocephalicus*. In addition, the *brachiocephalicus* is attached firmly to the *pectorals*. Its attachments and fascia also pull on the neck vertebrae. In other words, it's not accurate to say that the *brachiocephalicus* is actually able to move the foreleg forward all by itself. Many muscles are involved with this forward movement, although they are not designated as the "movers" of the forelegs. The muscles and fascia blend with one another and form an interrelated network.

Here's what this means: when a leg moves forward, it's not just the leg itself that's activated, but rather the entire musculoskeletal system is more or less involved through the fascia. This also holds true with injury and tension: all the surrounding muscles are affected. Surely, you can imagine that when this limited range of motion remains, it won't take

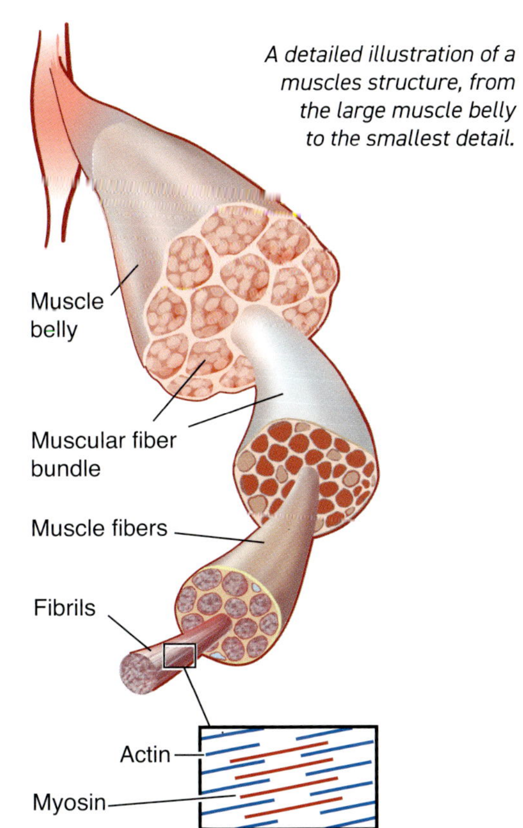

A detailed illustration of a muscles structure, from the large muscle belly to the smallest detail.

long before the entire musculoskeletal system is involved and the horse will soon demonstrate an altered gait.

When stimulated, muscles possess the ability to pull together. As a result, they can affect the parts of the skeleton to which they're connected, either moving them against each other or holding them in position against an external force. They enable movement, are involved with maintaining balance and also "carry" some of the body's weight.

By way of distinction: tendons are a part of the muscle. In contrast, ligaments are not connected to the muscle.

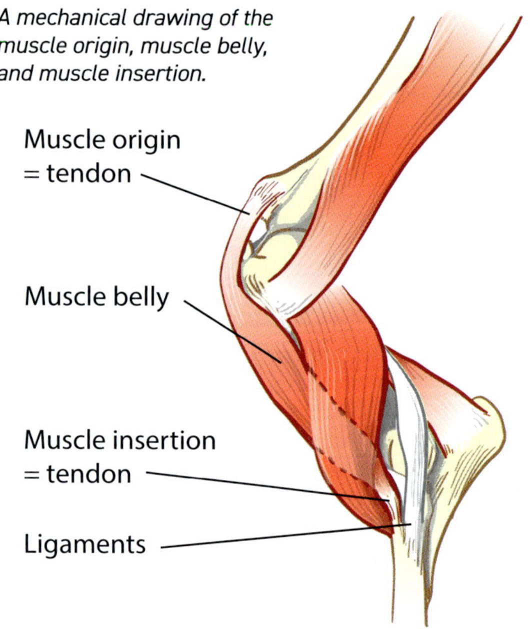

A mechanical drawing of the muscle origin, muscle belly, and muscle insertion.

■ Connective Tissue/Fascia

When you go to the butcher and look at the various offerings, you'll notice a grey skin on the meat. That's the connective tissue, which is also called fascial tissue. This system of surrounding connective tissue, strands and layers forms a complex whole-body network.

This is your body's unsung hero. For a long time, the fascia was believed to just be a filler in the body, but fortunately, in recent years, science has brought it more to the foreground. High-tech examination equipment such as ultrasound and micro-cameras yield more and more astounding knowledge about its important functions in your body. Fascia is now classified as its own organ. This means, if you separated out all other tissue of the body, the fascial tissue remains as a connected part. In other words, the fascia forms a suspense network that pervades the entire human and animal body. That's what the name implies: fascia means "bind" or "band" and "binding together" is exactly what this important organ does.

The connective tissue varies in strength: it can range from very, very thin to a thick layer; as for example, in a horse's superficial and deep flexor tendon (where it is as thick as a finger). There is fascia throughout the entire body, from head to hind hoof, which penetrates and encloses the bones, muscles, muscular connectors, organs, blood vessels, and nerve pathways. You find fascial tissue as tendon plates, as ligaments and tendons, and as "coverings" for the muscles.

Fact: Muscles and fascia form one unit.

Fascial tissue is comprised from 60 to 70 percent water. This fluid works like a lubricant between the layers of fascia, so that the muscles can glide over one another without rubbing. The fascia connects multiple joints and muscles together at the same time: straight, crossing, diagonal, and spiral in form. So, too, organs are characterized by fascia, which surround them and keep them in the correct position within the abdominal cavity.

Although the fascial tissue is seemingly thin and inconspicuous, the structure is extremely strong and has considerable influence on the horse's stability and mobility. In addition, the fascia gives the body its form. It also possesses receptors and sensors, making it one of the most important organs in

Physical Therapy for Horses

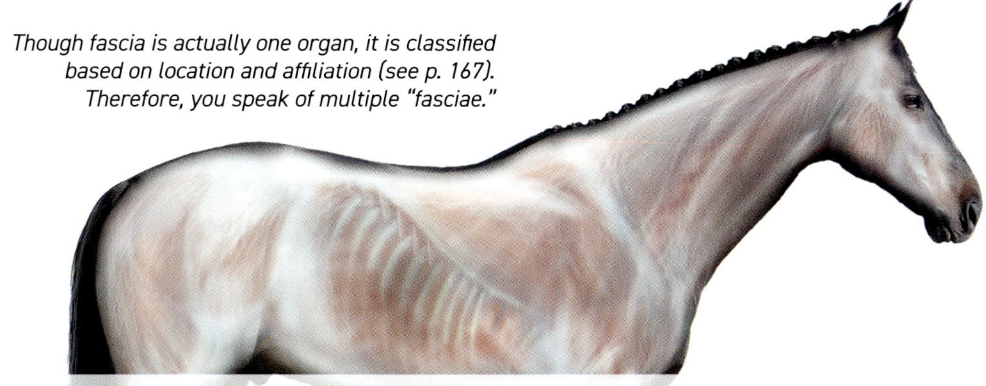

the body for communication. It's also involved with metabolism. As you can see, the fascial system is a multi-faceted and highly important organ.

Unfortunately, such a complex organ is also ripe for dysfunction. Among other things, the fascia can get stuck and this changes its structure. An adhesion can come about through injury, over or underuse, stress or too much pressure on the tissue (for example, from a saddle that doesn't fit). When the fascia is stuck, the fluid between the layers of tissue disappears. In consequence, the fascia changes, gets matted and toughens. In a horse with chronic back pain, there's always a change of the large, thick fascia of the back. This limits *losgelassenheit* in movement; it prevents, first, the lifting of the back, which again limits the forward and backward movements of the limbs.

Fascia is currently a fast-growing area of research as we've recognized that it plays an important role in health and in the resistance of disease. So, today, we know that it can be an important factor in chronic back pain in humans, for example.

Fascia is one uninterrupted unit of tissue in the horse's body from front to back, but also from outside to inside. This explains why the source of a problem and its symptoms may appear far from one another.

Fascia plays a leading role in the development and maintenance of strength (see sidebar). Fascia takes part in the development and distribution of power and has an essential function in stabilizing the spinal column and the joints of the body.

In physical therapy, osteopathology, chiropractic, and acupuncture, we've long attributed the fascia with a central role. Through the massage, mobilization, stretching, and stabilizing exercises that are described in this book, we can have an enormous influence. A horse with a healthy "fascia net" is more prepared to perform and less likely to get injured.

It's easy to recognize an adhesion of the fascia in the hindquarters. It's common to see this in dressage horses. A trigger can be overstressing the muscles, such as when horses are ridden too long in collection. You can observe the skin of the hindquarters forming wrinkles while moving. When the hindquarters are palpated, you can feel hard areas in the musculature. Here, too, the skin adheres and you won't be able to "lift" it from the underlying layer of skin.

■ How the Fascia Works

Example: When the horse lands during a canter stride (with the standing leg), the fetlock of the landing leg moves toward the ground and all the connected structures are stretched as a result. This includes the flexor muscles, deep and superficial flexor tendons and the ligaments (especially the suspensory) of the lower limbs (see photo, p. 26, left). As this takes place, energy is absorbed as it would be by a spring, in order to subsequently return it. The forces that are influencing the lower limbs and the "spring back" are in direct relation to one another.

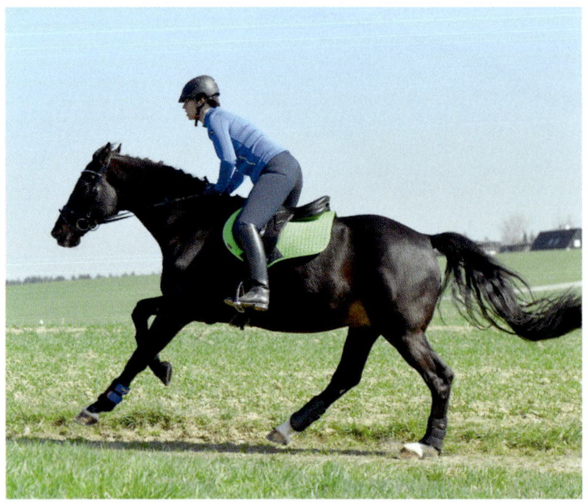

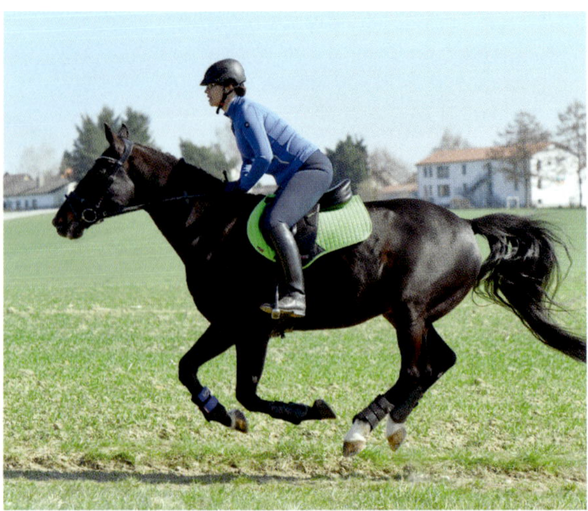

This means, the deeper the fetlock sinks toward the ground, the more energy the soft tissue must take up and likewise the greater the force released by the "spring back." This principle applies for horses that have normal, not weak, fetlocks (see photo, p. 4, left).

This "catapulting back" of the fetlock joint can be compared to a ball: it meets the floor, becomes deformed and takes energy back from this. The ball wants to return to its original form. Through the energy that's set free with this, the ball lifts again from the floor and springs back up (see right side photo, above). This elastic force enables the horse to move with minimal output of energy and also with big and long strides. This applies to horses in all disciplines.

For these mechanics to take place, it's essential that the connective tissue structures remain elastic. We can achieve this with our horses in that we stimulate the tissue with diverse inputs; for example, through cross-training and varying the horse's workload while riding over a variety of ground/footing.

Fact: The fascia and especially the tendons possess the ability to build up elastic tension, or force, recharge the energy and set it free as quickly as a catapult.

■ Muscle Function

We differentiate between dynamic muscles and static muscles.

● The Dynamic Muscle = Mobility Muscles

These muscles establish the motor function, speed, and power of a movement. As they can pull together (contract) very strongly, they're the hard workers among the muscles (they have little to do with fine motor function). You find these muscles more in the extremities of the hindquarters and the superficial muscles of the spinal column. A large distance between the origin and insertion is characteristic of these muscles; this means, they are long muscles with a large belly.

● The Static Muscle = Stability Muscles

These muscles are short, lie close to the joints, and often have a connection with the joint capsule and ligaments. They are responsible for posture and stability. You'll find most static muscles close to the spinal column. In contrast to dynamic muscles, these muscles are rich in nerves and can execute an extremely accurate motor function. These muscles are enormously important to the rider, as their function takes over when it comes to the development of motor sensitivity. Without motor sensitivity, you can't practice the riding arts. It's through these muscles that you school a horse's fine motor function. They teach the horse to respond to your body language. The better these muscles are developed, the less physical exertion a rider will need to execute a movement.

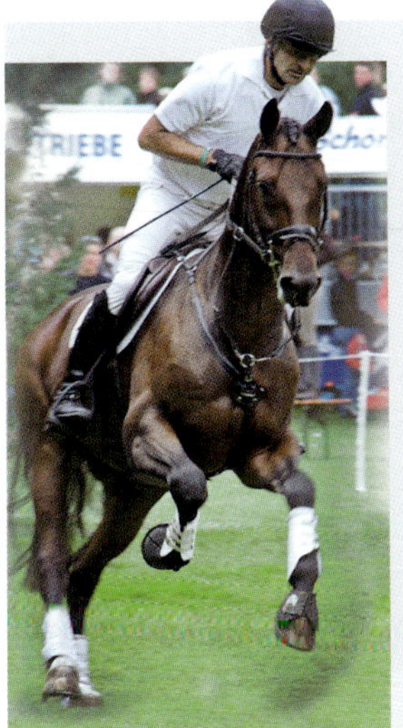

Example: With muscles that respond well, a shift of the weight alone will be enough. The sensitive muscles of the back notice the shift, send this information via the central nervous system and this returns a signal to the necessary joints and muscles.

Fact: With young horses, the static muscles are not yet very developed; therefore, young horses must first be schooled to the aids before they can respond to them with sensitivity.

■ Types of Muscle Fiber

As a reminder: the skeletal muscles are also called striated muscles because of their cross-striped musculature. A muscle is comprised of many muscular fiber bundles, which in turn are made up of many muscle fibers. There are two types of muscle fibers: Type 1 and Type 2.

These different types of muscle fibers work differently:

● "Slow-Twitch" Muscle Fiber—Type 1

These muscle fibers contract slowly and they require a rich supply of oxygen. Therefore, they can work well for a long period of time. You'll find more "slow-twitch" (slow) muscle fibers in heavier horses, such as draft horses, that are required to perform aerobically (work that requires additional oxygen). So, too, stabilizing muscles are comprised more of this type of muscle fiber. They deteriorate quickly when the horse is taken out of training due to injury, for example. Unfortunately, it's difficult to rebuild these muscular fibers. It's been scientifically proven that the stabilizing exercises in chapter 9 are helpful for building up this type of muscle fiber.

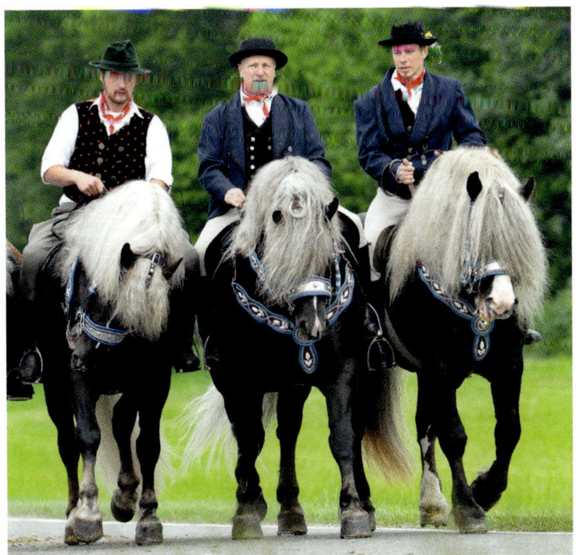

With such a leap, every muscle in the musculoskeletal system is engaged.

These horses aren't fast, but they can work for a long time and have a lot of power.

• "Fast-Twitch" Muscle Fibers—Type 2

These are once again divided into two groups.

High-Oxidative Muscle Fibers (Type 2A)

These muscle fibers have a high myoglobin content. Myoglobin have the capacity to take in lots of oxygen, which is important for powerful, long-lasting performance. You'll find these high-oxidative fibers in horses that must perform at a maximum over longer distances, such as event horses.

Low-Oxidative Muscle Fibers (Type 2B)

These muscle fibers have a low myoglobin content (more white). They can execute "explosive" contractions and don't need much oxygen, but they can't maintain this maximum power work over a long period of time and will tire quickly. The muscle masses of Quarter Horses and Thoroughbreds consist of up to 80 to 90 percent Type 2 muscle fibers.

Most muscles are mixture of all three types of muscular fibers. The percent of distribution of white and red muscle fibers is determined by genetics.

"Fast-twitch" fibers can actually change into "slow-twitch" fibers but the reverse is not possible. To explain more clearly, a sprinter can become a good marathon runner, but a marathon runner can't become a good sprinter; a Thoroughbred can become a good endurance horse, but a cold blood can't become a good racehorse.

A contraction happens when a nerve signals the muscles. This process is controlled by the brain and spinal cord. There's a more detailed explanation in chapter 4, "Nervous System," p. 86.

■ Types of Muscle Contractions

We can distinguish between three different types of muscle contractions:

- Isometric—holding (without movement)
- Concentric—pulling together/contracting
- Eccentric—stretching

Isometric Contractions

Strength develops while the muscle length stays the same; therefore, this is a muscular activity without movement. This means, the muscles are tensed to maintain strength. As this type of muscle work only happens deliberately (controlled by the reasoning mind), the horse can't execute this form of training for himself. The muscle activity required for high collection of the neck vertebrae or in a canter pirouette comes closest to isometric muscle activity.

You can test out how it feels to work isometrically. Hold your arms out at a 90-degree angle from your body and see how long you can hold this position (without moving your arms). You'll soon notice that gravity is pulling your arms down; they'll get heavy and the supporting muscles begin to "burn." If you continue to hold this position, you'll begin evasive movements in order to get relief for the upper arm muscles.

This work is truly challenging for the musculature, as the blood vessels are compromised through the constant contraction, which means less oxygen and nutrients are getting where they need to go. Please consider this when you work your horses in collection—it takes so much strength and can quickly lead to acidification and, thereby, weakening of the muscles.

For example, a danger lies in working with auxiliary reins (see chapter 12, "Preventive Measures," p. 200). If the horse is forced into one position, the muscles must actually work isometrically. And you've now seen for yourself how quickly that begins to "burn" and how painful it can become. Believe me—your horse feels the exact same way. Because of the "lever effect," your horse can't defend himself.

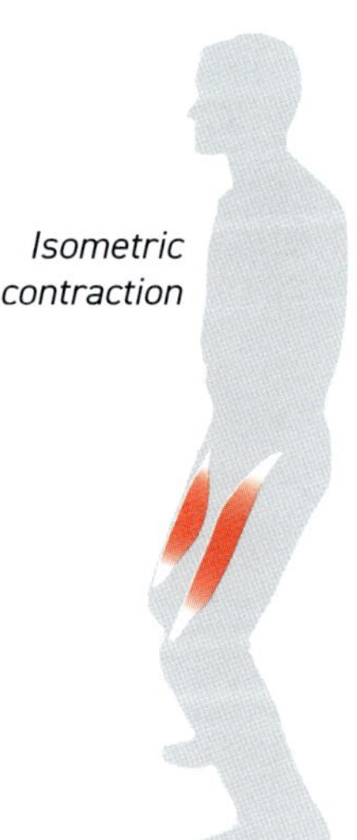

Isometric contraction

How can you tell if your horse is working to his limit? With auxiliary reins, you'll unfortunately have fewer chances to recognize that your horse is trying to "lift out of the frame" or lie on the bit, as the draw reins or similar are preventing him from escaping the forced position. You're forcing your horse into work for which he perhaps does not have the strength or stretching ability. Is that fair? The affected muscles will then be under-oxidized and over-acidified, and your training session becomes pointless. Therefore, my request: Please don't use auxiliary reins; they're not doing anything for the rider. In fact, it's a self-defeating practice! (For more on this, see p. 211.)

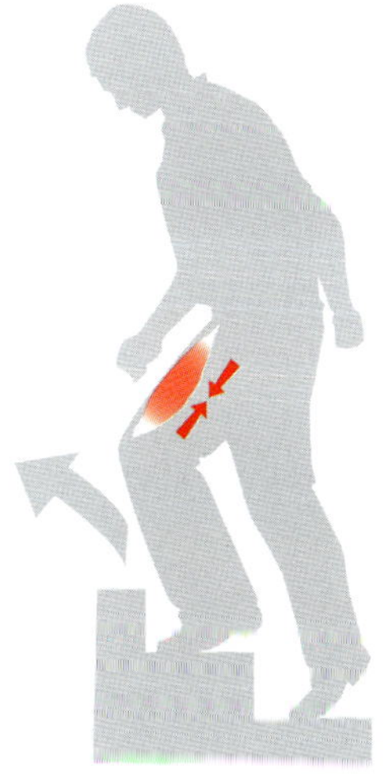

A concentrated contraction.

Concentric Muscular Activity

Concentric muscular activity means that the muscle contracts: it pulls itself together. When you walk up the steps, your quadriceps muscle (which lies on the front side of your upper thigh) contracts (see illustration); when your horse moves uphill or jumps over an obstacle, his stifle extensor works concentrically, meaning the origin of the muscle and its insertion get closer together.

Eccentric Muscular Activity

In this work, the muscle must stretch and at the same time brace against outside forces. The origin and insertion move away from one another. You'll experience this type of muscular activity when you walk downstairs (see illustration) or when a horse goes downhill. The eccentric muscle activity is the most effective way for building up muscular strength, as here the muscle must utilize many more muscular fibers than it does when the muscle is contracted.

With concentric and eccentric muscular activity, you'll always find a switching back and forth

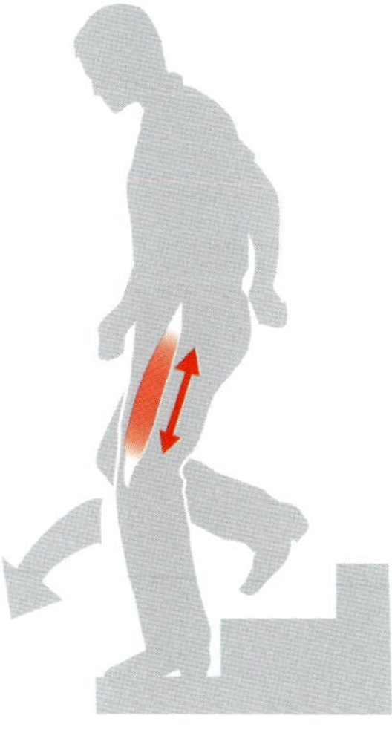

Eccentric contraction.

between tensing and relaxation in the muscle. When the muscle is engaged, the blood vessels are compromised; when it is relaxed, these are opened up so new nutrients and oxygen can be delivered and waste and carbon dioxide can be removed. In this way, the muscle is well-supplied by this "muscular pump." In isometric work, there's no movement in the muscles, so there's also no engagement and relaxation phases and no muscle pump. But, inside the muscles, engagement and relaxation can take place. This means, not all muscle fibers must contract at the same time so they can engage and relax within the muscle itself, and in this way, metabolism can continue to function.

Take note: It's not only the muscles that are responsible for strength, fascia is also involved in muscular activity.

◼ Stress Limits

In order to extract energy for the muscles from nutrition, you need oxygen. In a workout where the absorption of oxygen and workload are balanced, it's possible to demonstrate endurance for a long period of time. This balance of metabolic process to workload is referred to as "Steady State." In this phase, significant amounts of lactic acid are building over a long period of time. You have this in endurance sports, for example, distance and trail riding. The horse works aerobically. With this form of work, you can't bring about peak performance.

If you come upon the maximum performance limit of the horse, meaning you go past this "steady state," the oxygen delivery is no longer enough. The affected muscles must now work anaerobically. This phase should only last a short time before the lactate (salt from the lactic acid) builds up, acidifying the muscles, which means they start to "burn" and get painful. You'll inevitably soon see a rapid reduction in performance (the horse has no more strength).

Fact:
Aerobic: Metabolism occurs with enough oxygen supply.
Anaerobic: The affected muscles are not getting enough oxygen. Burning must take place without enough oxygen. This type of calorie burning can't be sustained for long. But you know that—the fire in the fireplace won't burn without oxygen either (white muscular fibers, Muscle Type 2B, see p. 28).

Example: A racehorse, that only gallops quickly over 500 meters, can bring his maximum performance and work in the anaerobic phase, as this is just a short track. But if he runs 2400 meters, the tempo must be lowered in order to stay within the "steady state" limits; otherwise, his metabolism will come out of balance. You've certainly experienced this yourself at least once. You need to get to the bus so you start running as fast as you can. When you're halfway there, it gets difficult to breathe and you can't maintain the tempo. You don't have the strength left and your muscles "burn." You've reached your "steady state" limit and you're working anaerobically. If you'd started out running more slowly, you'd likely have reached your goal more quickly as your muscles would have worked continuously and, therefore, could have worked longer. Obviously, this "steady state" zone differs from individual to individual. Through ongoing training, you can increase the point at which you enter an anaerobic phase. In this way, you and or your horse can improve fitness.

Why am I sharing this theory with you? I find it important that you're informed about your horse's work limits when you ride him, as much muscular tension and many injuries to the musculoskeletal system occur because of incorrect usage. If you work your horse too long in the anaerobic phase, his body will be stressed and build adrenalin, which inhibits the flow of oxygen. In addition, alternate muscles will take over for those that have become exhausted and acidic.

The Bottom Line

"Wrong" muscles take over tasks for which they are not intended, which means the training goal will not be reached. The stress on a muscle is accompanied by the stimulation of muscle growth. But, the muscle can actually only grow when the demand made is in accordance with its natural function.

This maximum workload is observable in all horses, regardless of whether you're watching racehorses or dressage horses.

Of course, endurance, event, and racehorses will reach the anaerobic phase faster. That's not so bad, as long as the horse is only there for a short period of time. You utilize the anaerobic phase in order to achieve fitness. However, you should observe your horse closely and recognize signs of fatigue, including increased respiration and elevated pulse, but also other signs: the horse lying on your hands, inconsistent rhythm, teeth grinding, getting tense, or noticeable hard breathing.

Dressage horses also move frequently back and forth between aerobic and anaerobic zones. With dressage horses that work with a high degree of collection, you're getting closer to isometric work. This work is really difficult for the musculature, which then requires lots of oxygen.

The more difficult the work, the more muscle fibers will be engaged. This is interesting to you as the rider: the harder the work and the more you reach the anaerobic zone, the more breaks your horse will need. These breaks are crucial during work: one to

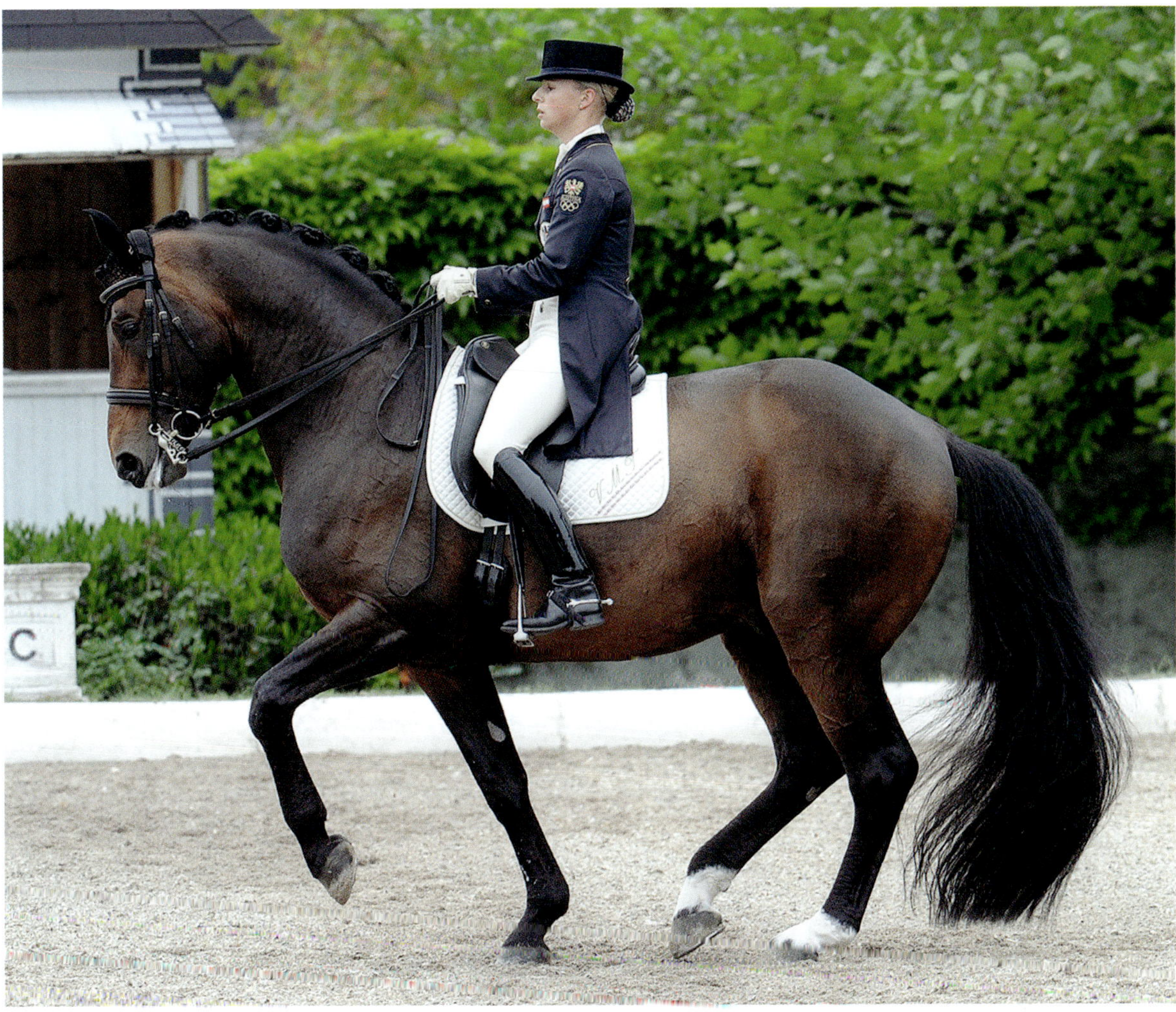

four minutes of walk on a long rein, regardless of the horse's level of fitness and the difficulty of the work. This means, if you have a horse that is being rehabilitated from injury, he will need a longer break than a horse in normal condition that has been in light work. You'll see that your horse will return to being ready to work much more quickly when you allow him to take breaks.

■ Sore Muscles

We all know what it feels like to have sore muscles and you know how uncomfortable that is. Believe me, horses find it just as uncomfortable as we do.

Exactly What Is Muscle Soreness?

In the past, we believed sore muscles were the result of overworked muscles collecting lactate, which couldn't be transported out of the muscles during work. This hypothesis has since been disproven, as muscle soreness first occurs much later, after the work has taken place, when the lactate levels have already returned to normal.

Scientists have determined that muscle soreness frequently occurs in untrained athletes and/or from strength training because not enough lactate has been produced.

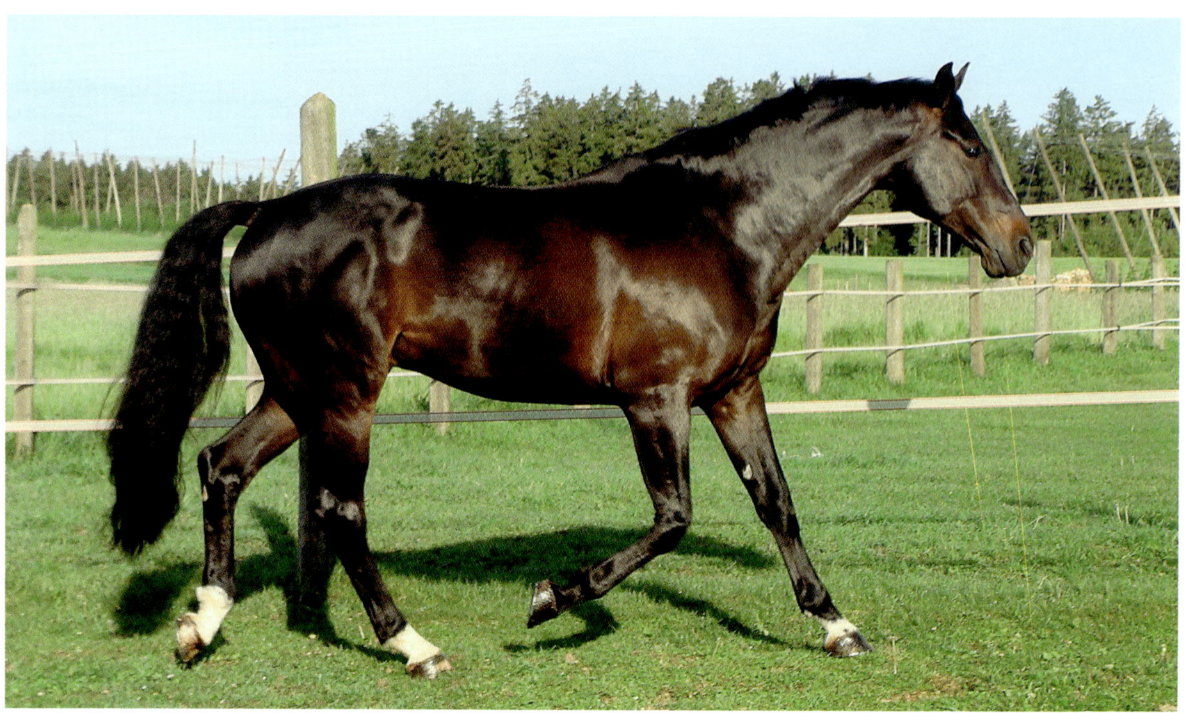

There's Much More to Muscle Soreness

When the muscles are powerfully engaged, the stress causes small tears in the muscular tissue. Lymph builds up as it enters the small tears in the tissue. The muscle swells and pain can be felt when it stretches—muscle soreness.

■ Muscle Tone (Basic Engagement)

Every horse has a basic engagement to his muscles, a tone. By tone, I am referring to the constant, slightly contracted tension that exists in all normal skeletal muscles. This basic engagement changes: when the horse is in his stall (standing), the muscular engagement will be less than when he's in movement. But not only that, the tone changes based on the horse's mood. When the horse feels good, fresh with energy, the tone is higher. So, too, when he's alarmed about something (in flight mode). A tired, lower energy but also relaxed mood leads to a reduction in tone.

Tone has a direct influence on the activity of muscular fibers. This has advantages and disadvantages for us as riders.

Horses that move a normal amount will move better and have higher muscle tone. This includes horses that have, for example, mild ataxia (a coordination problem) or weak connective tissue. This means, they innately have too much movement. So, too, an unstable stifle joint will be less of a bother if there's a higher level of base tone. The musculature then works like a corset and provides the horse with more stability.

A disadvantage of higher muscle tone is that due to the stronger activation of muscle fibers and muscles, lameness can be hidden. What looks like an "advantage" at first should not be "ignored" for reasons of health. It's worth mentioning that horses with higher tone will have more of a tendency to have tight muscles as a result.

As a rider, please be very attentive to the fact that there's a fine line between positive and negative muscular engagement (tension). Negative tension takes place when a horse recognizes danger. He "gathers himself" and you have the feeling that you're sitting on a "bomb." The rider can also cause this negative tension by riding with too much pressure. It may look spectacular and the horse may become more impressive, but when the entire schooling session is ridden this way, it's at the cost of the horse's *losgelassenheit* and over time will lead to chronic tension. Eventually, it will also lead to problems with the musculoskeletal system, such as adhesions and matting of the large fascia of the back.

■ Muscular Interplay

When a bend in the elbow joint takes place, it does not only involve a contraction of the flexor muscle (the executing muscle) of the elbow. The counterpart (antagonistic muscles) of the elbow flexor must stretch and give, so that a bending can take place. At the same time, the elbow flexor ensures that the bend is not too strong.

A movement does not only take place in a joint, but rather happens as part of a chain. This means,

when the horse wants to turn his head right and toward the back, multiple right-side muscles contract. This muscular interplay can take place all the way to the base of the tail.

Via the nervous system, the agonist (the executing muscles) gets the signal to contract. The antagonist (counterpart) received the opposite information: it should stretch. In the agonist, the reaction happens as the proteins, actin and myosin, glide into one another. Thereby, the muscle contracts and the muscular engagement (tension) is heightened.

Calcium and magnesium are required to separate the actin and myosin back out. Once this pair is broken up, the muscle can go back to its original state. If these minerals are insufficient, the muscles will have a hard time relaxing and tension will remain.

It's only possible to reach optimal performance and thereby *losgelassenheit* in movement when there is seamless cooperation among all the muscles in the body.

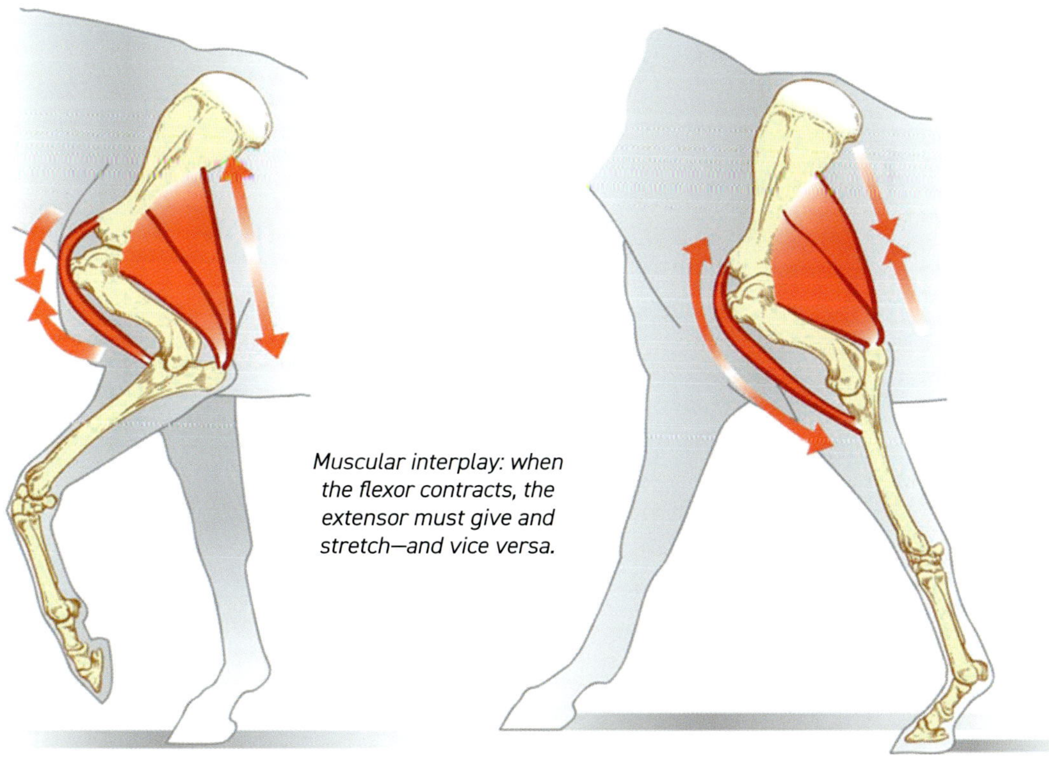

Muscular interplay: when the flexor contracts, the extensor must give and stretch—and vice versa.

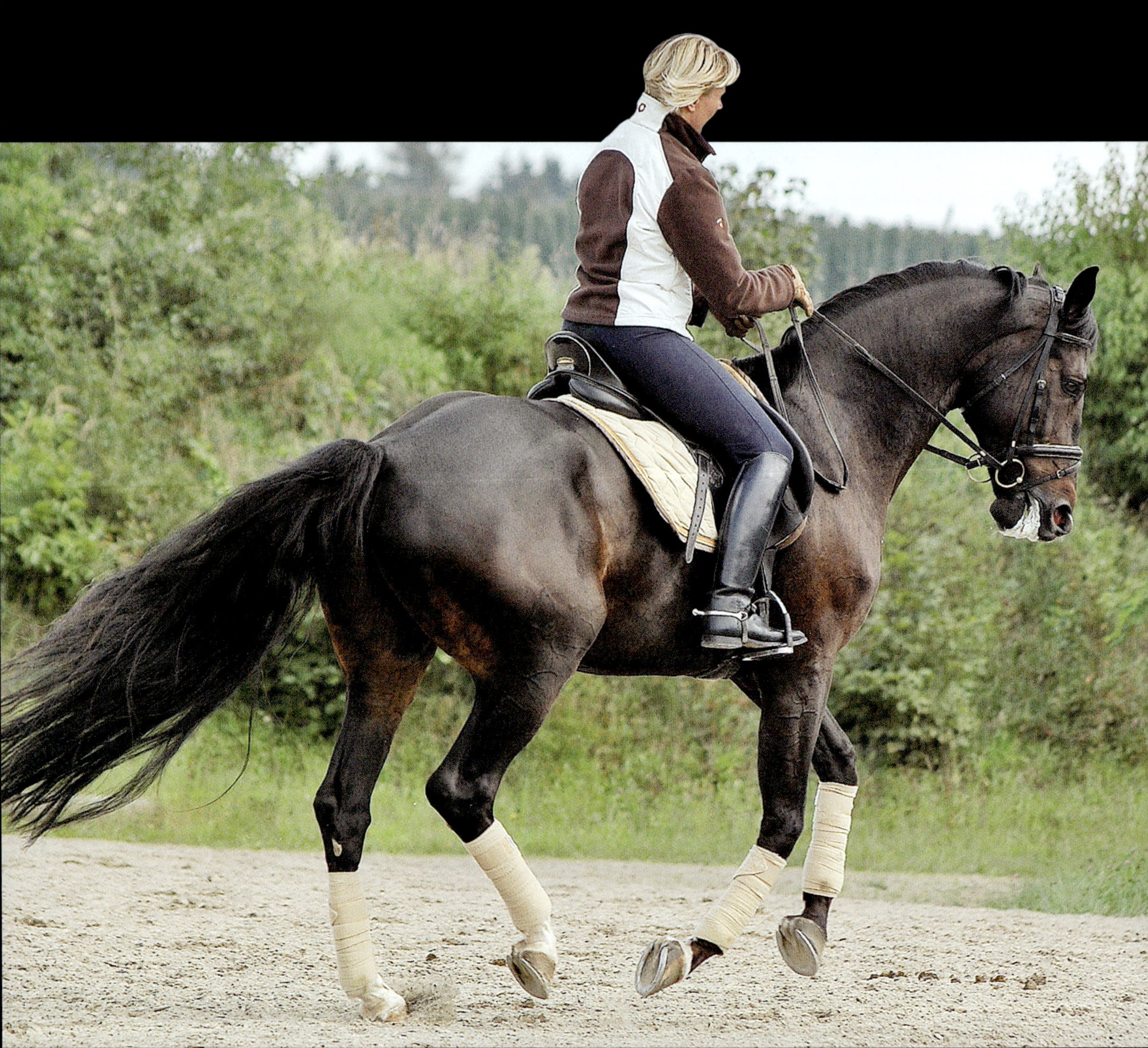

Chapter 3

Biomechanics

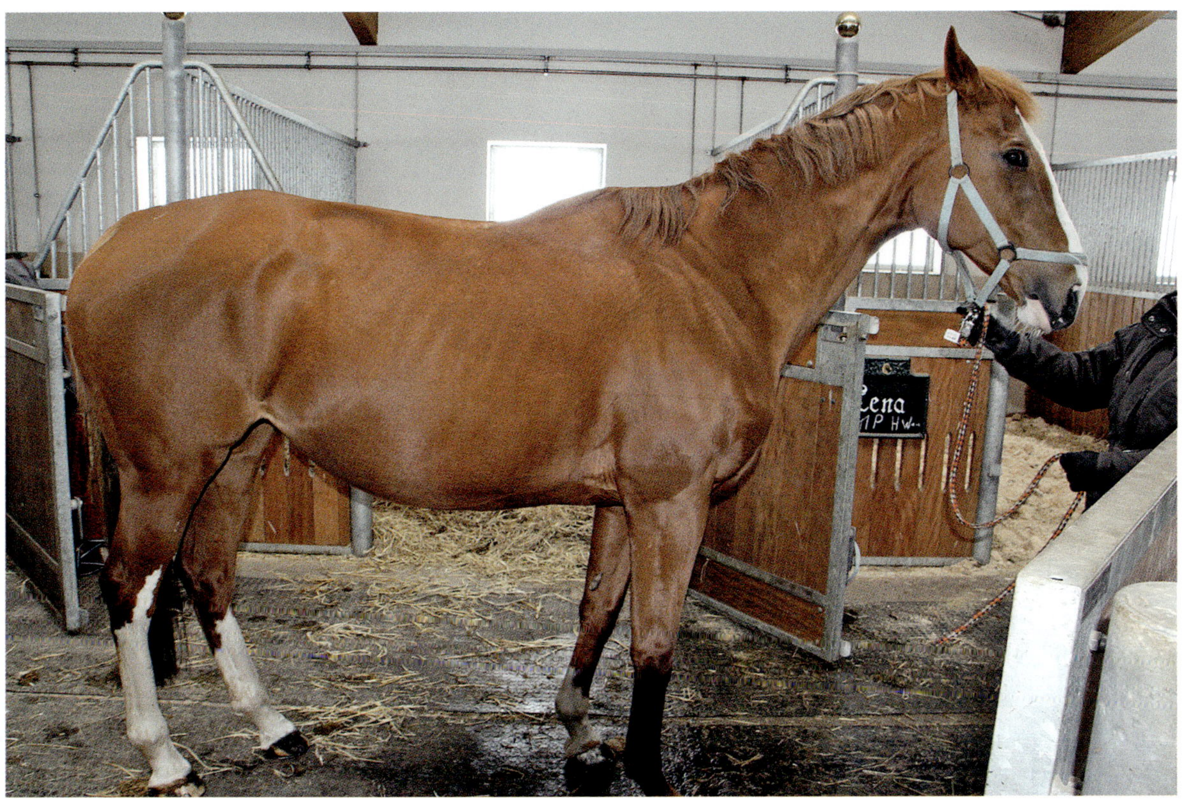

A poorly muscled horse with a pronounced underside of neck. You can clearly recognize the dip in front of the shoulder blade and that the muscling of the hindquarters has developed inadequately. The abdominal muscles are equally weak. This muscular development allows you to conclude that the horse cannot push from behind, come through his back, or carry his own neck when he's ridden.

"Biomechanics" or functional anatomy? These are concepts you've surely heard of at least once. How do they influence us and why is it useful for a rider to know more about them?

First, a short explanation of terms. *Biomechanics* refers to the function and structures of the musculoskeletal system. It incorporates knowledge from subjects such as anatomy, biology, physics and mathematics. But, no worries! You don't need to be a scientist to understand biomechanics. When the basis for an examination is precise observation and analysis of the horse's movement, with the goal of recognizing what's normal and what isn't, a basic knowledge of biomechanics is absolutely indispensable.

With deeper knowledge about anatomy basics, movement patterns, and the interplay between bones, joints, and soft tissue (muscles, ligaments, tendons), you're also better able to assess a horse's movement, his capacity, and, thereby, when he's overstressed. This helps avoid injury. And, ultimately, it also optimizes performance.

Biomechanics also helps people to recognize more quickly when the horse isn't moving correctly or has adopted a compensatory posture. The practiced eye recognizes compensatory movement patterns early on, with the goal of improving a weak spot and not disproportionately overstressing other parts of the body. If the horse has adopted compensatory movement patterns, it will follow that he is seeking relief and has developed a changed way of going. This also changes the natural balance of his muscle mass (an increase in "incorrect" muscling and

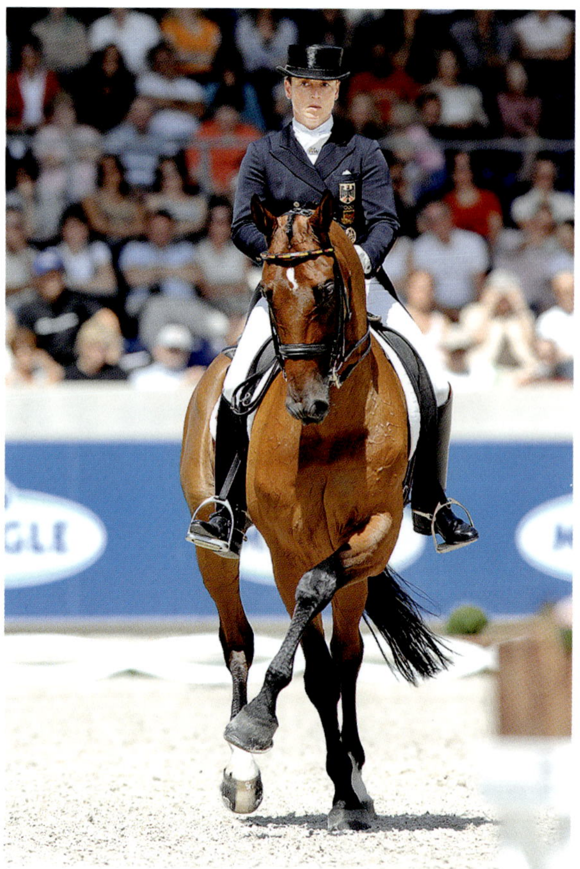

To execute this movement, the entire musculoskeletal system must be supple.

muscles. The musculature covers the skeleton in multiple layers. Its purpose is first to move the horse, second to stabilize the musculoskeletal system, and third to distribute the stress on the body. The short muscles (for example, the *musculi multifidus*), which are directly on the spinal column, work together with ligaments and joint capsules to support the spinal cord (stabilizers).

The stratified muscles have their origin and insertion on bones or fascia and travel over one or more joints. By contracting (pulling together of the muscles), the following movements of the joints are initiated: bending, extending, pulling to the inside or outside, turning toward the inside or outside, lifting or lowering. When there's a movement of a joint, there's always interplay with a muscle(s). During movement, the joint is led and protected by the muscles on all sides. The capacity of the joint to move is determined by its construction, the arrangement and tightness of the ligaments, and the pulling direction of the muscles.

From a mechanical perspective, it's important to know that movement does not only take place in the joint and its surrounding muscles. Movement always has a "domino effect."

Example: If the horse wants to bring his foreleg forward, the muscles work synergistically. This means, many muscles from his neck to his underarm are involved with bringing the foreleg forward.

decrease in "correct" muscling). This will result in more limited range of motion and the decrease in performance will lead to problems under saddle and frustration. The inevitable result can lead to damage of the musculoskeletal system.

To understand anatomy as an important part of biomechanics requires study of the body's structure, which is composed of bones, ligaments, vessels, nerves, and muscles. In this chapter, I will go over *functional anatomy* with you; this means I'll explain the interplay between the different body parts and make more tangible the individual important muscles—their functions and problems.

It's the muscles (and fascia) that initiate movement. For this task, the horse has about 260 stratified

Now, to the detailed sections of this chapter. In order to give you a better overview of biomechanics, I've divided the horse's body into different parts:

- Head
- Spine
- Cervical spine
- Thoracic spine and rib cage
- Lumbar vertebrae
- Hindquarters
- Forehand

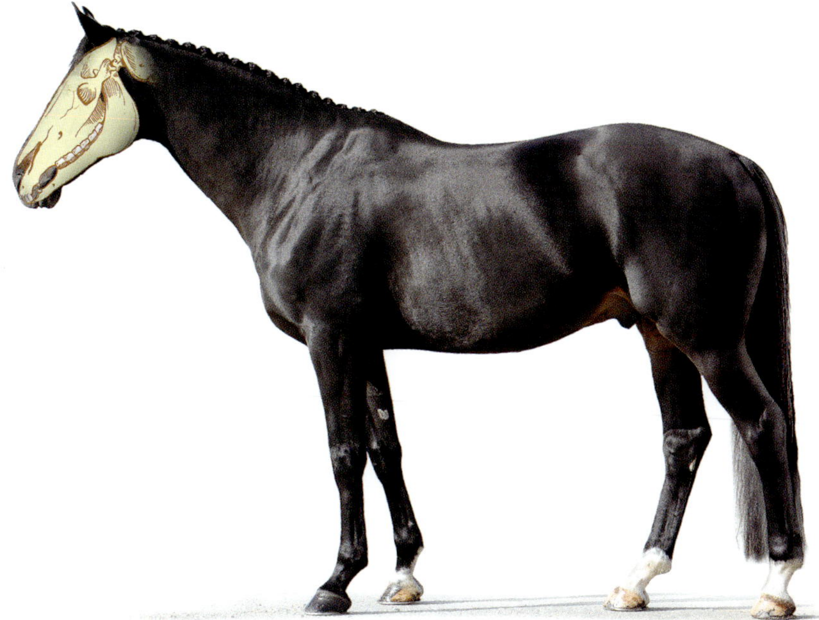

The Head

Although the head is not considered a direct part of the musculoskeletal system, it still has enormous impact on movement. Problems in the head area can trigger many symptoms in the musculoskeletal system.

Skull Movement (Cranial Rhythmic Impulse—CRI)

The skull is comprised of 29 mostly flat bones, which are bound together by sutures. These sutures are actually not true joints; they bind the bones together and look like a zipper. The skull has about 100 of these "bone binders." Because of the sutures, the bones of the skull can move lightly against one another. You can actually also feel on your own head how the skull widens and comes together again, approximately 8 to 12 times per minute. This mechanism is known as CRI.

CRI stands for *cranial rhythmic impulse*. It's a standalone impulse that begins in the mother's womb (so before the first breath) and only stops after death.

A short explanation: in the brain and spinal cord, you have brain/spinal fluid, which is known as cerebrospinal fluid. This fluid operates with a wave-like, fluctuating movement, from the pelvis to the brain. You can best feel this movement, which has 8 to 12 cycles per minute, in the head or the pelvis. Every movement of the body has this rhythm. The skull gets bigger and smaller, at the same time that the sacroiliac moves up and down, all while the limbs turn to the inside and outside. The entire body, including the organs down to the hoof, stretch and pull back together, with you hardly being aware.

Why Is This Rhythm So Important?

Together with the other rhythms of the body, this holds the body's structures in balance and keeps the organs' functions intact.

If there's a blockage in the head, spine, or pelvis, this can have an immense effect on the CRI. Therefore, it can also have an immense effect on the entire organism. When the skull's movement becomes restricted, perhaps triggered by trauma, (which may come from being tied, an impact, or a fall), or by tension, the result can be a change in personality or disorders of balance, vision, or hearing. In addition, back pain, organ disorders, and lameness can be triggered secondarily by limited movement of the skull bones.

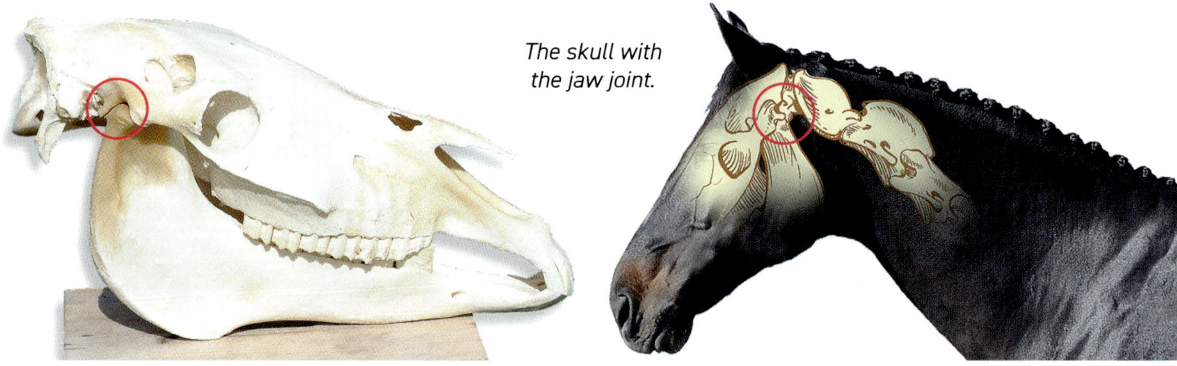

The skull with the jaw joint.

Jaw Joint

The jaw joint is the largest joint in the skull. It joins the lower jaw with the upper jaw. Here, the joint surface does not fit together optimally: it truly doesn't have a head and socket. This unfavorable structure is improved by a piece of cartilage, a disc. Luckily, through this construction of the jaw joint, it can execute the large, three-dimensional movement required to chew.

The jaw joint is moved by five muscles. The largest is the outer masticatory (chewing) muscle, which very beautifully runs along the cheeks—visible, wide, and flat. Because of its large movement, the jaw joint can compensate well for dental problems, for example. Having said this, when it comes to long-lasting problems (such as hooks on the teeth), the compensatory ability has the effect of limiting the movement of this joint and causing tension in the jaw muscles. This can even lead to dysfunction of the craniosacral system (skull to pelvis). The jaw joint has an enormous influence on the activity of the hindquarters. Potentially, you'll first notice dysfunction when the horse begins to lie on the bit, hide behind the vertical, tilt his head, and no longer accept contact. *Losgelassenheit* disappears, too. Finally, without *losgelassenheit*, the activity of the hindquarters shrinks. The horse is no longer able to accept weight onto the hindquarters, to flex and lower the joints of his hind end, which means he can't develop optimal power in the hindquarters. Therefore, the impulsion from back to front is no longer as "impulsionful" as it could be. As a result, the tongue (hyoid) bone muscle and the *brachiocephalicus*[2] muscle also get more tense, which can, in turn, limit the horse's ability to move his front limbs forward.

The reaction can also take place in reverse; for example, the jaw joint can be affected by a blockage in the hindquarters. Here, a chain reaction is caused in the subsequent soft tissue and joints and this leads to symptoms far away from the source of the problem.

Playing with the tongue (sticking it out or getting it over the bit), head shaking, or teeth grinding[3] are also signs that there's tension in the mouth region and it's likely you'll also find disorders in other parts of the body.

Fact: Even small changes with a horse's teeth can trigger massive problems in his musculoskeletal system.

Hyoid (Tongue) Bone

The hyoid bone is located in between the two lower jaw bones and is connected to the skull. The hyoid bone has muscular and tissue (fascia) connections to the larynx, the head (the auditory canal), the upper cervical vertebrae, the sternum, and shoulder joint. The long and short tongue muscles are needed to swallow and to maintain balance. (Pay

---

2 The *brachiocephalicus* muscle runs from the upper arm to the head.
3 Teeth grinding must not be confused with teeth chattering.

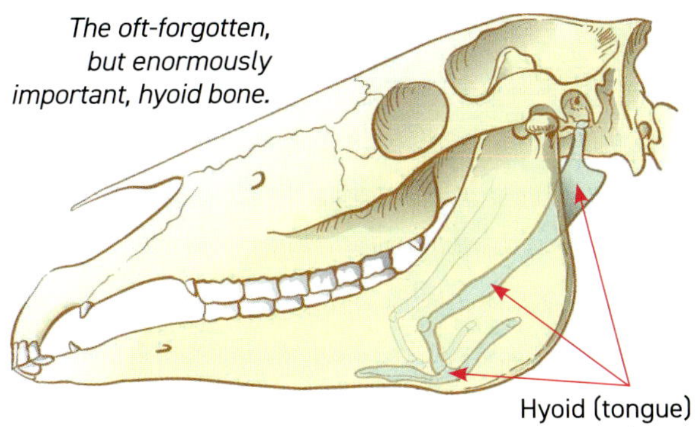

The oft-forgotten, but enormously important, hyoid bone.

Hyoid (tongue) bone.

attention to your tongue sometime when you're trying to balance!) Disorders in the areas described above are muscular in nature and can lead to multi-faceted problems:

Example: Hooks on the teeth can also lead to tension in the hyoid bone muscles. Because of this tension, the hyoid bone may turn slightly. It is believed that as a result of this rotation, the brain receives false information about the body's position, as there is pressure on the inner ear. The ear is the equilibrium center, which is why the connection from hyoid bone to the head can lead to balance problems. Jumpers that are insecure at the jump may have a problem in the connection of this joint.

With cribbing, the sternum-tongue bone muscles (*m. sternohyoideus*) will be badly overburdened. Because of the described soft tissue connection, cribbing can result in major blockages for the first and second cervical vertebrae, as well as disorders with swallowing and a dry cough. In addition, increased muscular tension and volume in the sternum-lower jaw muscle (*m. sternomandibularis*) are recognizable. These horses can also develop breathing problems, as these muscles originate in the sternum and tension here limits the movement of the sternum. The mobility of the sternum is an essential factor of breathing mechanisms.

You also should not underestimate long-term emotional stress. This can lead to tension of the jaw muscles and misalignment of the jaw and hyoid

bone joints. This dysfunction and the pain that follows leads to problems in other areas of the body. The reason is the joints are positioned in relation to one another; a misalignment of one joint has a negative influence on other joints.

A good sign of a relaxed jaw and tongue muscle is good saliva production. As is chattering of the teeth, which is often mistaken for grinding of the teeth and, therefore, interpreted as a negative. In fact, teeth chattering (as long as the noseband permits it!) is a good sign of a relaxed jaw. It's important to allow chattering, especially during upper-level dressage movements (piaffe and passage). The head and lower jaw are important components of the forward movement of the forelegs. During this, the lower jaw must be able to "move with"—it must be relaxed in order to fully achieve this movement.

Fact: Teeth that have not been professionally pulled cannot only lead to local pain and, therefore, cause problems under saddle, but also can cause blockages from the poll all the way to the hindquarters.

The Spine

Be honest—do you actually know exactly where your horse's spinal column is located? If I were to ask you, could you draw this directly on your horse? Thankfully, we have the drawings in books, as putting them directly on the horse is not actually that easy. However, it's a huge advantage to you to be able to differentiate bones from muscles. Likewise, as a rider, you should know what you have in front of you, under you, and behind you!

The entire spinal column is formed from a connected chain of bones. It begins at the head and ends about 50 individual bones later at the tail. In a normal horse, it is almost three meters long. The vertebrae are connected by short and long ligaments and the intervertebral discs. The spinal column looks like a long, moveable pipe.

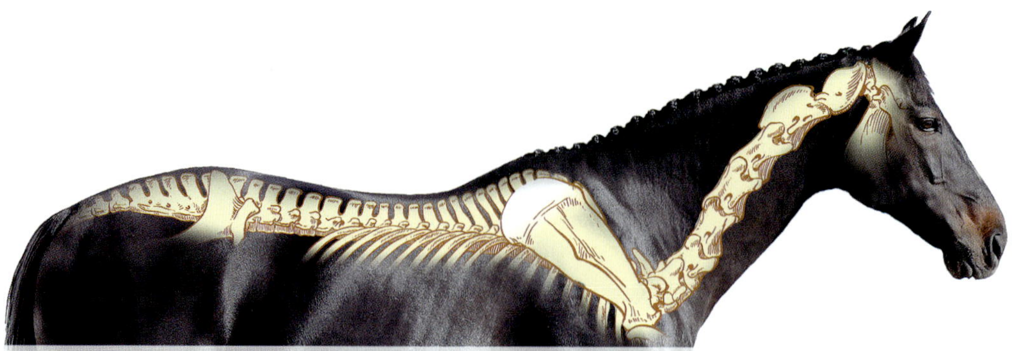

The spinal column serves as a stem for the entire body; it is the protector of the spinal cord and serves as a distributor of the nerves to their other areas of responsibility. It delivers the power that originates in the hindquarters to the head. For you as a rider, one of the spine's functions is to carry you.

The spinal column is divided into five parts and normally consists of 7 cervical, 18 thoracic, 6 lumbar, 5 sacral, and 15 to 21 coccygeal vertebrae. The different parts have different movements; together, they have a three-dimensional movement, they bend and stretch and execute longitudinal bend as well as left and right turns. In between each bone, aside from the poll (head-atlas-axis connection), there are intervertebral discs. The thicker these discs are, the more movement in that area of the spinal column. Horses, in comparison with other animals such as dogs and cats, have at their disposal a relatively stable and strong trunk. To a certain extent, the mobility of the limbs is dependent upon the mobility of the spinal column. The mobility of the spine is dependent upon the tone of the deep muscles of the spinal column, the ligaments, and the elasticity of the discs. This construction makes the horse a good long-distance traveler. This makes sense for the horse as he requires less energy to move and stabilize his vertebrae. Therefore, he can apply his energy purposefully to the large muscle groups of the forehand and hindquarters.

Take Note: Thanks to relatively stiff thoracic and lumbar vertebrae, the horse is able to carry both you and his large organs almost effortlessly.

By comparison, when you watch a dog or a cheetah sprint, it's possible to recognize that the spinal column of these hunters moves a lot more than the spinal column of a horse. The power required to move the muscles of the spinal column and limbs is costing the predators a lot of energy. This energy is used up very quickly, which means these animals cannot run fast over long distances.

Nature has taken even more into account: in contrast to dogs or cats, horses have immensely large internal organs, which also need to be carried.

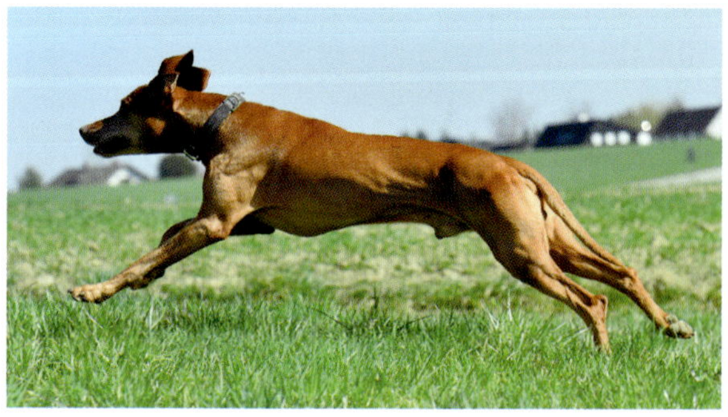

Horse and dog stretched out at a gallop.

Physical Therapy for Horses

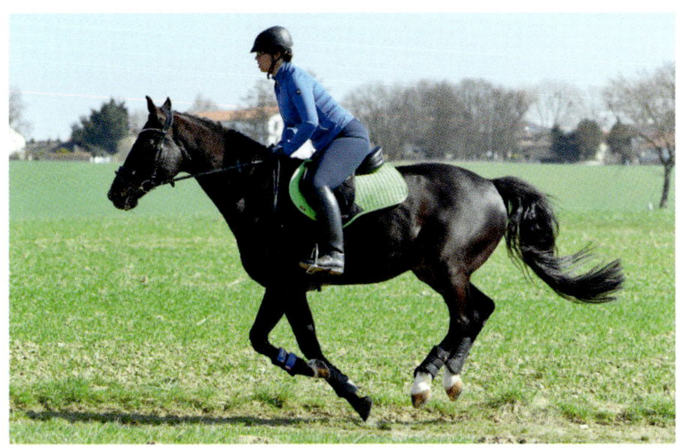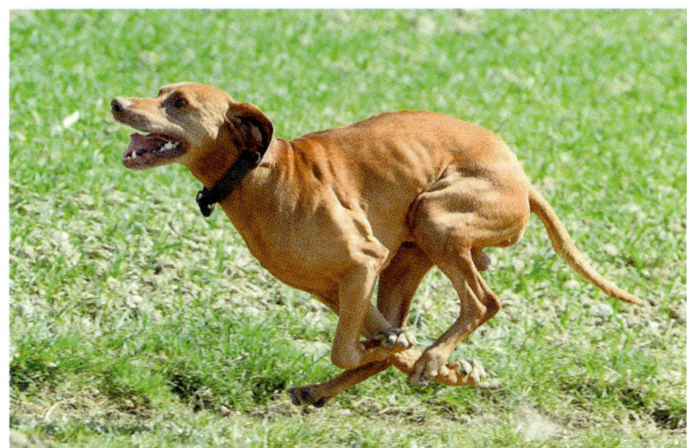

Horse and dog at a gallop with the hindquarters gathering under the body like a spring. Here, you see the difference between horse and dog in the curvature of the spine.

Their relatively stiff spinal columns help them to stabilize this weight against gravity.

Let's first take a look at the individual vertebrae in the various regions of the spine:

- The cervical vertebrae do not have pronounced transverse or spinous processes.
- The thoracic vertebrae have long spinous processes, but no transverse processes.
- The lumbar vertebrae have long transverse processes, but less pronounced spinous processes than the thoracic vertebrae.

The shape of the topline is, therefore, not formed by the vertebral bodies. In the neck, it's the nuchal ligament and musculature that's responsible, while in the thoracic and lumbar regions, it's the length of the spinous processes.

The withers are formed by the spinous processes of the second to ninth thoracic vertebrae. Thereby, it's normally the fifth to sixth spinous processes that

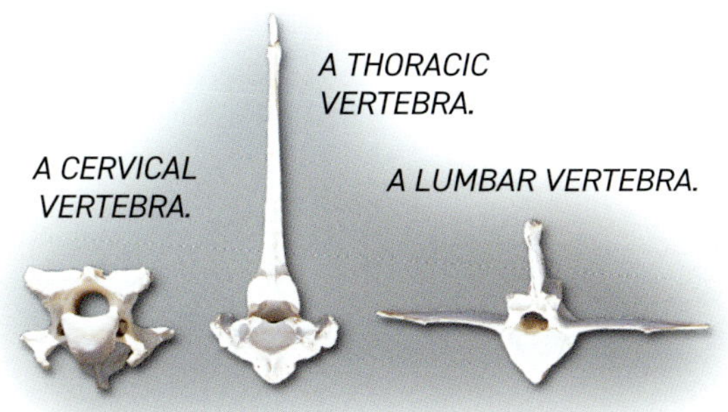

forms the highest point of the withers. In horses, these can be up to 30 centimeters (almost a foot) in length. In this area, they are tilted toward the back. However, at about the fourteenth or fifteenth thoracic vertebrae, they get shorter and point more upward, so that they stand more vertically in this area.

At the sixteenth vertebra, the spinous processes begin to tilt slightly toward the front of the horse and continue to get longer until about the third lumbar vertebrae. The last three are shorter again.

The spinous processes on the sacrum again lean toward the back.

Fact: The length of the spinous process of the withers is an important factor for the effortless carriage of the head and neck through the nuchal ligament and the musculature, which begin at the withers.

And just why are these directional differences among the spinous processes so important? These different tendencies have a substantial advantage for the carrying ability of the back. More on this subject coming soon!

Fact: The third lumbar vertebra has the longest spinous processes among the rear thoracic and lumbar vertebrae. Because of this length, it often stands higher and shows itself as dominant over the other spinous processes. As a result, this vertebra is often diagnosed as blocked, which may not always be the case. Often, this spinous process is easier to see, when the back/gluteus muscles lose mass.

The Curve of the Spine

When you look at the horse from the side, you see the neck has a beautiful curve and the head is the highest point. The withers are approximately the same height as the croup and round upward. The saddle area swings downward and is slightly lower.

Many believe the path of the spine is identical to the topline (as it is in people). But, that's just not so! When you look at the horse's spinal column from the side (meaning the path of the spinal column joints without spinous processes, muscles and ligaments), you can recognize curves that run completely differently from the topline.

- A lift between the head and the third cervical vertebra.
- A hollowing from the fourth cervical vertebra to the tenth thoracic vertebra, although, from the fourth thoracic vertebra on, the rest form practically a straight line. In this curve, the seventh and last cervical vertebra is the deepest point.
- Again, a lift from the eleventh vertebra to the coccyx (tailbone).

The lift in the spinal column lends itself to accommodating for movement/locomotion, and allows a clearly larger range of movement. The hollowing part of the spinal column is responsible for stability and, therefore, is restricted in its ability to move.

The Nuchal Ligament

As already explained, the nuchal ligament forms the topline of the neck and is the foundation for the crest. It's a very strong, elastic band, which runs from the occipital bone (poll) to the withers. At the withers, it connects to the spinous processes of the third to the sixth thoracic vertebrae. From here, the band changes; it is anchored to the highest point of the spinous processes (upper spinous processes) almost all the way back to the pelvis. The farther it gets toward the pelvis, the thinner and less elastic it becomes (see illustration below).

In the neck area, the laminar portion of the nuchal ligament has an important function. It has direct contact with the second cervical vertebra to the second spinous processes of the thoracic vertebrae. Thanks to the length of the thoracic vertebrae, the band remains passive, but very effectively carries the horse's neck and head and keeps them upright, without requiring much muscular power. This construction is tightly connected to the neck musculature by fascia.

The nuchal ligament and the lamellar portion of the nuchal ligament, along with the upper spinous processes, are of great importance to the mechanics of the spinal column.

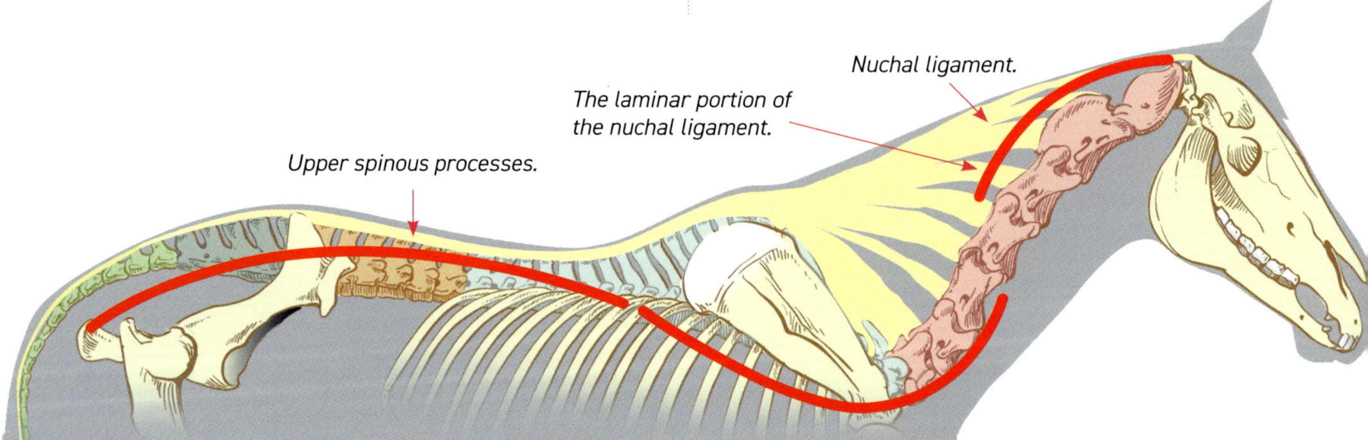

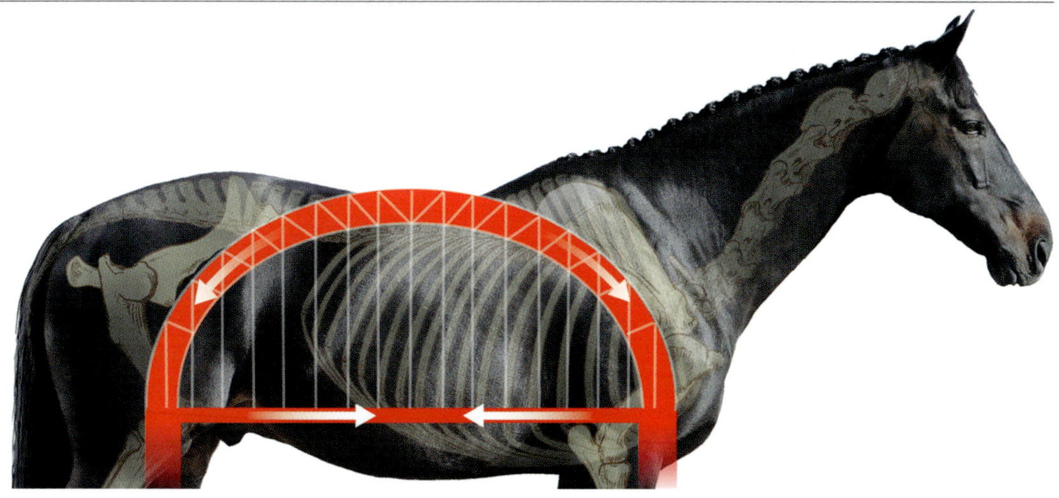

The horse's carrying construction can be visualized as follows: the entire trunk forms one unit, whereby the spinal column forms a bow, while the rib cage, sternum, and the musculature in this area form the string that tightens the bow. When the abdominal muscles contract, a pressure builds in the trunk, whereby the spinal column experiences a compression that lifts it upward.

The Horse's Carrying Ability

Over time, much consideration has been given to the question: What about the horse's physical construction allows him to carry us? In this regard, the talk ranges from house and roof construction to bridge construction. The "Bowstring-Bridge-Concept," which takes as its model a bow and arrow, comes closest regarding the statics of the horse:

Moreover, for the biomechanical concept of back function, the influence of the head and neck movement is important. When the head lowers, the nuchal ligament pulls on the withers, the spinous processes straighten up, the upper spinous processes are also stretched, and these effects combined lift the back to the middle of the saddle area. Then, the loin-pelvic muscles and abdominal muscles are responsible for the remainder of the spinal column. When they engage, the pelvis straightens up, the upper spinous processes get a pull from the back (therefore, the different directionality of the various spinous processes) and the back lifts.

The exact opposite takes place when the horse lifts his head up and the back muscles strain. The spinous processes of the withers lose the pull from the nuchal ligaments, tip farther toward the back, and the back sinks. In the pelvic area, the exact same

happens. Through the lifting of the head, the abdominal muscles lose their optimal engagement and the pelvis tips. The hind limbs can no longer step underneath (because of too much tension on the extensors of the limb—see "Muscles That Move the Leg Back," illustration, p. 74). The rear thoracic and lumbar vertebrae fall.

As you see, the nuchal ligament has a major influence on the carrying ability of a horse's back. With this knowledge, it's also clear why young horses and horses rehabilitating from injury should be ridden in a green horse frame—long and low. First, through forward-downward riding, you develop the "passive" carrying mechanisms[4], with which the trunk can carry weight and the limbs can move freely. This "passive" carrying should translate over time into active carrying. This means, your goal when riding is to strengthen the musculoskeletal system in such a way that the muscles are carrying the weight. Only when the muscles get strong enough, will the horse be able to adapt a more upright frame and shift his center of gravity and weight toward the back. The prerequisite muscular

---

4 Passive carrying = carrying with the help of the nuchal ligament and upper spinous processes. Active carrying = carrying through muscular strength.

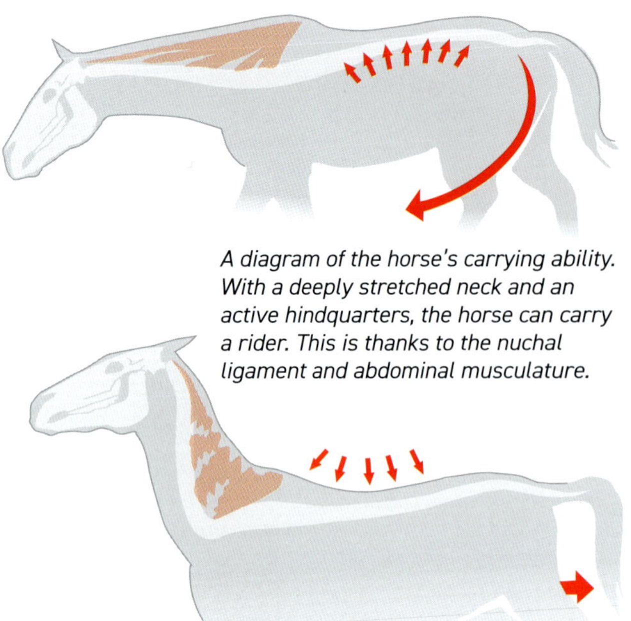

A diagram of the horse's carrying ability. With a deeply stretched neck and an active hindquarters, the horse can carry a rider. This is thanks to the nuchal ligament and abdominal musculature.

strength and the expectation for work must always go hand in hand. The following still holds true: do the right work at the right time!

Fact: The vertebrae (thoracic and lumbar), in conjunction with the ribs and sternum, are the center point of biomechanics for the horse.

Example: A common mistake that is made with young horses is that they are asked for too high of a carriage and too much collection, too soon. By bringing them to a collected frame too early, the neck and back muscles lose their stretch and the horse must engage muscles that are not actually intended to carry weight (such as the *longissimus dorsi* of the back). Instead, the job of the *longissimus dorsi* is to stretch the back and to carry forth the power of the hindquarters, from back to front. When this musculature needs to help with carrying, the back is pushed down/drops and the horse's *losgelassenheit* will immediately be lost—as described above. The horse no longer has a swinging back; the development of power and transference of power from the hindquarters, over the back, to the forehand becomes restricted. So, too, the mobility of the limbs suffers and the horse moves with "tense steps." This way

of going looks truly spectacular, but the stress of it can't be distributed throughout the body. The stress instead stays stuck in the limbs, and over time, can lead to overload and injury.

As a functional unit, the back is an important center of biomechanics in the horse. It can only function optimally when the horse is developed calmly, with enough time and without any tension. When the horse has enough strength and stability for a movement, it will be easier for him to learn and execute.

Fact: Multiple factors influence the whole system. But to keep it simple: it's the contraction of the abdominal muscles, together with the loin muscles, that lift the back, while the contraction of the back muscles and individual gluteal muscles hollow the back.

The Movement of the Spinal Column

Between the individual vertebrae, there are three directions of movement. Therefore, the following movements are possible: lifting/hollowing of the back, longitudinal bend, and rotation. The range and direction of movement are dependent upon which area of the spinal column is involved in the movement. Fundamentally, the mobility of the neck is clearly higher than in the thoracic or lumbar vertebrae, with the exception of the transition between the last lumbar vertebra and the sacrum.

Longitudinal bend and rotation consist of smaller movements and, most of the time, happen simultaneously. We talk about a combined movement. How large the combined movement is depends upon the position of the spinal column—meaning whether it is lifted or hollowed (see illustration left). Without this combined movement in the spinal joints, the longitudinal bend would be significantly limited; horses would be clearly less mobile.

Example: When your horse bends to the right around the inside leg, there is always a lateral inclination together with a turning of the affected vertebrae.

Everyone must know the feeling of riding on a circle and the horse carrying his head high and dropping through his back. The horse is not bending around the inside leg and, in terms of longitudinal bend, he feels hard and stiff. But, if you ride a volte with forward-downward stretch, the longitudinal bend feels bigger and more supple. This difference has a natural cause, for which there's an explanation.

The foundational movements of the back are lifting and pushing away (dropping), whereby the lifting of the back allows a larger range of movement than dropping of the back does. So, the mobility of the spinal column is influenced by its position.

If the spinal column is in a more lifted position (kyphosis) as it would be by a forward-downward stretch, the vertebrae and joints glide lightly apart from each other. Thereby, the contact to the joint surface is reduced, which favors mobility. In turn, the movement is limited by ligaments and muscles. In this position, the vertebrae are more mobile, which is why you should strive for this when riding. The deep, stabilizing muscles of the back are more effectively engaged, the long muscles of the back can relax again and again in this position, and both muscle groups optimally move and stabilize the back. The rider feels this in the saddle: the horse's spinal column swings, the horse travels over his back, and it gives the rider the good feeling that she can "sit into the horse." Genuine collection is only possible from this position, as the effect is that the pelvis is straightened up and the hind legs can then work in the direction of the horse's center of gravity and, thereby, take on more weight.

However, if the spinal column is in a dropped position (lordosis), certainly due to a lifted head and pushing away of the back, the vertebrae are closer to one another. This movement will be stopped by the bony structures, such as the spinous processes, and the close connections of the joint surfaces. Now, the vertebrae have a clearly lessened range of movement than they did in the lifted position, which, therefore, also makes them more stable. When the back is dropped, the vertebrae lose their mobility, locking up, so to speak, and the deep stabilizing musculature is no longer engaged. This has the disadvantage that, over time, this muscle group will become ever weaker. For you as a rider, it's uncomfortable; the back is tight and you're thrown out of the saddle with every trot stride. When the back is tight, it is physiologically impossible for the horse's pelvis to straighten upward and the hind legs can no longer swing up under the horse's center of gravity when he moves.

At this point, it must also be stressed that the lifted and dropped vertebrae form a symbiotic relationship that can only function together. The commonly held impression that lifted is "good" and dropped is "bad" cannot be sustained. The horse needs this mobility in his spine in both directions.

My Tip

To gymnasticize the musculoskeletal system as well as build up the musculature, you should ride your horse forward and downward. The reason is the vertebrae will be in a lifted position and, therefore, have more mobility, which allows the muscles to strengthen and stretch. Thereby, the horse's mobility, stability, and strength will all increase.

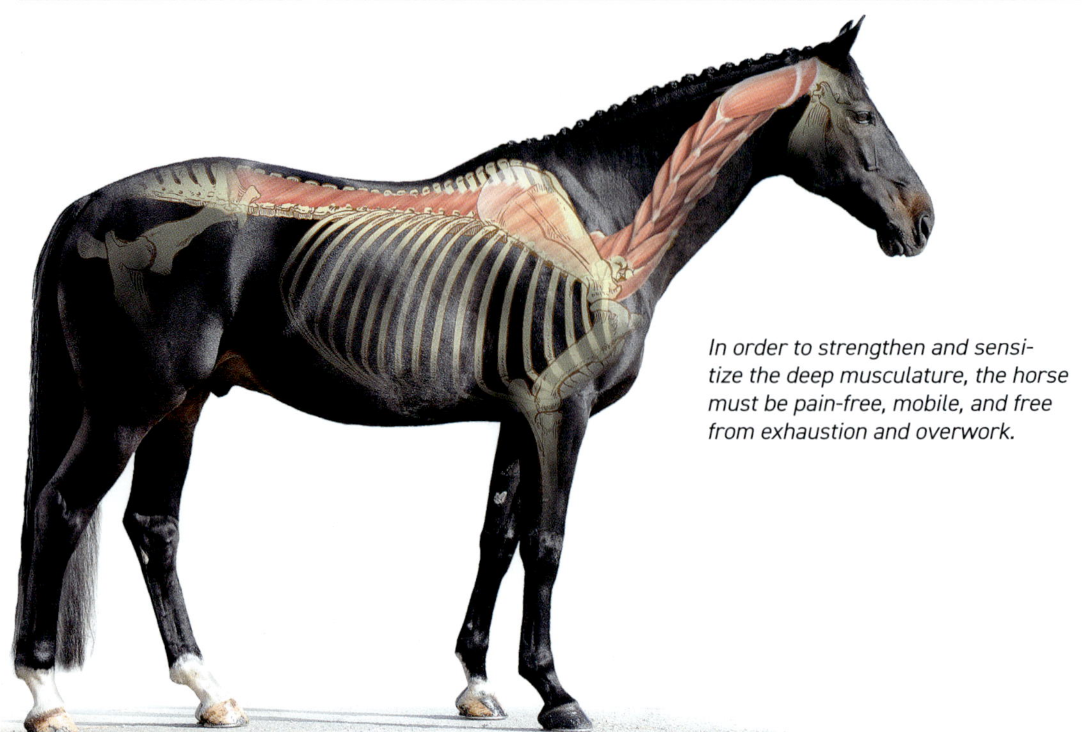

In order to strengthen and sensitize the deep musculature, the horse must be pain-free, mobile, and free from exhaustion and overwork.

The Muscles of the Spinal Column

◼ The Deep Short Muscles of the Spinal Column

The deep, short muscles of the spinal column cannot be seen but are so important: the small, short backbone muscles. These short muscles are located near to and above the whole spinal column—from head to sacrum. These muscles run from vertebra to vertebra. They can execute small movements such as stretching, longitudinal bend, and turning of the spinal column, but their most important job is to stabilize the spinal column. As described in chapter 2 (p. 46), these muscles are primarily comprised of Type 1 muscular fibers. They work involuntarily. These muscles react automatically and are not consciously controlled. They're guided and controlled by the joint position, posture, position and situation. They are richly supplied by numerous proprioceptive and highly sensitive nerves. The large, long muscles of the spinal column can first contract only when the deep, short muscles of the spinal column have stabilized. For example, a horse can only develop his trot (medium and extended) in conjunction with the strength of the deep muscles of the spinal column (and abdominal muscles).

The proprioceptive nerves are important for information regarding the positioning of individual vertebrae to reach the central nervous system. With the help of these nerves, the vertebrae are monitored in their position, stabilized and muscular engagement (tone) is regulated.

As a rider, you use these deep, short muscles of the spinal column to improve communication between your horse and yourself. Through heightened sensitivity in these muscles, the horse can better understand your body language and you can apply your aids with more refinement. For example, you can trigger a response through only a slight shift in your weight or engagement of another body part.

Fact: It's been determined that in people with back pain, this deep musculature begins to deteriorate within 24 hours. Three days later, this muscular atrophy is even recognizable by ultrasound. This knowledge can also be applied to horses.

Because you can't see these muscles and, therefore, can't assess them visually, they're often neglected or not considered important. But often these muscles cost the horse mobility, stability, coordination, and rideability. The higher the movement or performance required, the better trained and more sensitive these muscles need to be. Although we riders tend to give the long muscles of the back the most attention (likely because we can see and feel these muscles), it's really the deep, short muscles that are first affected by overwork, trauma, poor saddle fit, or incorrect riding. When they remain tense over a long period of time, a blockage is inevitable. The activity of the back is limited and, over time, the *longissimus dorsi* will also be affected.

Fact: When the stabilizing musculature tightens up, the vertebral joints move closer to one another. Thereby, they become less mobile and the back stiffens. The horse loses his elastic gait; for the rider, the back feels like a "piece of wood" and the trot will become difficult for the rider to sit.

■ The Large, Long Muscles of the Spinal Column

The long back muscles (*longissimus dorsi*) are, as the name implies, the longest muscle of the body. More importantly, it's one of the most significant muscles for a riding horse. It stretches along both sides of the spinal column, from sacrum and pelvis to the occipital bone, but it's also divided into several

parts. Like a twisted dishcloth, this muscle runs through your horse's back and lies above the deep, short muscles of the spinal column. Because the muscular fibers can only contract in their direction of travel, the job of the back muscle becomes clear: it is the lifter of the head and neck, and the stretcher (downward) of the lumbar and thoracic vertebrae.

In the trunk area, the *longissimus dorsi* has multiple, diverse functions: at walk and trot, the long back muscle does not work at the same time on both sides of the spinal column. An interplay should be recognizable.

Example: At the trot, when the left hind foot lands on the ground, you can see an engagement of the back muscles on the left side of the body. That gives the horse the possibility to shift weight from the diagonal forehand toward the hindquarters, thereby freeing up these limbs to move forward. As this takes place, it should always be possible to see an interplay of the back muscles in rhythm with the movement.

At the canter, it looks different. Here, the muscles on both sides of the back work at the same time in order to lift the forehand. This is easily recognized when watching the horse jump from behind or in a canter pirouette.

The longissimus dorsi *can only contract optimally when the deep musculature of the back is able to stabilize the spinal column. A perfect pirouette depends upon the horse being able to stabilize his trunk.*

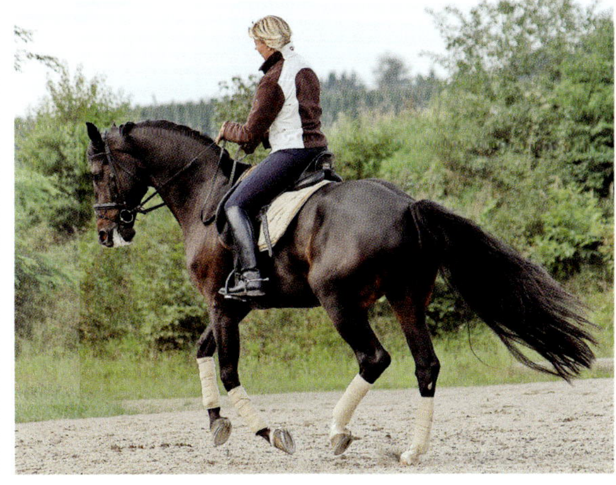

Together with the loin muscles, one of the important jobs of the long back muscles is to transfer the power of the hindquarters forward all the way to the head. However, if there's too much tension, the movement stimuli/forward impulse remains "hung up" in the musculature and can't reach its goal. This horse will become uncomfortable to sit, as the stretched spinal cord (in a hollowed position) is locked and, therefore, can't swing. In addition, tension in the long back muscles automatically leads to tension in other areas; for example, in the gluteal and hamstring muscles, which are connected to the back muscles.

Always keep it in the back of your mind that the *longissimus dorsi* can get tired quickly and cannot tolerate continuous engagement. For example, if the workload is too stressful due to intense collection that's too much for the deep, short back muscles and abdominal muscles to stabilize, the long muscles of the back must aid in stabilization. This is not their job!

My Tip

In order to loosen tense back muscles, it's helpful to do multiple transitions between canter and trot. Lateral movements can also work wonders. When the hind leg crosses under the belly, it triggers a stretch of the long back muscles and gluteal muscles. Through the repeated stretch, the back muscles will also relax in time.

Fact: The longissimus dorsi *is a "movement muscle," which was not created to carry a rider.*

◼ Abdominal Muscles

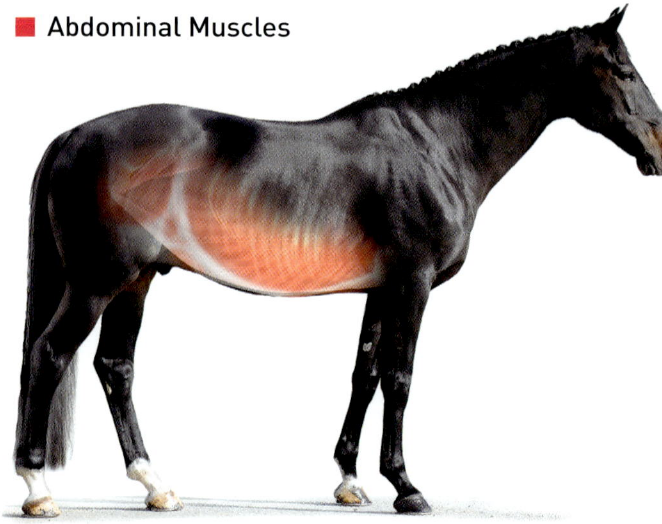

The four abdominal muscles, two straight and two diagonal, lie over one another in such a way, that they function as a hammock for the internal organs.

As the horse stands on four legs and has only a relatively short sternum as the sole bony part of his underside, it's clear that strong fibers are at work here to carry the internal organs. For four-leggeds, this task must be accomplished by the abdominal muscles, the underlying muscles, and a sinewy disc. All of these structures are moored in such a way that they form a diamond pattern, functioning like a hammock, and in this way, they can carry the internal organs effectively.

The abdominal muscles function like a corset around the trunk. Through the contraction of the abdominal muscles, pressure is increased in the abdominal cavity. This pressure is pushed upward, through the intestines, and in this way supports the spinal column. Engagement takes place in the small vertebral joints, which the spinal column needs to stabilize further.

The two straight and two diagonal abdominal muscles also have other functions, beyond carrying the internal organs. They're also important to the horse's biomechanics.

The outer, inclined abdominal muscle (*m. obliquus externus abdominis*) is important for the mechanics that allow the underside of the pelvis to contract and move closer toward the sternum. In addition, it has an indirect connection to the femur, so that it is involved with the hind legs moving forward.

When the horse moves at a trot, he brings his diagonal limbs forward simultaneously; for example, front left and right hind. Thereby, the two sloped muscles assist, in that they provide a diagonal stability to the trunk. At canter, the horse has a moment of suspension, during which the abdominal muscles stabilize the trunk and bring the sternum and pelvis closer to one another. During the standing phase, the abdominal muscles relax as the loin muscles take over the task of stabilizing the spinal column.

If the extensors of the hind legs are relaxed and prepared to stretch, and if the pelvis is upright, the hind legs are able to come forward under the horse's belly. From here, stretching and strengthening of the hind legs follows. No matter what discipline you ride, you use the forward-driving aids (legs) to activate this mechanism.

One thing is clear: the area of the lumbar vertebrae must be mobile. This area must be able to lift up in order to enable an optimal contraction of the abdominal muscles. If this area is tense, which is often the case, the abdominal muscles and/or the loin muscles cannot operate to bring the sternum and pelvis closer to one another. As a result, the horse is no longer able to achieve true collection.

When under great strain, the abdominal muscles are also a part of the respiratory system. Through contraction, they help press air out of the lungs. They're also involved when the horse blows out. Through contraction, the air is pushed out of the lungs. This is a sign of *losgelassenheit* and contentment.

The abdominal musculature is also very important for the biomechanical function in the horse's body.

Therefore, they should get extra attention. Among other things, you can do targeted abdominal training from the ground (see chapter 9, "Stabilizing/Strengthening," p.166). Under saddle, you can best activate these muscle groups through canter work and all lateral movements. Just riding in walk and trot is less strenuous and, therefore, does not develop the abdominal muscles.

Fact: Without abdominal muscles, there's no activity of the back!

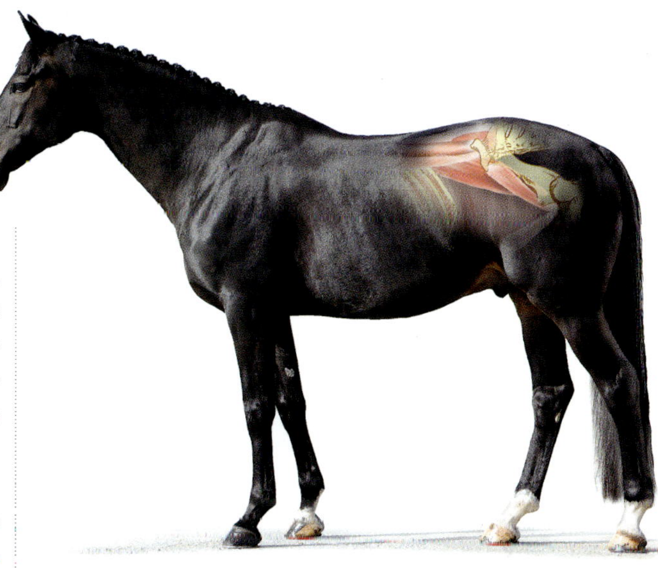

Loin Muscles

Unfortunately, the internal loin muscles (*m. iliopsoas*) cannot be seen from the outside. Therefore, few take these seriously. But, together with the *longissimus dorsi*, these muscles belong among the most important for the riding horse.

Fact: The loin muscles are the only muscles to be found under the rear thoracic and lumbar vertebrae. One of the loin muscles is the "filet muscle" and, therefore, the fleshiest muscle of the body, so a pure "movement muscle."

The loin musculature has multiple functions. It bends the hip joint, since it attaches at the thigh, thereby bringing the hind leg forward. In addition, it holds in place the posterior area of the chest and the entire lumbar region during the moment when the horse uses his hind legs. When the saddle and the rider's weight come onto the horse's back, there's a heightened engagement of the muscles in this area. A main reason for warming up is to loosen this muscle group. The best loosening exercise for the loin muscles is posting trot.

Fact: You can't have an active hind end without a loose loin muscle that is able to contract.

Symptoms of a tense, tight loin muscle are a dragging toe and/or a delay in the hind legs coming forward. These horses can also have problems stretching their hind legs toward the back when the farrier wants to hold a leg up a little higher. With these horses, you'll see a stiff back behind the saddle area. Over time, a roached back can develop. When the loin muscles are really tense, it can even cause the pelvis to become crooked. Eventually, the toe on the affected limbs will point outward. A further problem is that the nerves responsible for stimulating the *quadriceps* muscles run through the loin muscles. When there's tightness, these nerves are compromised, and you may see symptoms in the stifle joint/patella. This can hinder or block the hind legs from coming forward.

By the way, the engagement of abdominal and loin musculature becomes evident to the rider when the horse searches for the bit and the contact. What this means is that it's only when a horse is moving onto the bit correctly that the abdominal muscle chain is strengthened, the long muscles of the back are stretched and relaxed and he is slowly developing the ability to carry himself. Therefore, riding with connection has a special importance. The stronger the horse's belly and pelvic musculature gets, the less the horse will tend to lean on the bit. The horse will become light in the hand and the

interplay between back and neck extensors becomes effective and harmonious. It takes two to three years to achieve *losgelassenheit* and an improvement in balance. Young horses that are ridden with a high degree of collection don't actually have enough strength, stability, and balance; therefore, they can quickly fall into compensatory movement patterns. The soundness problems that result may show up much later when the horse has a sudden drop in performance ability or there's irreparable damage to the musculoskeletal system. Many talented horses will never reach their performance potential because as young horses they were pushed too hard, too fast and/or they were not trained according to the physiological training scale.

Fact: The entire spinal column is one dynamic unit and the rest of the body can only function when this body part is in a state of biomechanical balance.

Fact: Studies have shown: horses with back problems are lame more often than horses that don't have back problems. In addition, it's known that these horses show an altered way of going, along with drop in performance and limited mobility in back and pelvis.

When the horse contracts his abdominal muscles, the pelvis and sternum are drawn closer together, like a bow, as the engagement of the tendons pulls the two points closer together. Through this contraction of the underline and stretch of the topline, the hind legs can reach farther forward in the direction of the horse's center of gravity. A prerequisite for this mechanism is balanced trunk musculature. The abdominal and loin muscles must have the ability to lift the back and the deep, short muscles need enough strength to stabilize the back in its lifted position (see illustration, p. 43). If they can't do this over the long term because of back pain and/or muscular atrophy, the long muscles of the back and the rib musculature must compensate by being constantly contracted. This contraction becomes so strong that the abdominal and loin musculature have no chance of lifting the back against the gravitational force and tension in the topline and can no longer straighten the pelvis. Thereby, the expectation of supple relaxation and rhythm in the riding horse is lost (see chapter 3, "The Horse's Carrying Ability," p. 43).

A Blockage in the Spinal Column

Fact: Limited movement in a horse's back is often the reason that a horse is demonstrating poor performance.

You're riding a volte to the right, but the horse won't bend. It feels as if the horse is carrying a pole inside him. He's stiff from front to back. He can't actually have a blockage in every vertebra in his body, can he? No, that doesn't happen, but a blockage anywhere in his spinal column is enough to cause such symptoms. For example, a blockage in the poll can limit longitudinal bend and supple movement throughout the horse's entire body.

For many riders, the solution to such problems is to ride on through the stiffness. And perhaps the horse does feel better at the end of the schooling session. Thereby, the horse gives you the feeling of suppleness since he is a movement artist. He can execute superb movements of evasion. But, then the next day, he's just as stiff or even stiffer. This is when your alarm bells should be going off—something isn't right here.

Over time, the structures that execute compensatory movement are harmed extensively because they're executing movements for which they were not intended and for which they don't possess the mobility or strength. In other words, the musculoskeletal system is overburdened.

And obviously, you can loosen and relieve stiffness and the need to move in part through riding. But that only works when you approach your horse's limits of movement without using methods that are too forceful or too strong (for example, auxiliary reins or a harsh bit). Yes, it's your goal to ride the

horse toward suppleness and stabilization, thereby making him more supple and agile and relieving minor blockages.

Cervical Vertebrae

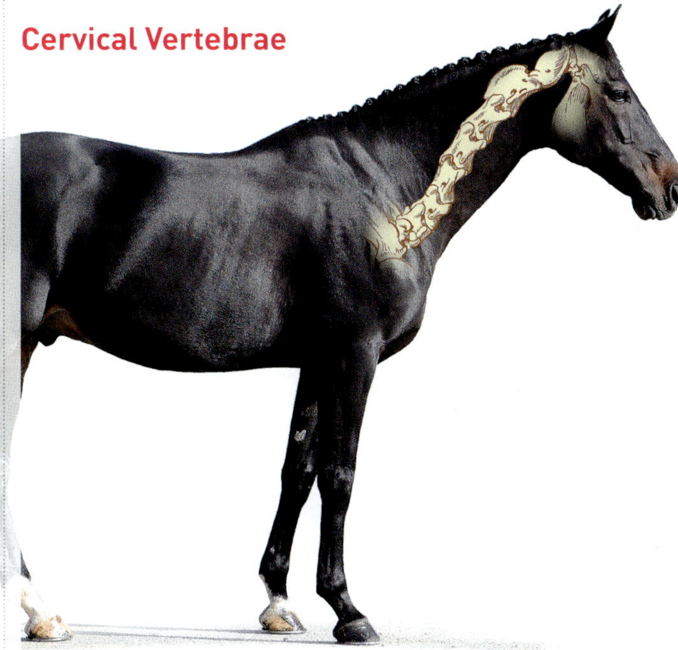

Your horse is standing relaxed in his stall, tail toward the door. He hasn't even realized that you've entered. You speak to him and he turns 180 degrees, but without moving his feet. As this takes place, you see that the trunk stays almost completely still; almost all of the movement takes place in the front part of the body—the head and poll. I'll now discuss how this is possible.

The cervical vertebrae area 1 is the most mobile section of the horse's entire spinal column and is comprised of seven powerful bones. The vertebrae are tightly bound to one another and have large joint surfaces and thick intervertebral discs. As they don't have any lateral "fences" (such as ribs and large spinous processes), they possess great mobility. This is important so that the horse can survey his entire environment easily. He can lift his head, drop it down, look toward the back, scratch his leg, or even reach back to scratch or caress his croup.

Because the vertebrae are very complex and different from one another in their movement capabilities, I have divided them into two parts:

- **Poll**—Occipital bone/First and Second Cervical Vertebrae (Atlas–C1/Axis–C2).
- **Neck vertebrae**—Third Cervical Vertebra (C3) to First Thoracic Vertebra (T1).

The Poll

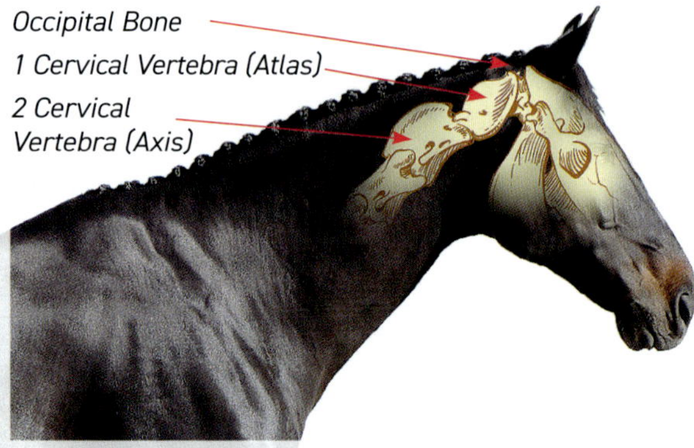

You enter your horse's stall. The horse sniffs you, greeting you with his mouth, perhaps searching for a treat in your pocket. Observe how much his poll moves as he does so. Bending, stretching, longitudinal bending, turning, and sliding sideways. Here, it's clear that this body part possesses great flexibility.

The poll is also referring to the first cervical vertebrae, so is comprised of the occipital bone, first cervical vertebra (C1–atlas) and second cervical vertebra (C2–axis). From an anatomical perspective, the first two cervical vertebrae are very distinct in form. C1 vertebra is short and round, has large articular cavities all the way to the head, which allow gigantic movement. Characteristic are the two side wings, which you can really easily feel (see illustration above). C2 is longer and narrower in form. It does not have a large connecting joint with C1, but rather a special "tooth" that sticks into the spinal cord and forms the connection to C1. Together, they offer great freedom of movement for the poll and head. In contrast, the joint connection from C2 to C3 is relatively fixed, as it must work like a counter pole to give the cervical vertebrae stability.

■ Biomechanics of the Poll

Observe your horse when he's searching on the ground for something to eat. He's stretched his neck and head down in a line. The movement of the head goes here and there and is executed with fine, small motions, in order to guide the mouth and its sensing abilities to the right spot. This refined movement of the head comes from the poll. Visually, the horse's neck is like your arms, his poll your hand joints, and his mouth your fingers. Accordingly, there must be lots of mobility in his poll in order for his head and neck to be able to be adjusted precisely.

Now, let's get to the joint movement in the poll. Between the head (occipital bone) and C1 (atlas), you have the so-called "yes" joint, which is responsible for the bending and stretching of the head. Your horse can almost stretch his head as an extension of his neck vertebrae. You can observe this stretching movement when your horse stretches over his window or stall door, when he's grazing, or when he's galloping. The opposite movement is the bending of his head.

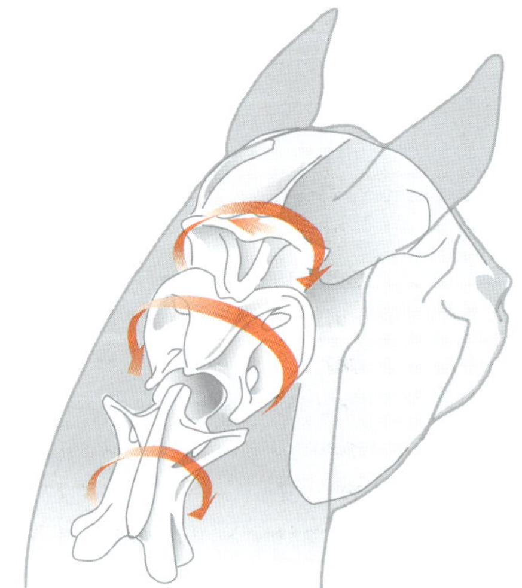

This is how the vertebrae turn during a volte to the right. This movement must always be available to achieve correct positioning in the poll.

In addition, there are two small, but enormously important movements, which take place in all turns that ask for longitudinal bend. Here, by exception, there's a sideways glide (and no longitudinal bend) in the joint between the head and cervical vertebrae, combined with a light turn. These two movements must happen together in order to bring about a larger amplitude of movement.

> *Fact: In order to understand this movement in action, let's now ride an imaginary volte to the right. You want to see the inside eye and the inner rim of the nostril.*
>
> *In order to make room, the occipital bone glides toward the left and turns lightly to the right. In contrast, C1 turns to the right (see photo, p. 52, right). Through these mechanics of the poll, you can see the inside eye and inner rim of the nostril in a vertical line, with a correctly positioned horse. It's the muscles and ligaments as well as the joint surfaces that allow and execute these movements.*

Between C1 and C2, you find the "no" joint. It executes a sideways swinging of the head (as if shaking the head "no"). This means, the main movement is the turn from right to left. This joint is the only joint in the entire spinal column that does not execute three-dimensional movement.

Why am I explaining the biomechanics of the neck to you? Because I find that with this knowledge, you'll better understand the possibilities available to your horse and you can incorporate this knowledge into your daily work. The horse lets you know which movements are possible in the different joints. You recognize when he wants to execute an evasive movement and you can counteract more quickly.

■ The Poll Muscles

Many of the long neck muscles, which originate in the trunk, shoulder, or beneath the cervical spinal column, have their point of insertion on the head or neck. Obviously, they have influence over the movement of the poll. They are also co-responsible for balance and the movement of the entire body.

There are also small, short muscles, which are responsible for the precise adjustment of the head. These muscles are found only in the poll between the occipital bone, atlas, and axis. They allow the stretch, lateral tilt, and turn in this area.

These poll muscles are intended to move; they are not intended to carry the poll high and can't work static and eccentric for long. "Static" means to hold/stabilize, and "eccentric" refers to working in a stretched posture. But this is the type of engagement needed from these muscles during collected work. Therefore, you should pay attention to these muscles. Otherwise, they can quickly get overtired, triggering tension in this area.

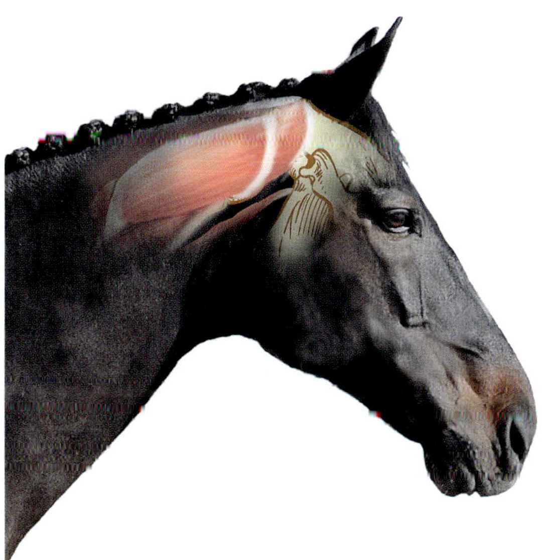

When kept in a stall, a horse stands for much longer periods of time with his head raised than he would if he were in a pasture eating grass. Standing with his head raised for a long time like this, without the small three-dimensional movements, leads to increased stress of the poll muscles. Please consider the fact that hay nets and racks that are positioned up high only make the stress worse, as the horse must always stand with his head up and constantly make an unnatural upward movement in order to get his hay. In conclusion—horses are not giraffes!

The following symptoms are signs of stressed and fatigued poll muscles: the horse no longer wants to be touched in the area around his ears, he becomes head shy, pulls the reins out of the rider's hands, demonstrates little nodding movements when ridden, begins playing with his tongue and—worst case scenario—starts with head shaking.

> *Fact: In nature, the horse carries his head directly above the ground, about 16 hours a day, in order to procure the nutrition he needs. He moves slowly forward, while his head remains stretched toward the ground. In this position, his poll muscles are stretched to a maximum and unburdened. His neck vertebrae also get a "pleasant pull."*

My Tip

Regardless of your riding style, you should always work your horse in intervals; this means repeatedly allowing for a few minutes of walk on a long rein in order to prevent and avoid tension and injury to the entire musculoskeletal system. You will experience the benefits of allowing your horse to recover mentally and physically.

> *Fact: When a horse begins to nod his head during work, it's a sign his poll musculature is weak. This nodding is to evade/experience relief.*

■ Blockages in the Poll

As I've already described, we would like to be able to see the horse's inside eye and the inner rim of his nostril when he's positioned. When we can't, this is a sign that the rider is not giving the correct aids or possibly is using the rein too strongly. Also, the horse often has a blockage in his poll. The blockages that we encounter most often are found between the head and the first vertebra of the neck. Thereby, the sliding and turning of the head opposite the first cervical vertebra is blocked. When you're riding, you'll notice this as the horse can't release in his jaw and can't be positioned. When riding it will become obvious that your horse can't relax and position himself at the poll. He's crooked at the poll. You can't see his inside eye or the rim of his nostril at the same time. This blockage can have an immense influence on the entire musculoskeletal system and your horse's well-being. Unfortunately, you won't always find the associated symptoms in the neck; it's more common, in fact, for these poll problems to manifest in the hindquarters. On the topic of "blocked poll," I could describe numerous secondary symptoms in the entire body. Here, I'll limit myself to the most important, which are found in the head region.

This is also the blockage that has the biggest influence on the horse's overall well-being. Due to muscular tension, blood flow in the direction of the head is compromised. This leads to reduced circulation and delivery of nutrients in this area of the body. So far, I have yet to read about horse headaches in any of the subject literature, but I have often seen and treated horses with headaches. These horses want to be left alone, but can act either aggressive or apathetic. I most easily recognize this pain in their eyes. These horses have small, compressed eyes. Often, the massage techniques described in chapter 7 (p. 122) do the trick to relieve this pain. And you can surely believe me when I say, it's a beautiful feeling to recognize when the horse begins to relax, the eyes open wider again, and the gaze is more relaxed.

These blockages can also affect the sensory organs of the head. For example, you may see oversensitivity of the mouth, so that the horse won't accept the bit, or oversensitivity in the area of the ears, which can present itself as constant head shaking.

Through fascia, the second cervical vertebra has close contact with the jaw joint. Blockages in this joint can bring forth a symptom such as irregular wear on the teeth. It begins with muscular tension in the jaw muscles, from which problems develop such as difficulty accepting rein contact. In addition, these horses frequently pull the reins from the rider's hands when being ridden.

The Cervical Vertebrae (C3 – C7)

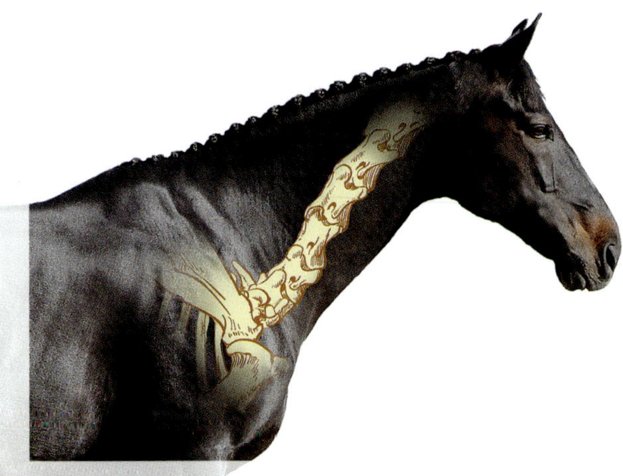

Through the movement dynamics of the cervical spine, the head stretches toward the ground and, likewise, can stretch high in the air. It can also bend left or right without a problem. From a mechanical perspective, the vertebrae in this region have many different movements.

■ Biomechanics of the Neck

You're observing your horse at pasture. He's carrying his head low while he's grazing or he moves it up and down gracefully while playing. A fly lands on his flank and bothers him. With a swing of his head, he manages to reach 180 degrees behind him, and that fly is gone! You best compare his neck to the arm of an excavator: his head is the shovel. The shovel's arm is highly mobile, in order to be able to get the shovel to the exact right place. This is just how the neck works: it has a large movement radius in order to be able to bring the head to every position. In its "normal position," there is a lifted curve (kyphosis) present in the neck. But from C4 to the tenth thoracic vertebra (T10), the spine is in a hollow position (lordosis) (see illustration on p. 42.) Through this lordosis the spinal column is more stable, but also less mobile. When the horse carries his head deeper,

the lordosis lifts up: the deeper the head drops, the more vertebrae are positioned in kyphosis. Through the lifting (kyphosis), the sideways longitudinal bend increases, and the spine becomes more mobile.

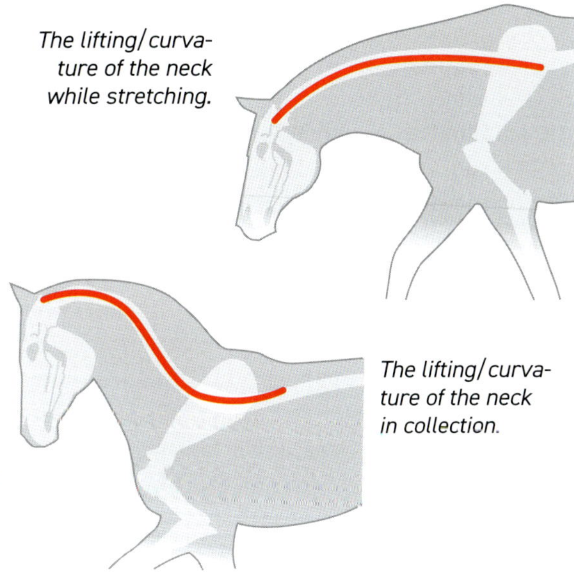

The lifting/curvature of the neck while stretching.

The lifting/curvature of the neck in collection.

You can best observe these positional differences in the neck region when a horse is being ridden. Ideally, you should ride your horse forward and downward in the loosening/warm-up phase. One reason for this is related to the position of the cervical vertebrae. The more forward and downward the head is carried with an active hindquarters, the more the lordosis in the cervical region is lifted. For you as the rider, this means the longitudinal bend is larger and the neck muscles can be warmed up more easily. In this position, the cervical spine has more mobility.

However, if you ride, let's say, a collected half-pass to the right, you'll see that the spinal column is now in a "compromised" position, always staying in kyphosis. The longitudinal bend is happening mainly just in the poll. In the lower neck vertebrae, you see now the "hollowed" position (lordosis). Therefore, the longitudinal bend is not so strongly expressed, but the spinal column is much more stable in this position.

Fact: If your horse should shrink behind the vertical when you're riding forward and downward, it's his reflex to lift the head and neck upward. There are two reasons for this: first to be able to "scan" the environment with his eyes and locate any danger. Second: in case the horse needs to quickly flee, he needs a stable spinal column; he gets this automatically when he lifts his head.

The movements available to the neck (C3–C7) are contraction, stretching, and longitudinal bend. A turning movement is much less common here, and is dependent on the position of the neck: when the neck is carried high, the longitudinal bend and turning are much less available as they are when the head is carried low. The "Bermuda Triangle" for your horse is the seventh vertebra. This vertebra is naturally highly mobile, but also highly susceptible to loss of mobility. Here, important nerves exit to supply the forelimbs. From the neck area, you get the large range of movement that meets up with the relatively "movement deprived" thoracic spine. In addition, this vertebra is connected through a joint with the first rib. All of these influences combine to make the C7 a highly sensitive part of your horse. To complicate matters, this junction lies deep under the shoulder blade, where it's well-protected but also, unfortunately, difficult to examine using traditional medicine. However, with the help of the manual techniques offered by physical therapy and osteopathy, it's possible to diagnose movement anomalies in this area.

■ The Neck Muscles

The muscles of the neck lie in multiple layers. A small anatomical reminder: the small, short muscles that lie along the spinal column are primarily responsible for the stability of the cervical vertebrae. The long muscles, which run over multiple joints, are responsible for movement. I'm now going to take a close look. The following applies to all of the neck muscles I'll discuss in this chapter: they are not connected to the forelimbs.

There are actually additional muscles that lift, stretch, or contract the head and neck, but these muscles actually have their origins in the shoulder blade or upper arm. I'll describe those later in this chapter (see p. 76). Generally, you can say that a large part of the neck musculature lies above the cervical spine and is tasked with stretching and carrying the neck and head. To serve as a "helper" for carrying the head, you also have the nuchal ligament (see p. 42).

There are a couple of muscles that are not actually utilized much when the horse is being ridden well. These lie on the underside of the cervical spine. Their job is to lower and bend the head and neck.

■ Head and Neck Extensors (Lifting)

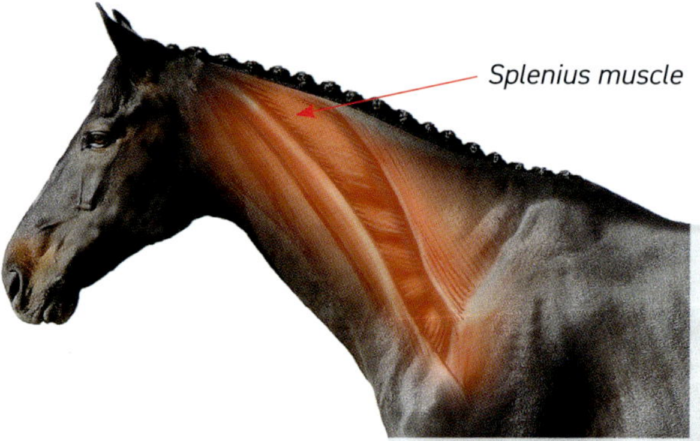

The main job of the head and neck extensor is to carry, stretch, and lift the head, poll, and neck. Many of these muscles are also involved with the longitudinal bend when there's contraction on one side. The muscles that lift and extend are primarily positioned between the cervical vertebrae and the upper portion of the nuchal ligament. On both sides of the laminar portion of the nuchal ligament, these muscles fill out part of the large in-between space.

For a riding horse, these head and neck extensor muscles should ideally take over more and more the function of the nuchal ligament; namely, to carry the head and neck. One of the most important muscles involved in this task is the *splenius muscle*.

Physical Therapy for Horses

It's easy to both see and feel this muscle under the skin. This muscle is one of the strongest neck lifters the horse has. When the horse is galloping, it's this muscle that initiates the distinct nodding movement of the head. But this muscle's most important task of all comes in during collection of the riding horse. This muscle gives the horse the power to carry himself, and thereby, also the possibility of shifting his weight from his forehand toward his hindquarters. The more strength this muscle develops, the more able the horse is to achieve an elevated carriage.

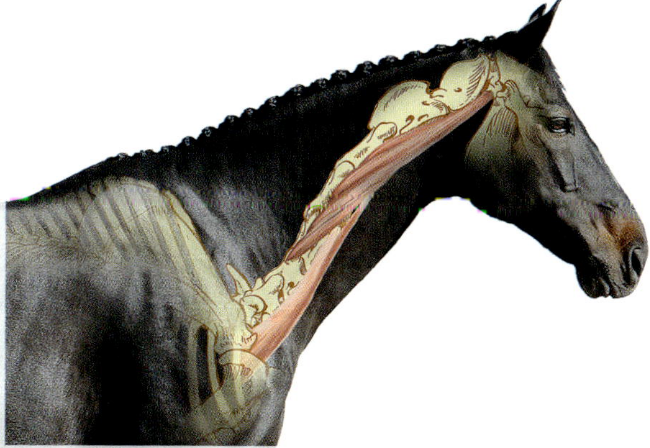

■ Head and Neck Flexors (Lowering)

These muscles are found nearby to and beneath the cervical spine; they flex the head and neck and work together with the neck extensor muscles during longitudinal bend.

The first muscles that I'd like to introduce are the strong "rib holders" (*scalene* muscles). They lie in the deeper muscle layer, in part protected by the shoulder blade. Their origin is on the first ribs and their insertion is not far from there—namely from C4–C7. These two muscles both have the same task: during inhalation, they lift the first ribs, which helps this muscle during inhalation. In addition, during correct collection, they lift the cervical vertebrae upward, and when one side contracts, the *scalene* muscles execute longitudinal bend in the neck.

These are muscles that you need to give lots of attention to when riding. Under certain conditions, they can cause a horse to be "rein lame." This refers to something you see only when a horse is ridden. When the rein is taken up, these horses demonstrate uneven rhythm in the forehand. There can be multiple causes, but unfortunately, the cause is very frequently hard hands on the rider's part. The reason for the uneven rhythm is that the neuroplexus (*plexus brachialis*) runs between the two *scalene* muscles. When the *scalene* muscles are tight, it leads to compression on this sensitive bundle of nerves and to loss of mobility where they attach in the neck. This leads to every bend of the neck irritating the neuroplexus and eventually to the disruption in rhythm. The danger lies therein that tension in the *scalene* muscles can lead to permanent lameness.

Other diagnoses in the forehand can also stem from the *scalene* muscles; for example, navicular disease or lameness without clinical diagnoses.

It's not only a mechanical reduction in movement that results; the horse's inhalation is also reduced as the first rib suffers because of tension in the *scalene* muscles.

Fact: Unclear lameness can have its source in the cervical vertebrae.

When a horse is well-ridden, you actually won't be able to see or feel the contracting muscles in the direction of the poll and head, such as the long head

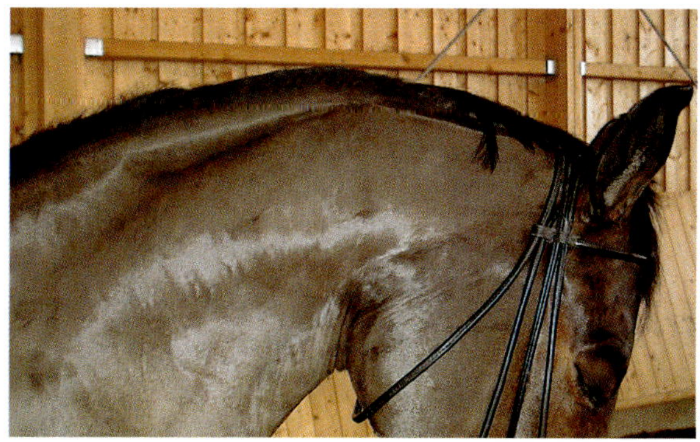

Here you can clearly see the "false bend" in the poll.

muscle (*longus capitis*). When they engage, they make the neck and head stiff and strong. If you're able to see them, it's an indicator that the horse is not coming forward correctly from behind and/or that the rider is holding too tightly with her hands.

Because the rider's hand is forcing the muscular contraction, the horse bends his head and neck so much that he comes behind the vertical.

Over time, this incorrect riding will also be visible in that the horse builds a "false bend" in his neck. He'll develop a strong bend between C2 and C3. You'll then be able to see a clear lift in his crest in this area.

■ Blockages in the Neck

Your horse shows one or more of the following symptoms: breathing problems, lameness, uneven rhythm, stumbling, shortened gaits, positioning problems, changes in positioning of the lower limbs and hoofs, or he even attempts to rear whenever you track in a certain direction. All of these are symptoms that can be triggered by a blockage in the cervical vertebrae. I'll now elaborate on a few different origins of these symptoms.

The joint between C3 and C4 is susceptible to blockages and tends toward instability. Through an injury, such as a fall, it can become limited in function. The source of the problem is presumably the reversal of the kyphosis to lordosis (this means it goes from a lifted to a "dropped away/hollowed" position), which causes the junction of the joints to become a weak spot. In this joint, the blockage can trigger a disruption to coordination. Thereby, the spinal cord is compromised and the "communication" between the brain and the musculature of the hindquarters is interrupted.

When it's C5 and C6 that are blocked, the source of the problem is more often of a secondary type—for example, bad shoeing. Between C5 and C7, the nerve that controls the diaphragm (phrenic nerve) exits. Through a blockage in this area, the nerve can

become compromised. The connection between the central nervous system and the diaphragm worsens and the strong breathing muscles can't work optimally. In this way, the strongest respiratory muscle is weakened. It can follow that the horse's breathing also suffers.

Most disorders and blockages of the lower cervical spinal column are found at C7. An origin that can trigger many of the above-named symptoms I've already described under the section "The Neck Muscles" on p. 56. It's the tensing of the *scalene* muscles, which affects both the first ribs and also the last three cervical vertebrae. It's C7 that is the first to get blocked under this tension and also demonstrates the most symptoms.

From a rider's perspective, a blockage of C7 is clearly recognizable. The horse can't duck his neck in the direction of the blockage; it will even be positioned in the opposite direction. These horses aren't comfortable to ride, their trot is short and choppy, and they are often unwilling to move forward. The vertebrae and nerves can become so strongly painful, that they eventually even rear. These horses aren't evil—they are just in extreme pain. Those among us who have had a pinched nerve in the neck or experienced sciatica will know exactly what I'm talking about. It's exactly the same pain.

Fact: It's common to only encounter these symptoms on one side of the body.

For the horse, the neck is the balancing pole that allows him to keep his balance. If the horse wants to kick out with his hindquarters, he lowers his head/neck in order to bring his weight forward. If he collects or wants to rear, he automatically lifts his head in order to shift his weight back in the direction of his hindquarters. When he trips, he tries to use his neck to find his balance again. Every problem in the neck area will limit its helpfulness for balance and, therefore, bring the horse out of balance.

Thoracic Spine and Breastbone

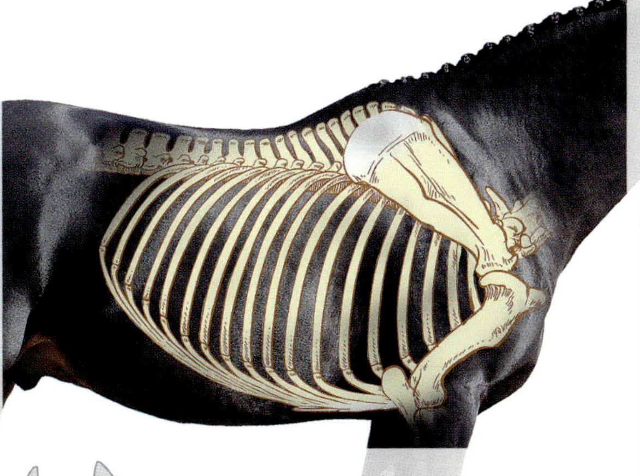

The thoracic spine is built like a ship. The breastbone resembles a keel, the ribs form the ship's side, the vertebral bodies form the deck, and the spinous processes are the mast. Inside, you find the most important organs necessary for life—the lungs and the heart. They lie bound together, protected between two arrows: the forelimbs.

Seen from the front— the thoracic spine and breastbone are constructed like a ship.

Biomechanics of the Thoracic Spine

Because the thoracic and lumbar vertebrae have the hard job of carrying the inner organs, this section of the spine is built more for stability than for mobility. When compared to the cervical vertebrae, the thoracic region is often described as "rigid" in terms of mobility. But that's not the whole truth. You can hardly believe that this construction of long spinous processes, small joints, and joints that connect to the ribs and breastbone actually allows for any mobility whatsoever. But the sum of the small movements of multiple joints really adds up to a lot of mobility here.

As previously discussed in the "Curve of the Spine" (photo on p. 40), a normal horse has multiple "curves" in his spine. One such curve is seen in the "hollowed" position from C4 to T10. From there, the spine again curves slightly upward through the lumbar vertebrae to the sacrum. The mobility of individual sections is dependent upon whether the whole back is in a lifted (contracted) or hollowed (stretched/extended) position. The most mobility of the lifted back can be found in the area of T17 and T18; the least movement is found in the withers (T3 to T9).

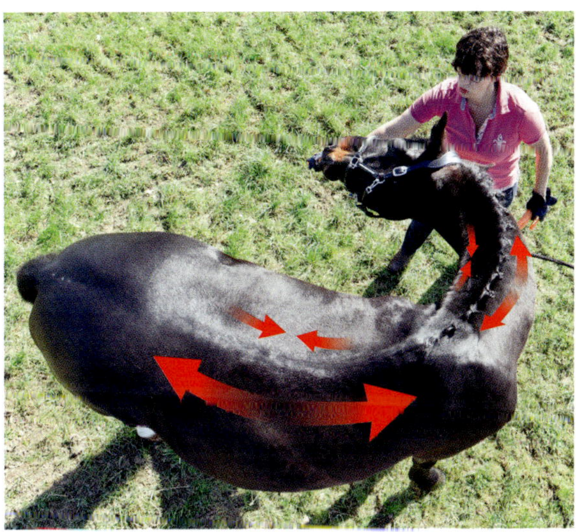

It's clear to see the longitudinal bend through the entire spine—the contraction on one side and the wonderful stretch on the other side.

With a hollowed (extended) back, the extent of the movement is smaller, as this will be limited by the spinous processes. In this case, the most mobile area will lie between T14 and T18. Here, too, the withers will have the least mobility. This can be explained by the fact that the downward tendency of the spinal curve is limiting longitudinal bend. You'll find the most longitudinal bend from T10 to the end of the thoracic spine, as here the spinal column stays in a slightly upward lift.

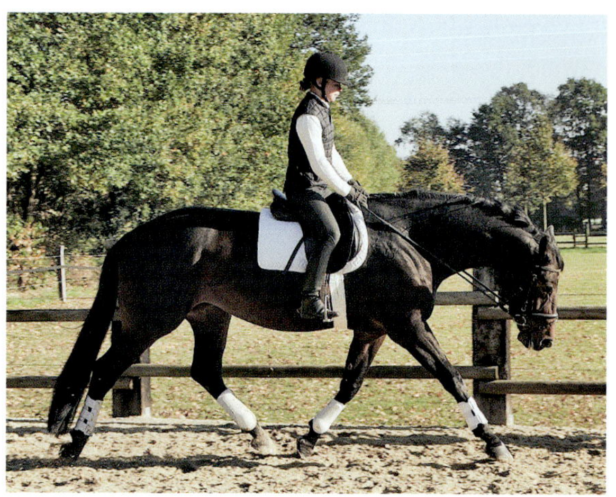

A horse that is moving nicely from back to front, toward the bit: With active hindquarters and in this forward-downward (long-and-low) position, the passive carrying mechanisms carry the rider. The horse has a free and powerful movement pattern and, therefore, he can optimally strengthen his musculoskeletal system.

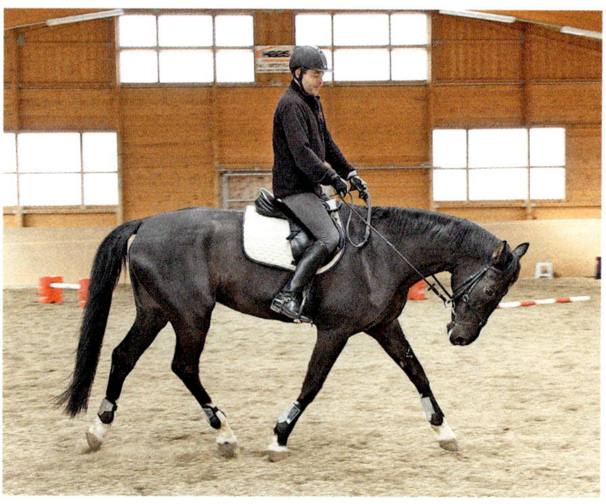

A horse that's being ridden forward and downward from the hand alone, without active hindquarters: Here, the carrying mechanisms are not functioning optimally. Because of inactive hindquarters, the pelvis cannot straighten up. The hind limbs work stiffly, and the horse has shifted his weight too much to the forehand. He's not carrying his head and neck himself, he's leaning on the rider's hand.

In riding, you want to reach the point that the back lifts, so that the horse is able to carry you. When riding forward and downward, this carrying happens "passively" with the help of the nuchal ligament and supraspinal ligament. By moving the head toward the ground, there's a pull on the nuchal ligament and the spinous processes of the withers are pulled forward (upright) and through the supraspinal ligament, which lifts the back. This process goes back to T14. Through the tipping of the pelvis, there's a pull on the band coming from behind, which then lifts the back upward from the fourteenth vertebra. This carrying mechanism only works when the abdominal muscles and the hindquarters are active. So, it's not enough for the horse to just travel with his neck extended and head low.

To get the optimal longitudinal bend, it's really important that the horse lift his back (kyphosis). From a mechanical point of view, this means the spinous processes separate from one another, the back is in kyphosis, and lateral inclination and turning happen in the same direction.

However, if you're riding your horse with a hollowed back, you cannot expect much bending through the ribs. The back stays in lordosis, the vertebrae turn in the opposite direction, and they will quickly begin to lock up. For you as a rider, this means that your horse will be stiff under saddle in terms of longitudinal bend; you'll have difficulties sitting his trot, and all three basic gaits are restricted.

Mechanically speaking, you can't separate the thoracic vertebrae, the ribs, and the breastbone. All thoracic vertebrae are attached to a pair of ribs, which are either directly or indirectly in contact with the breastbone through cartilage. There are 18 thoracic vertebrae and the same number of ribs. They run parallel downward toward the breastbone. The ribs' task is to protect the vital organs such as heart and lungs. However, they also must be mobile, which is why only the first eight ribs are in direct contact with the breastbone and the other ten are connected in part by a long thread of cartilage. These cartilage connections allow the ribs to expand outwardly during breathing, moving back and upward in order to give the lungs room. For this reason, the last ten ribs are also referred to as the "breathing ribs." The first eight are called "true" or "sternal" ribs.

Physical Therapy for Horses

Muscles of the Thoracic Spine and Breastbone

Because many muscles run along the entire spinal column, I've described the most important muscles of the thoracic spine in on p. 46. A gentle reminder: there are small, short muscles, which go from vertebra to vertebra and are mainly responsible for stability of the spinal column. In addition, there are long muscles of the back, which run from the back to the head and are responsible for movement. Not to be forgotten are the abdominal muscles, which are found in the trunk. In addition, there are muscles in the breastbone area (external and internal intercostals), which lie flat in between each rib and are responsible for inhalation and exhalation.

Fact: On the underside of the thoracic spine (toward the chest cavity), from T5 on, there are no muscles, but rather a ligament that gives the spinal column a certain stability from below.

Blockages in the Thoracic Spine

When there's a blockage in the thoracic spine, there will be a tendency for it to get stuck in a stretched out (hollowed) position. The horse can no longer lift his back. This phenomenon has clear disadvantages for rider and horse. It's now impossible for the horse to truly work over his back. These horses travel with head and neck up, the back hollowed and the hindquarters inevitably trail behind.

It's obvious that in this dropped position (stretched out), the back muscles tense up. Even when being groomed, the horse drops his back away, and he'll do the same during mounting. When ridden, the horse travels without enthusiasm or impulsion. These are only a few of the many signs.

When the back is hollowed, it also changes the joint articulations to the ribs, which are positioned to the sides of and between every thoracic vertebra. Remember the anatomy chapter: between each vertebra, there are nerves that provide for this area.

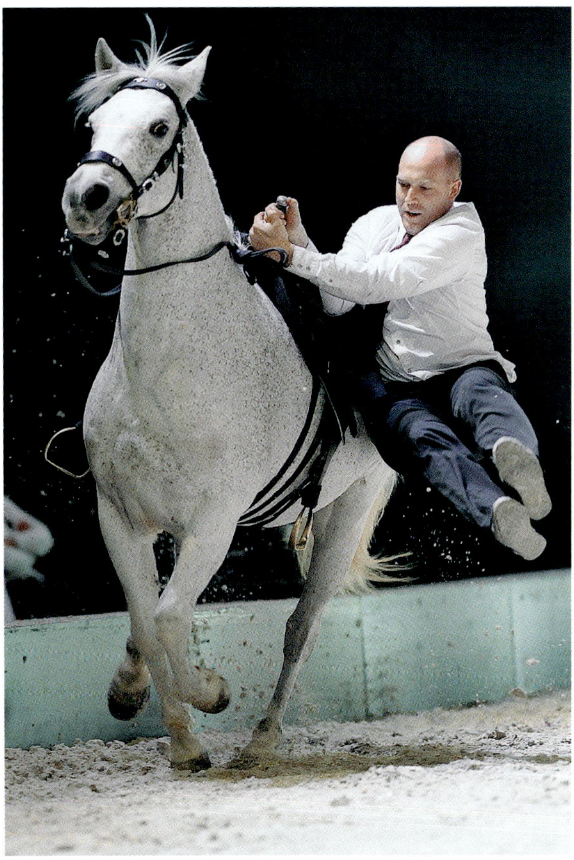

The horse carries his head high in order to stabilize his spine while in a more dropped away position (lordosis). Thereby, he is able to maintain his balance.

The nerves that are in the thoracic spine region primarily provide for the internal organs. When there's a blockage, the nerve endings can get smaller and this compromises the nerve. In addition to local pain, the symptoms can include functional disorders of the nearby organs.

Often, the withers must carry a heavy burden. The saddle or harness lie here and often don't fit optimally. Consequently, muscular tension and loss of movement in this area is triggered. So, too, mounting can be a source of blockages, especially when you mount from the ground without counterbalancing the saddle with a helper on the off side. When you mount from the left, the entire withers is bent longitudinally to the right and also twisted to the right, which causes immense pressure on the small joints of the vertebral bodies. If this happens often, it can irritate the nerves and trigger irreparable damage. You can avoid these blockages in the withers area by always using a mounting block. In this way, you'll apply more vertical pressure and avoid unwanted twisting of the withers. It's interesting to notice that many horses hold their heads high when being mounted. That's a suitable way to achieve strong lordosis in the withers and, thereby, stabilize the spinal column.

Blockages in the withers are easily recognized in your daily interactions with your horse. Even when you're retrieving him from his stall, he'll seem to "walk on eggshells." Very carefully and with short steps. When you're tacking up, the horse may act "girthy." The short-stridedness will improve over the course of the schooling session, along with the loosening of the back, but this horse will never be entirely relaxed.

With jumping horses, blockages in the withers are an especially big problem. They jump without engaging their back. So often, they'll race around the course, out of control, running out at jumps as refusing would be too painful. When rails are dropped, it's with the front limbs. In addition, the rider will "have lots of weight in the hand."

Some of the nerves that provide for the heart and lungs travel between the vertebrae of the withers. This means, blockages in this area can potentially cause symptoms in these two organs. But the reverse is also true: for example, a cough can lead to blockages in the withers.

When a horse has tension and limited movement in the deepest point of the back (mid-saddle area), you'll have the feeling when you ride that the horse is divided in two parts. The movement of the forehand and the hindquarters don't "fit" together and the impulsion of the hindquarters will brake beneath you. With horses like this, the liver may be undernourished and irritated. If there are gastric ulcers, you can also expect more limited movement

in the thoracic vertebrae. These horses are grumpy during girthing, as this applies more pressure to the stomach. When ridden, horses with stomach ailments will not lift the withers and back.

The joints between the vertebrae in the section of the thoracic spine that's farther back can also trigger serious problems in the organs. When a horse has recurring colic without a recognizable organic cause and/or the veterinary treatment doesn't bring about the desired outcome, the horse can be examined for blockages and muscular tension, as the last thoracic vertebrae have a connection to the intestines, where impaction colic occurs.

If the horse has been cast in his stall, it's possible that a reduction in mobility will follow, as a result of the immense pull/twist that has been put on the junction of the thoracic and lumbar spine, which is a weak spot.

In addition, when a thoracic vertebra is blocked, the rib that it is associated with is always affected. Naturally, the reverse is also true. The rib can become immobile through respiratory illness, improper stress (rider and equipment) or through trauma. The result, as always when there's a loss of mobility, will be an under-functioning of the affiliated structures. For example, when there's a blocked rib, the symptom that manifests could be a reduction of lung capacity or even a disrupted heart rhythm!

Fact: One thing is clear—the layman cannot resolve many of the blockages in the spinal column on her own. But it is important that you see the connections of the horse's entire body and recognize early on when you need the assistance of a medical professional.

Physical Therapy for Horses

The Lumbar Spine

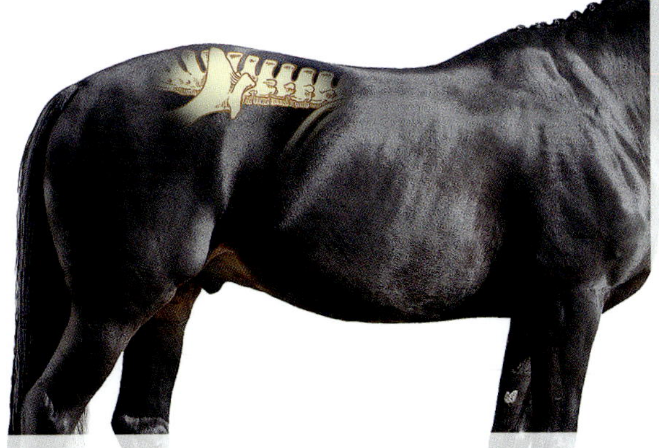

The lumbar spine builds a "bridge" between the hindquarters and the forehand. Formed by big, wide spinous processes, it's here that many large muscles attach.

Biomechanics of the Lumbar Spine

Observe your horse as he moves freely in the pasture. When he gallops, you'll see that the front part of the lumbar spine is more stable and still, while the back part of the lumbar spine moves up and down. And you can really recognize how the lumbar region and pelvis work together. The most mobile joint in this section of the spine can be found between the last lumbar vertebra and the sacrum. Here, the intervertebral discs are strongest, which is how the joint obtains its freedom of movement. In order to bring the legs far forward, there must also be a lift in the lumbar spine. When firing the forward impulse, the back is stretched and the legs are brought as far under the horse's body as possible, to gather the maximum amount of power. The last lumbar vertebra is meant for forward movement, mostly engaging in flexion and extension.

The lumbar vertebrae do not have a connection to the ribs, but they have very wide and long spinous processes. They limit longitudinal bend, but, through the combined movement (lateral inclination and turn are always simultaneous), you can always find enough longitudinal bend in this region. Thanks to this small but important turning, the horse has the ability to execute perfect lateral movements with his body.

Musculature of the Lumbar Spine

Because the lumbar vertebrae "hang in the air," it's advantageous for this area to have strong muscling along the underside. The lumbar spine is held and carried by the four muscles of the abdomen and the loin muscle. In addition, the supraspinal ligament also "carries" the vertebrae through a pull from the back (when the pelvis is upright). The muscles that are responsible for moving and stabilizing the lumbar vertebrae are described in the section called "Spinal Column" (p. 46).

> **My Tip**
>
> **The saddle should never be allowed to reach the lumbar region and sit back there because the lumbar vertebrae cannot carry any additional weight.**

Disorders of the Lumbar Spine

The mechanics of the hindquarters are dependent upon the mobility of the lumbar spine. When the lumbar spine can't lift, the hindquarters can't execute flexion, and the musculature that is necessary for forward movement cannot develop the necessary strength. This movement limitation can trigger other symptoms, as the following examples show:

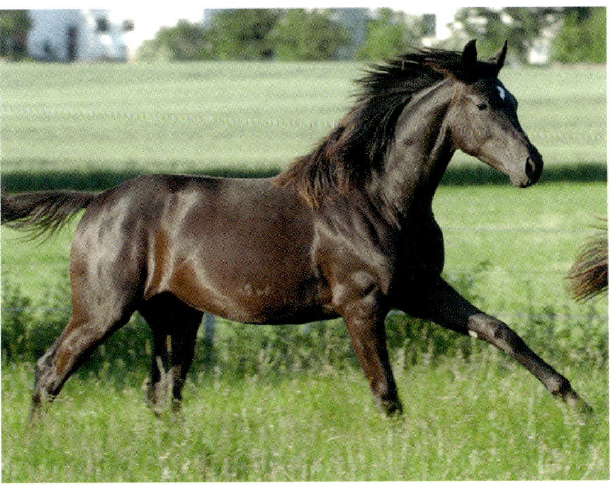

- Although the spinal cord only reaches the second lumbar vertebra (2L), nerves extend to the sacrum and provide for those internal organs that lie toward the back of the horse. The junction between the thoracic and lumbar areas is—like all junctions in the spinal column—a weak spot. This vertebral segment influences the horse's genitalia. Therefore, if a mare's circulation is limited, she may have inflammation of the uterus, whereas a stallion may experience testicular torsion. Geldings who have sticky scar tissue from castration may also have a blockage in this segment.

- The segment at L2 controls the kidneys, so that when there's a longer-lasting restriction of movement, it can actually change the quality and quantity of the urine. This blockage often occurs among Western horses due to the execution of sliding stops or among racehorses that must lift their backs to the extreme in order to bring their hind legs so far forward.

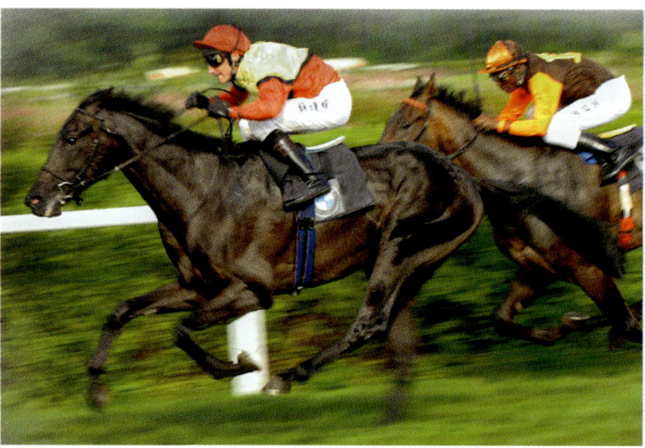

Due to the increased lift in the rear part of the spinal column, the horse is able to bring his hind legs far forward. Should the spinal column be blocked, the hind legs can't step under as far. This means that over a longer race, the horse would lose lots of ground and probably not be able to win.

> *Fact: If you can manage, with massage and stretching, to get your horse mobile and pain-free in the lumbar spine, it may be that you need to "put your glue on" when you're riding. After being blocked in this area for a long time, these horses often have the need to buck, even when the rider is on!*

- If your horse has chronic diarrhea that is not responding to traditional veterinary medicine, it's possible that a blockage in the transition from T18 to L1/2 is the source of the problem. In addition, a blockage of L3 can trigger instability of the stifle, causing the horse to frequently fall out behind.

- L4 and L5 can compromise the sciatic nerve. This triggers pain and leads to muscular weakness and uneven rhythm or even to lameness.
  The last lumbar vertebra before the sacrum is the most mobile. As this is a junction vertebra, it's especially prone to blockages. Possible symptoms that can result from a blockage of L6 relate to the bladder. These horses must often urinate, but don't do it completely. They always feel an urge to urinate, but don't release any urine.

With all thoracic and lumbar blockages, it's always possible to feel tension in the surrounding muscles. When the back is healthy, you should be able to take your flat hand—but with a firm pressure—and stroke the entire back, without your horse tensing his muscles or dropping through his back. If your horse reacts, there's tension, which automatically means a movement limitation!

Physical Therapy for Horses

The Limbs

The horse's limbs are equipped with bones that are long, but light in relation to their body weight. The big, strong muscles are found near to the trunk. The farther you get from the middle of the body, the less mass and weight the limbs have. From the knee and hock downward, you'll find no more muscles, but rather just tendons and ligaments. This construction gives the horse the possibility to move efficiently in terms of energy and elastically. Through the long muscles, and tendons and ligaments in the lower limbs, the mechanics work like a spring.

The horse's forelimbs are aligned for a supporting function and, thereby, are not generally much involved with forward movement. To be able to fulfill their supportive role, the forehand functions like a high-performance spring, which absorbs and stores energy in order to then set it free again.

The hindquarters possess massive muscles, which are responsible for forward movement. So, figuratively speaking, the horse does not have "all-wheel drive," but rather has "rear-wheel drive."

The Hindquarters

A racehorse is led into the start box. The signal is given, the door opens, and the horse can gallop off. But for a split second, the horse shifts more toward the back, instead of galloping forward. First, he lifts his head, thereby moving his weight from forehand to hindquarters, flexes all of the upper joints of the hindquarters, as if he's going to sit down, but then catapults himself forward with an insane amount of power. From 0 to as much as 37 mph (60 km/h) in three gallop strides, and that's only with a one-horsepower "engine"!

Riding can be like driving a Porsche. Both—horse and Porsche—have a motor at the back, and both have tremendously powerful motors. I'm now going to take the horse's "turbo motor" apart and look at it very precisely.

Because the horse is a flight animal, he needs speed and power to survive. The "motor" is comprised of big, fast, and strong muscles. (You'll feel this when you massage them!) It's not only muscular strength that helps the horse to develop his full ability, it's his entire hindquarters that are responsible for his fast and powerful flight.

When you look at the skeleton of the hindquarters, you can see that it's built differently from the forehand, where some bones stand vertically.

In the hindquarters, the cannon bone stands straight, but all other bones are angled. The angles of the bones are important to the hindquarters' ability to develop power and absorb shock. In addition, they are disposed with a fantastic apparatus of muscles and ligaments. One more difference from the forehand: the hindquarters have a joint connection to the trunk via the pelvic-sacral connection.

An essential construction for keeping the hindquarters upright is the two tendons that stretch between the stifle and hock joints, one in front and one along the backside. This construction is like a "frame saw" in design (see illustration, p. 66).

When a flexing of the stifle joint takes place, there's automatically also a flexing of the hock joint. Or vice versa, when there's an extension of the stifle joint, there will be extension of the hock. This means you cannot stretch the knee and hock joints separately from one another. This can make it so difficult—for example, during a lameness exam—to determine in which joint the lameness is originating.

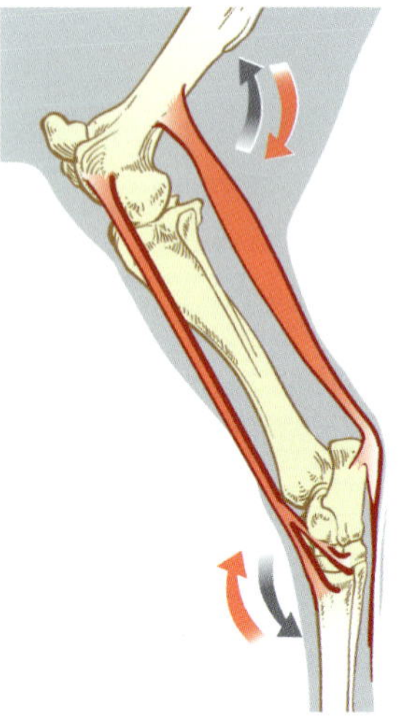

Because of this frame-saw design, the horse can support his hind limbs in an upright position.

The "flexing of the haunches" refers to an increased flex in the hip, stifle, and hock joints, which is a prerequisite for the development of power and has an important shock-absorbing function. Without the "frame-saw design" the horse would not be able to maintain flexion of the haunches. During flexion, the horse gets "smaller" in the hindquarters and, thereby, can take more weight onto his hindquarters. Only in this way is it possible for the horse to have a quick and

Extension ⟶

Flexion ⟶

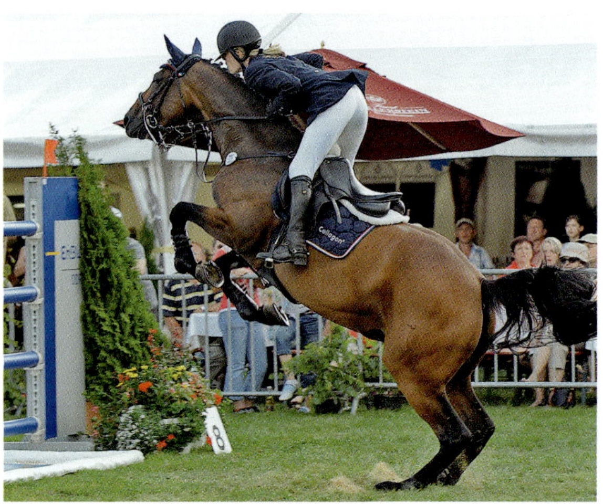

powerful reaction when he encounters danger or to collect himself under a rider, which is what you ask from the horse at the highest level of the Training Scale. Unfortunately, this is also the hardest part of training for every horse as the flexion of the haunches principally takes place through muscular strength. This means it takes a lot of power and effort from your horse. Try moving 10 meters in a squat position yourself. You'll notice how strenuous it is! The same is true for your partner, your horse.

The Sacroiliac Joint

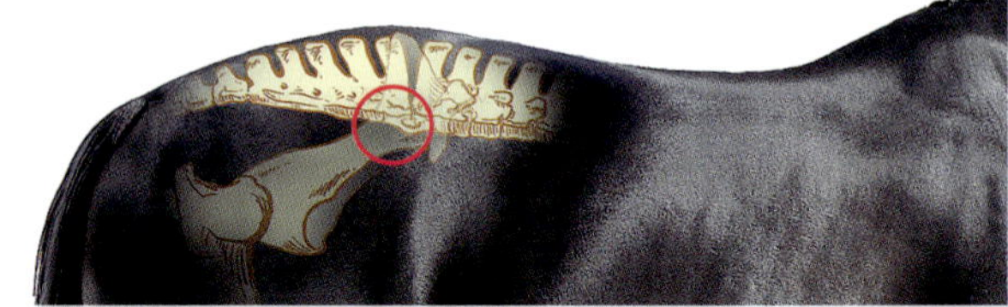

■ Biomechanics of the Sacroiliac Joint

From a mechanical perspective, the sacroiliac joint has the most difficult job of the entire musculoskeletal system. On the one hand, it must carry lots of weight, while on the other hand, it must absorb, compress, and deliver forward all the power that is developed in the hindquarters. For these two mechanical functions, the joint must be stable on one hand, mobile on the other.

The sacroiliac joint is, as its name implies, the joint articulation between the sacrum and the pelvis. The joint is also vulnerable to problems in other

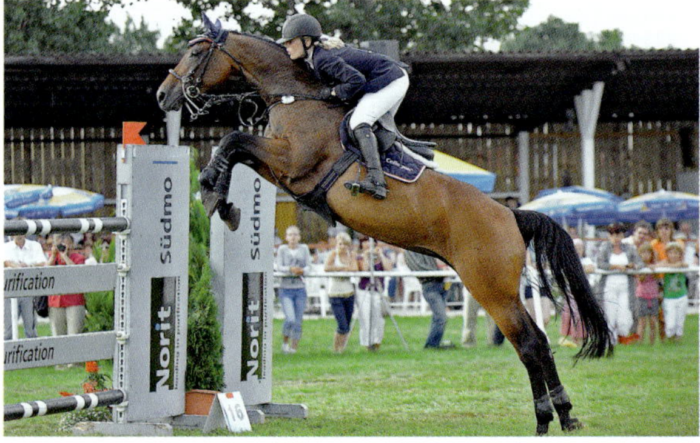

The higher the jump, the more the horse must flex his haunches in order to "catapult" upward and forward like a spring.

locations: this means, in this joint, you often see secondary blockages. Therefore, for you as a rider, the sacroiliac joint is one of the most important joints in the body, and you should keep an eye on it. I'm now going to explain the construction of this important mainstay of your horse's body.

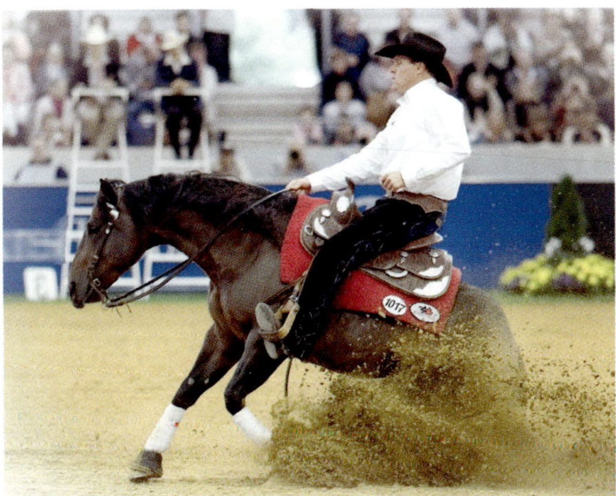

During a sliding stop, the sacroiliac joint is subjected to high stress.

● The Sacrum

You'll find the sacrum at the end of the lumbar spine. It forms, so to speak, an extension of the spine. The bones look like a cross—in fact, in German, these bones are called "*Kreuzbein*," which translates literally as "cross bone." The sacrum consists of five vertebrae, which fuse together when the horse is approximately five years old. The spinous processes of the sacrum tilt toward the back, which means in the opposite direction from the spinous processes of the lumbar area (see illustration on p. 66). Thereby, with the help of the long supraspinous ligament, the sacrum is well-formed for lifting, which is important to the horse's ability to lift his back like a bridge and, in turn, to carry weight.

● The Pelvis

The pelvis is formed by three bones, which only become fixed and resilient in the full-grown horse. The meeting point of these three bones (ischium, pubic, and iliac) forms the socket of the hip joint.

Together, the pelvis and sacrum form the sacroiliac joint, which forms the bony connection between the haunches and the horse's trunk.

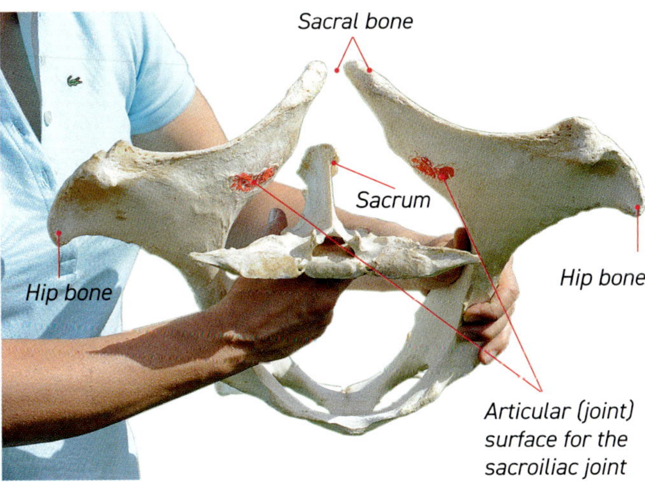

The sacrum and iliac bone photographed from below. The red point on the pelvis is the small flat articular/ joint surface of the pelvis. The sacrum sits between and the two "wings" of the sacrum form the articulated joint.

When the horse develops strength in his hindquarters, the sacroiliac joints become the center of forward movement. From this center, the pushing power travels over the spine in the direction of the forehand.

Observe this joint closely and you'll recognize two special characteristics. First, the joint surface of these two bones is really small in comparison to its function. Second, it's a flat joint, which means the joint does not get any stability from its construction. This differs from other joints, such as the hip joint, which has a pronounced ball and a socket. The flat, small sacroiliac joint is held together only by fixed ligaments. What exacerbates the situation further is that the sacroiliac joint has no muscling that directly support its stability and move directly with it.

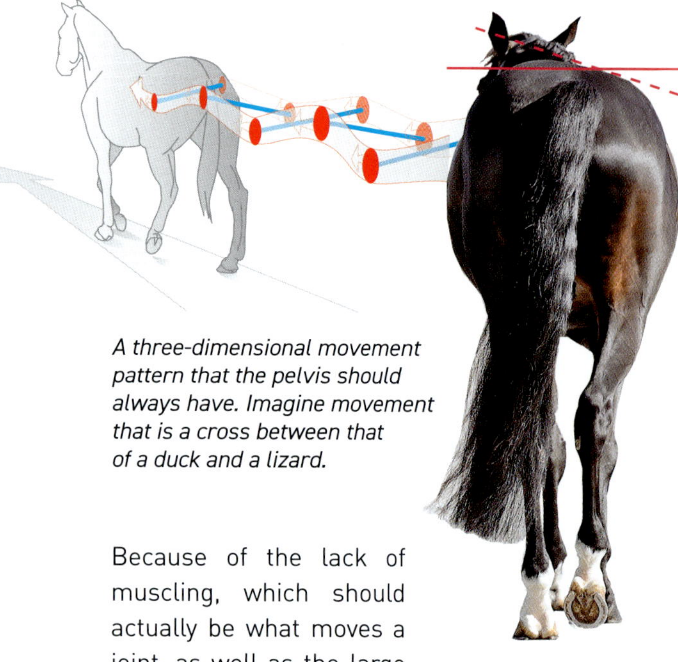

A three-dimensional movement pattern that the pelvis should always have. Imagine movement that is a cross between that of a duck and a lizard.

Because of the lack of muscling, which should actually be what moves a joint, as well as the large and tight ligaments, many experts have claimed that the sacroiliac joint is rigid and inflexible. This belief must be contradicted. It's in fact a very mobile joint, which you can well observe when your horse walks away from you. The whole pelvis makes a three-dimensional movement. Imagine movement that is a cross between that of a duck and a lizard: it's both a rolling and forward-moving way of going. Thereby, the iliac bones move opposite from the sacrum—over and under—independently of one another. You should be able to see this movement combination on both sides of the pelvis. If it's not there in either direction, you'll no longer have three-dimensional movement.

You can read more about how to better monitor and observe the mobility of the sacroiliac joint in chapter 5, "Observation" (p. 92).

■ Disorders of the Sacroiliac Joint

In practice, you often find injuries and blockages in the sacroiliac joint. They can have a primary source, for example, from trauma or injury. However, it's also unfortunately very common for the sacroiliac joint to be affected when there are blockages or disorders in other locations of the musculoskeletal system. The symptoms can result in a reduction of movement between the sacrum and the pelvis and/or pelvic misalignment.

When there's a blockage in the sacroiliac joint, the transmission of power from back to front is weaker. It's reduced and, thereby, the forward impulsion is greatly weakened. The horse does not carry through correctly with his hind end. So, too, can collection and tracking up of the hindquarters be reduced, which can cause uneven rhythm and eventually lameness. The pelvis then moves as a whole—no mixture of duck and lizard gait. To compensate for this loss of three-dimensional movement, there's more pressure on the lumbar vertebrae. In addition, these horses can't hold their true canter lead and often spring into a cross-canter. These horses also don't like to back up. They lose the longitudinal bend in the direction where the hip is lower. A further sign of a disorder in this joint: your farrier will find it difficult to bring the horse's back leg toward the back.

A misaligned pelvis changes the mechanics of the whole horse. When the horse's pelvis is misaligned on the right side, his whole pelvis on this side is lower, often also with a turn of the whole pelvis. This automatically will change the position of the hip socket and, thereby, also the fit of the femur in the socket. As a result, all the remaining joints of the hind limbs will also be falsely positioned. So, too, the engagement of the soft tissue is changed. The soft tissue will either have too much or too little engagement.

The spine is also harmed by a misaligned pelvis. It turns in the same direction as the lowered hip and the spinal column is blocked. Here again, the engagement of the soft tissues is altered. Most often, it's the lumbar spine that's affected, but a misaligned pelvis can also have a negative influence on the spine all the way to the horse's head.

Still another disorder of the sacroiliac joint is the twisting of the sacrum in relation to the pelvis. You

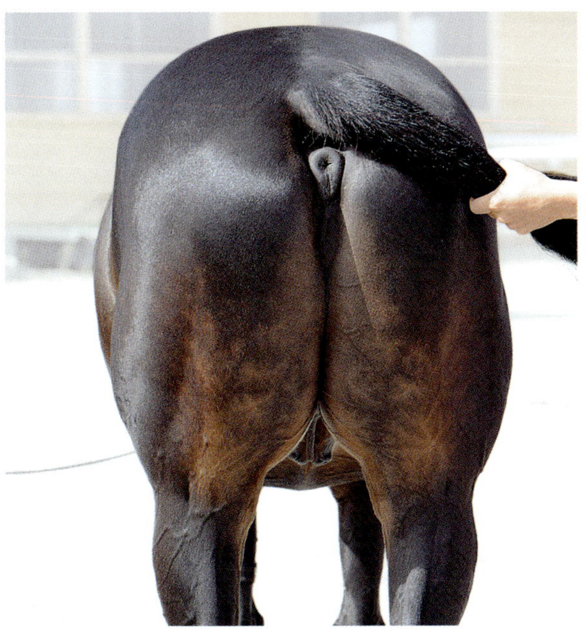

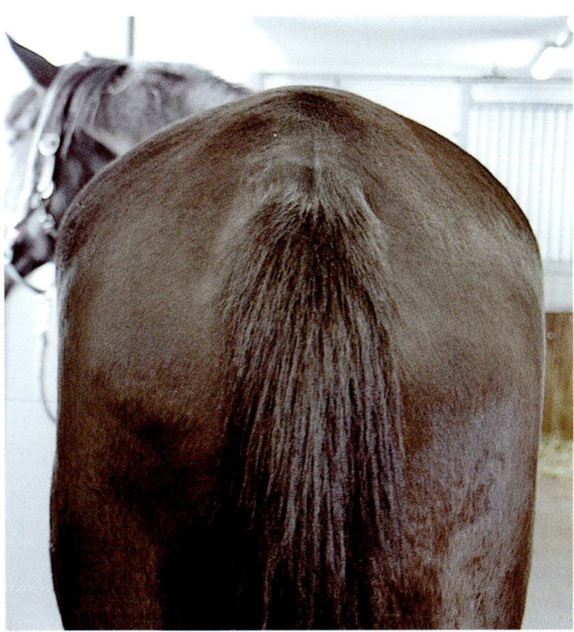

When you look at your horse's croup from behind, the topline should almost form a heart. (You can see this really well with draft horses.) Ideally, the gluteal muscles form the highest point of the croup with the two iliac tips (as in the photo on the left and see photo p. 101, right). With horses that have a problem in the sacroiliac joint, there's often a swelling. In the photo to the right, the iliac tips are the highest point because of swelling.

may not immediately be able to see this false positioning, but you will be able to feel it. The sacrum and the first cervical vertebra are connected, via a membrane called the *dura mater*, inside the spinal canal. A practical example will make this clearer: If the right side of the sacrum is lower, then the wing of the C1 vertebra on the right side is also lower. You probably won't recognize the source of the problem: the twist in the sacrum. However, you do notice a problem with positioning in the poll. The horse won't want to be positioned through the right side of his jaw!

Fact: Disorders of the sacroiliac joint are always accompanied by muscular atrophy of the croup muscles on the affected side.

A final example of a disorder of the sacroiliac joint is that the peripheral nerve cords become affected.

Through a blockage and/or an incorrect position of the sacroiliac joint, and the resulting changes to the affected engagement of ligaments and muscles, nerves can become pinched. For example, the sciatic nerve, which is as thick as a finger and supplies the hindquarters, can become compromised due to the tightening of the ligaments and muscles. Horses try to relieve the nerve, in that they push away through their back and thus tip the pelvis downward. As a result, the croup appears flat. The limbs are positioned toward the back or the horses stand with an extremely round back with their legs positioned far under the belly. Either way, they are trying to avoid the pull on the nerve. And, obviously, their way of going will be changed due to the inflammation of the nerves. Those among us who have lived through sciatic nerve pain know best what I'm talking about here!

My Tip

Few horse owners realize that their horse has a misaligned pelvis. Observe your horse regularly in order to be able to respond quickly when unevenness occurs (see chapter 5, "Observation," p. 92).

The Hip Joint

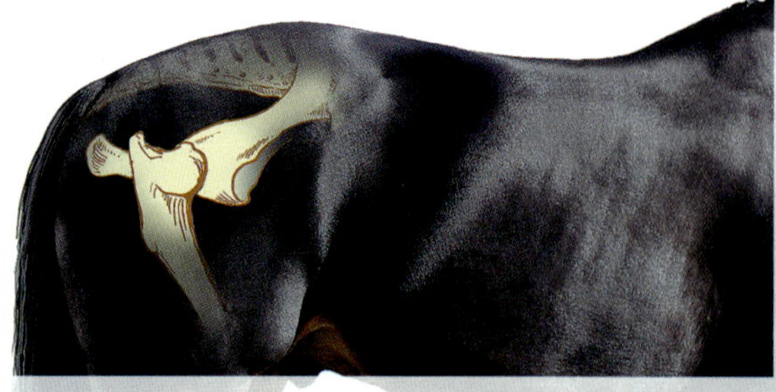

■ Hip Joint Biomechanics

The hip joint is one of the most stable joints in the horse's body. The large, solid femur finds perfect support in the pelvic socket and is fixed there by really strong ligaments. Although it's a perfect ball and socket joint, which actually has lots of mobility in all directions, its mobility is lost in favor of the stability of this joint's surrounding ligaments.

The hip joint can generously contract (flex) and extend (stretch). As you can see clearly during lateral movements, the horse can easily bring his hind limbs toward the middle of his body (adduction) and away from the middle of his body (abduction). So, too, a small twist of the femur to the inside or outside is possible. These last two movements of the hind limbs are primarily coming from the hip joint, although they are possible in all joints of the hind limbs (except for the fetlock joint). The expansive movement amplitude that we humans have in our hip joints is not available to the horse.

Example: In movement, it looks like this: when the horse brings his hind leg forward, the primary movement is contraction. Through the joint congruency in the hip joint and the longitudinal bend in the spine, the leg will come forward while it is guided slightly toward the center of the horse's body, slightly turned outward, and then stopped. This combined movement makes it possible for the hind limbs to come far forward.

In the standing phase (retraction), the leg is extended. Thereby, the limb moves away from the center of the horse's body and slightly turns toward the inside. At the end of the extension, the limb is thereby pushed away from the center of the horse's body, to avoid the limbs from touching. Here, too, the leg can better extend through the combined movement.

This three-dimensional movement in the hip joint can be seen only through the transfer of weight and the longitudinal bend of the spine. There should not be a visible twist of the limbs.

By the way, we humans execute the same movement pattern when we walk—it's a three-dimensional gait!

Fact: These combined movements are important in order to be able to execute the full range of motion/ movement. If any of the hip movements are blocked, the horse won't be able to execute maximum extension and contraction of the joint.

■ Disorders of the Hip Joint

If there's a loss of this combined movement in the hip joint, the horse will execute an evasive movement. Instead of turning his hip joint, he makes an avoidance movement with his entire limb. You can observe that the hoof on the ground at the end of the standing phase is turned toward the inside (and the hock tips away toward the outside). A source of this damaging evasive movement can be a shortening of the soft tissue in the hock area. The horse must, therefore, execute the evasive movement as his whole leg has turned. For the joint beneath, this turning is a much higher stress to bear. So, too, an instability and/or muscular weakness of the hindquarters can trigger these symptoms.

You can easily determine this reduction in mobility during lateral movements. Horses that have hock problems don't execute these exercises correctly because lateral movements require maximum turning and sideward movement from the hock joint.

Just like you, horses can suffer from irritation of the sciatic nerve. The source of the problem can be a

Physical Therapy for Horses

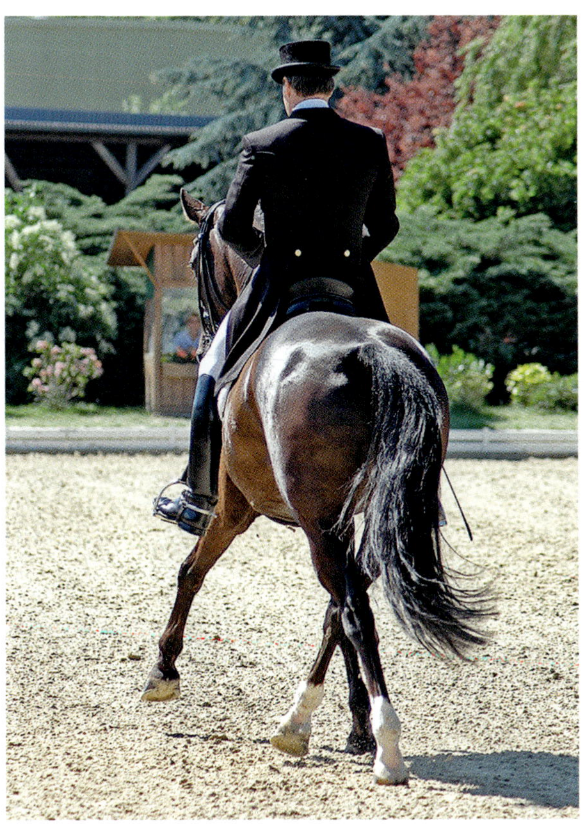

Correctly moving hindquarters: Here, the pelvis tips downward and, in doing so, creates the condition for the hind leg to come far under the center of the horse's body. This is possible thanks to the mobility of the hock, sacroiliac joint, and back.

compression of the nerve in the sacroiliac joint, but also in the area of the hip joint. The nerve runs directly behind the hip joint and muscular tension can cause too much pressure. When tight muscles cause compression, the nerve cannot optimally glide, and this triggers an irritation of the nerve. What follows is pain and reduction of movement.

Fact: Because the hip joint is very stable, it mainly incurs blockages through a trauma (like slipping) or a secondary disorder in the body, such as a blocked jaw or shoulder joint or blockages in the lumbar spine.

The Stifle Joint

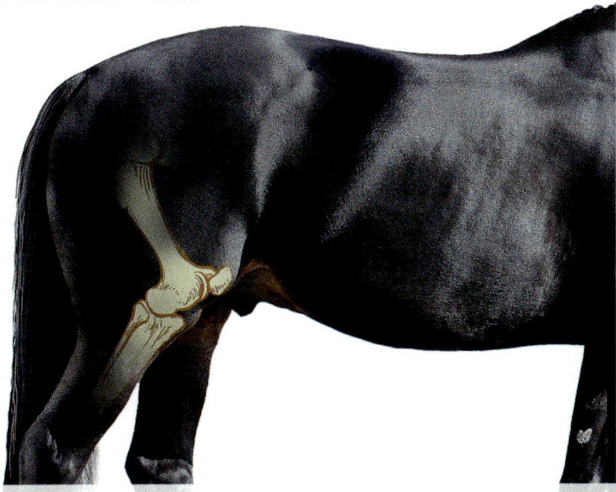

■ Biomechanics of the Stifle

We always talk of one stifle joint, but from a biomechanical perspective, there are actually two joints if you consider the connection to the patella (knee cap). The femur and tibia form one joint and, together with the femur, the patella forms a second connection.

The joint surfaces between the femur and tibia are not congruent; this means, they don't fit together. Therefore, this joint has two *menisci*, which provide the important balance between stability and shock absorption. But all of this is not enough to maintain stability for this wobbly construction. Therefore, the stifle joint is also surrounded by many strong ligaments.

As with all joints of the hind limbs, contraction and extension are the most important movements. To a moderate degree, the stifle joint can turn inward and outward and also make a small movement toward and away from the center of the body, but its capacity for movement is much less than that of the hock.

■ Disorders of the Stifle Joint

Many horses have an unstable stifle, which is noticeable under saddle when they "fall out" with their hindquarters. This is especially common among young horses going through a growth spurt. The stifle ligaments are not yet stable enough and the muscular strength necessary to maintain the stifle is not yet available to the horse. After the growth spurt is over, this symptom will disappear. With older horses that always fall out behind, I see a connection to the muscling of the hindquarters. In particular, the *bicipital* and *quadriceps* muscles catch my attention. The reason is that both these muscles have a connection to the stifle ligaments and the engagement of these muscles controls these ligaments. I've noticed that with many horses that fall out behind, these muscles are simply too weak. Experience has taught me that the stifle joint can become more stable through purposeful training of the surrounding muscles. The falling out of the hindquarters will then disappear.

On the front side, you find the *quadriceps* muscle of the upper thigh (see p. 73, left). Through tendons, it's tightly connected to the patella. A locking of the patella is an important component of the horse's standing mechanism. Among other things, the *quadriceps* muscle is responsible for its locking and releasing. If the muscle is suffering from tension or lack of strength, it can make this task a lot more difficult. Eventually, it can lead to a suspension of the patella, in which case the horse will no longer be able to move forward.

A blockage in the junction between the thoracic and lumbar vertebrae can be the source of symptoms in the stifle joint. You can see the connection between the two regions of the body. Therefore, with horses that often have stifle-area problems, you must also carefully monitor the correlating sections of the spine.

In addition, tension in the lumbar musculature (*iliopsoas*) can limit the mobility of the patella. The nerve that is responsible for triggering the *quadriceps* muscle runs between the *lumbar* muscles. If this muscle is tight, it compromises the nerve, which in turn weakens the connection between the central nervous system and the *quadriceps* muscle. The muscle loses its strength.

The Hock

■ Biomechanics of the Hock

The horse's hock consists of seven perfectly interconnected bones (including the outer splint bone), which are of great significance for movement. Because of its angled shape, this joint can powerfully support forward impulsion, while also working as a good shock absorber. Because of the shape of its rolling ridge, where movement (contraction and extension) primarily takes place, there's hardly any three-dimensional movement. But, during contraction, the cannon and toes are guided slightly to the outside. This guiding-to-the-outside is easily recognized when you bend the hind limbs.

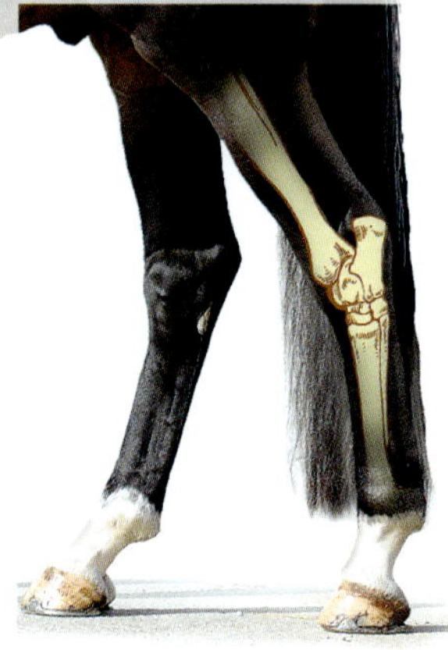

■ Disorders of the Hock

Blockages in the hock can bring about a reduction of the maximum range of movement. Unfortunately, this disorder won't stay local. Because of the specific "frame-saw" construction of the hind limbs, loss of movement here will also limit the mechanics of the stifle joint. The construction of the hind limbs also makes it difficult to differentiate as to whether it's the stifle or the hock that's blocked. Therefore, I need to examine the mobility of both joints.

The Joints of the Lower Limb

The construction of the joints of the lower hind limb are comparable with those of the forelimb. The only exception is that the hind limb cannon bone is somewhat longer, and the toes are angled more steeply. The toe-extensors and toe-flexor of the forehand are described in "The Forehand" on p. 76.

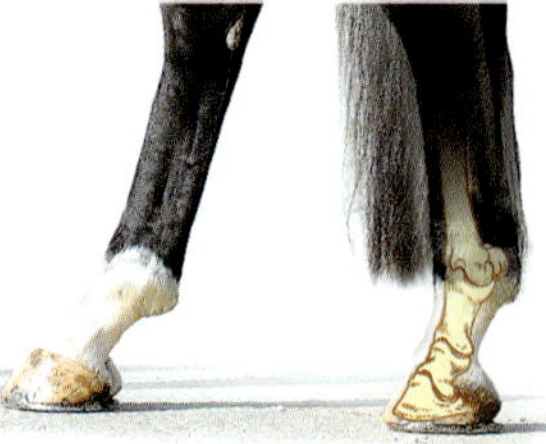

Physical Therapy for Horses

The Musculature of the Hindquarters

Because the hindquarters are the motor, this is also where drive comes from. This drive originates with very powerful muscles, which are layered over one another in multiple pieces. Many of them have more than one muscle belly, which reach over multiple joints, allowing them to develop a lot of power. In a Warmblood of typical muscling, this muscle mass can be up to 30 centimeters (about a foot) thick above the pelvic bones. Deep inside, there are small, short muscles. With so many muscles, it's easy to understand that the deep muscles cannot directly be felt or massaged. The farther toward the surface that you get, the more volume the muscles possess. I'm going to divide the muscles of the hindquarters into the following groups:

- Muscles that move the hind leg forward.
- Muscles that move the leg backward.
- The gluteal/croup muscles.
- The adductor muscles.

■ Muscles That Move the Hind Leg Forward

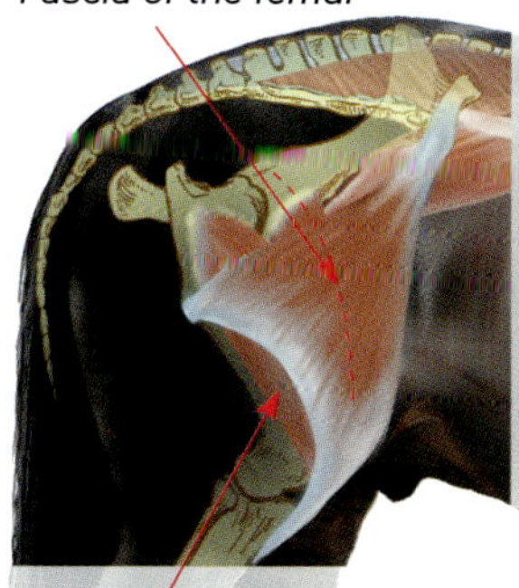

Fascia of the femur

Quadriceps muscle

From this group, I want to draw your attention to the *quadriceps* muscle of the femur (m. *quadriceps femoris*), which protects and stabilizes the stifle. Thereby, it has the most important task when the horse demonstrates correct collection. As the name implies, this muscle has four parts, which together travel outward from the pelvis and femur in the direction of the knee. There, they surround the patella as a unified tendon and further attach to the tibia. This muscle extends the stifle, holds the patella in its place, and helps in part to contract the hips.

This muscle has a tremendous influence on the ability of the hindquarters to flex and lower. The deeper the horse lowers his hind end, the more this muscle must work to extend. In other words, the quality of the hind-limb joint flexion and collection is dependent upon the strength of the *quadriceps* muscle of the femur.

This muscle quickly comes out of balance when the static of the leg is out of order, such as when the heel is too short. This leads to an altered engagement, which limits the sliding as well as the locking and unlocking of the patella.

● Tensor Fascia Lata (m. *tensor fasciae latae*)

This muscle (see the illustration to the left) is important to the stifle's ability to extend and stabilize, like the *quadriceps* muscle. As the name already implies, this muscle is responsible for the tone of the fascia of the femur, which surrounds the stifle joint. As described in chapter 2 (p. 22), many large muscles (responsible for movement) lie over multiple joints and, therefore, they often have multiple functions. This is equally true here: when the muscles move the hind limb forward, this also simultaneously contracts the hip joint.

The tensor fascia lata originates at the hip bone (iliac crest). If the horse has, let's say, a misaligned pelvis due to tension or a trauma/ fracture to the hip bone, this muscle can no longer work optimally. As the entire mechanics of the hindquarters is disrupted, it also can lead to instability of the stifle.

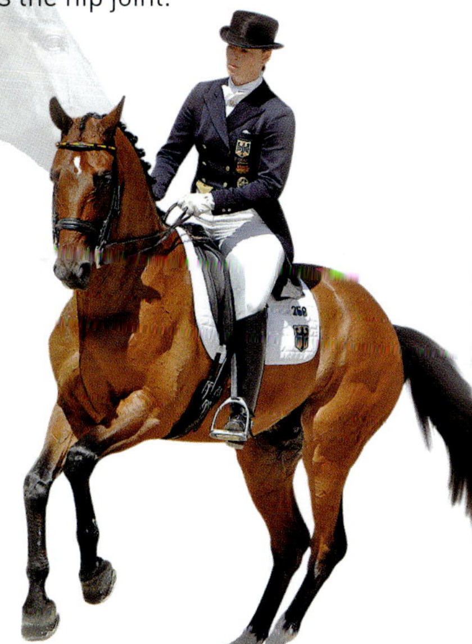

Fact: Executing a pirouette is significantly more difficult for the muscles of the hindquarters than an extended trot, as the pirouette moves in the direction of static work. In extended trot, the horse must develop lots of power, but in the extension, he has moments of "recovery" when the hind legs are floating forward (see "Types of Muscle Contractions," p. 28).

■ Muscles That Move the Hind Leg Back

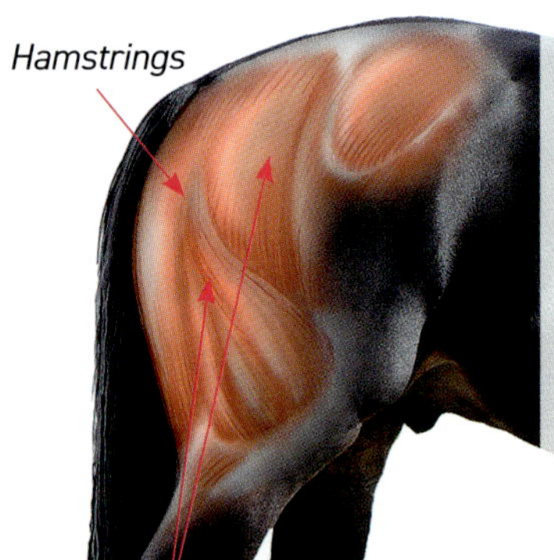

The extensors of the hind limbs are three powerful and long muscles, which are found at the way back of the horse and run over two to three joints.

From a mechanical perspective, it's the contraction of these muscles that moves your horse forward. During the pushing phase, all three upper joints are extended with the help of these muscles. Although they actually only reach the stifle joint, these two muscles have connective tissues, fascia, and tendons that insert at the point of the hock.

The two hamstring muscles (*m. semimembranosus, m. semitendinosus*) are always affected when the back muscle is tensed. Then, the horse will not like being brushed or touched. By very persistent tension, they'll move away from the slightest pressure and even threaten to kick. When you ride, you'll notice that your horse won't reach toward the front. As a result of this tension, the horse will no longer lengthen his hind leg beneath his center of gravity during the moment of suspension, so this moment is shortened. Therefore, the forward impulsion is no longer as powerful as it should be. When the horse drags his toe along the ground, this can be a sign

My Tip

When the hamstring muscle is tensed, you should massage your horse's back! Without even directly touching the horse's long hamstring muscles, you'll see how relaxed and loose they are after you massage his back. There's a close connection between the hamstring muscles and the back muscles. You can see this effect in reverse as well.

that the hamstring muscle has not developed enough engagement to lift the toe off the ground.

The femoral biceps muscle (*m. biceps femoris*) is a multi-function muscle. It contracts the hip joint, extends the stifle joint, and in turn, contracts the hock joint. Although it is called biceps (indicating two heads to the muscle form), it actually has three heads and is the largest muscle of the hindquarters. The biceps are closely connected with the stifle joint and provides it, along with the sacroiliac and hip joints, with the all-important stability. If this muscle is weak, the horse may "fall out" behind, especially during transitions.

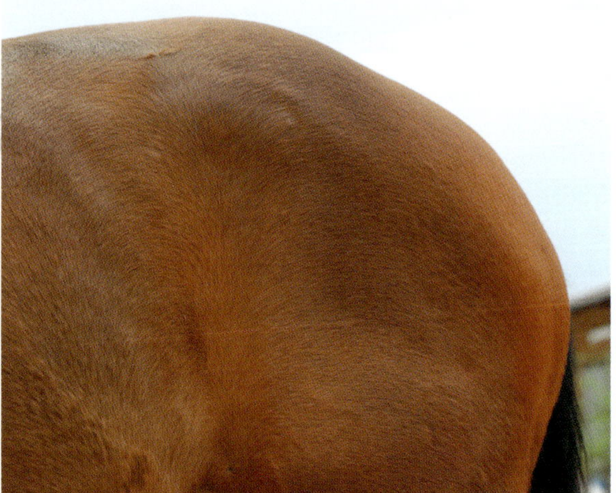

It's easy to see the strong hamstring and weak biceps muscle. This horse may have problems with stability of the stifle or sacroiliac joints.

These are the muscles that form a beautiful, round hindquarters. There are three gluteal muscles: a deep, middle, and superficial. They all originate at the femur and have diverse tasks. To make this even more complicated: one muscle extends the hip joint; another flexes it; but all three work together to bring the leg away from the center of the body (abduction), as you'd see in lateral movements.

The largest muscle of the hindquarters is the *gluteus medius*. One point of origin is on the *longissimus dorsi* and together they lift the

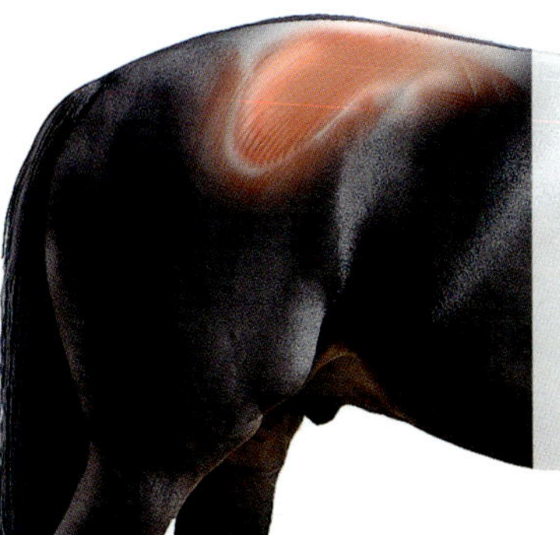

forehand; for example, when the horse is galloping or jumping. This muscle has an extension—a "tongue"—that stretches over the entire lumbar spine region and connects with the *longissimus dorsi*.

A diagnosis that I frequently make is a tensed back under the saddle area. There's clearly accumulated tension in the *longissimus dorsi* and the tongue of the *gluteus medius*.

This tension is so pronounced that I can see and feel it clearly. Erroneously, the tensed musculature is often mistaken for a well-muscled back.

Tension in the gluteal muscles leads to a blocking of the lumbar vertebrae when they try to lift. In turn, this influences the loin muscles, which are positioned along the underside of the lumbar spine. It's their job to lift the back, but they are not strong enough to work against the gluteal and back muscles. Eventually, because of tension in the *gluteus medius*, the horse can no longer lift his back.

Fact: The gluteal muscles reach T16 or T17, so the end of the saddle area, and cover the entire lumbar spine region. When you palpate and massage this area, it's likely to be the gluteal musculature that you're treating and not, as is often mistakenly assumed, the long muscles of the back, which lie under the gluteal musculature.

At canter or gallop, the gluteal muscles will be called upon to varying degree, in relation to the tempo. A racehorse touches down upon his hind limbs differently from a dressage horse, for example. The dressage horse brings his hind legs under his center of gravity and sets them down there. Therefore, more will be asked of the gluteal muscles of the dressage horse and they are, therefore, very important for his ability to shift his weight toward the hindquarters.

In contrast, the racehorse gallops at a higher tempo. His gallop strides are quicker, longer, and flatter. Therefore, the hind legs are not moving so far in the direction of the center of gravity and less will be asked of his gluteal musculature.

The *gluteal* muscle, like the *femoral biceps* muscle, is composed of various muscle fibers. Its superficial area is comprised primarily of fast-twitch (Type 2) muscle fibers, which are responsible for movement, whereas the deeper part has slow-twitch (Type 1) muscle fibers, which are important for stability.

My Tip

Don't forget about the superficial gluteal muscle. It will give you a lot of info about how well the horse is tolerating his current load. If the required level of collection is too high, this muscle will tense up immediately, first taking on volume and will feel hard. If you continue to ride with this high degree of difficulty, the horse will begin to move evasively and, over time, the croup will flatten, and the musculature will become irregular.

■ The Inner Upper Thigh Muscles (Adductors)

When you stand behind your horse and move his tail to the side, you are looking directly at his adductors. This muscle group fills out the inside of his upper thigh. It originates at the pelvis and inserts in various points along the inside of the upper thigh, the patellar

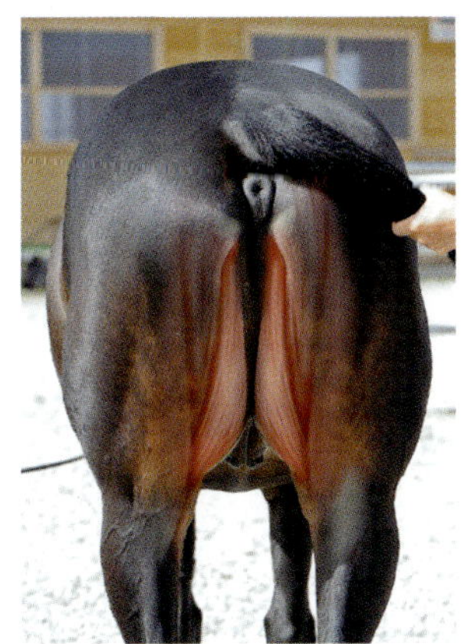

ligament, and the lower thigh bone. Its action can be wonderfully observed during lateral movements, as these are the muscles that pull the hind leg toward the center of the body. In addition, these muscles help to bring the leg forward and back.

Because the skin on the inside of the upper thigh is very sensitive, many horses don't like to be touched here. In my experience, there's often tension at hand, especially when the croup muscles, as counterparts to the inner upper thigh muscles, are painful and/or underdeveloped. As a result, the lateral movements are not even, the strides are short and they develop a "hobbling," which stretches the muscles. Therefore, lateral movements are uncomfortable for the horse. A further characteristic among horses that have a shortening here is that they travel close with their hind legs.

The Forehand

Watch a horse on a show jumping course—it's fascinating to see the mechanics of the forehand when the horse lands after a jump. First, a foreleg touches ground, taking on the entire weight of horse and rider, then the other limb follows. Consider the weight that this foreleg, extended straight out, must receive—according to the laws of physics, this foreleg should splinter like a piece of dry wood! But, thanks to the fantastic construction of the forehand, it doesn't splinter. Now, I'd like to offer you a glimpse into this magnificent construction.

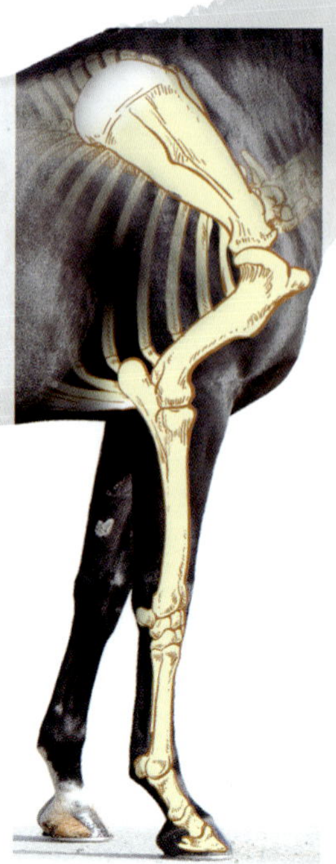

The genius of this construction lies in the fact that the forelimbs have no connection to the skeleton. The forehand is attached to the trunk by ligaments and muscles only. In a figurative sense, you can image the forelimb-trunk construction as follows: the forelimbs are two fixed poles and the trunk is like a boat that's rocking between them. When the connecting cables (the muscles and ligaments) hang freely and loosely, then the boat (the trunk) can move back and forth freely (see illustration on p. 59, bottom left).

This "jetty" connection makes it possible for the shoulder blade to execute broad gliding movements in every direction; for example, upon landing after a jump. The impact doesn't affect the limb, because of the sliding movement, it's able to capture the energy and pass it along to the neck and back. But, obviously, it's not only the shoulder blade that captures the energy. There are still other fantastic constructions of the forehand that support this shock absorption.

According to nature, the horse's forehand is meant to carry and is, therefore, only minimally involved in forward movement. To achieve its supporting/stabilizing function, the forehand works like a high-performing spring, which can absorb and store energy and then set it free again. On average, it carries about 60 percent of the horse's body weight, along with the head and neck. In addition to shock absorption, it also works to balance and receive the impulsion of the hindquarters. Because of the strong forces at work here, the forehand is more prone to injury than the hindquarters. In order to avoid injury, it's essential to have a forehand that is stable, but at the same time, mobile.

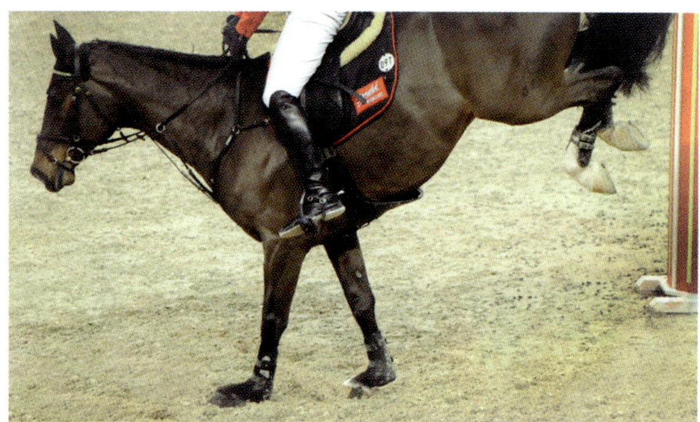

Upon landing, the forehand must take on the entire weight of horse and rider and absorb the impact. It's easy to recognize the elasticity of the forearm muscles. You can see how low to the ground the fetlock moves.

Physical Therapy for Horses

Biomechanics of the Forehand

Horses are runners and consequently evolution has equipped them as follows: they possess a narrow chest and vertically positioned shoulder blades. Through this configuration, the shoulder blades become part of the limbs. The advantage: the forehand is much longer as a result.

The largest movement pattern in all joints of the forelimb is contraction (flexion) and extension (stretching). In all joints, with the exception of the fetlock, you'll also find small movements: one toward the middle of the body (adduction), one away from the middle of the body (abduction), and a small twist toward the inside and outside. The fetlock joint is unique. Because of the way it's formed, the small movements are limited, but in turn, it is extremely capable when it comes to contraction and extension.

Apart from the shoulder joint, all joints have strong ligaments, which give the forehand stability despite its extreme mobility, and keep the movement in check.

In order to cover the subject of the forehand as clearly as possible, I've differentiated between:

- **The Upper Forehand**—Shoulder blade, shoulder, and elbow joints.
- **The Lower Forehand**—Knee, fetlock, pastern, and coffin joints.

■ The Upper Forehand

● Shoulder Blade

Because the horse does not have a collarbone like we do, there is no boney connection between the forelimbs and the skeleton (the trunk). The shoulder blade forms this connection and is, so to speak, a "phony joint."

The shoulder blade is a large, flat bone, which is slightly curved on the trunk side. The shoulder blade has a bony extension toward the withers, which almost reaches them. It supports the sliding movement.

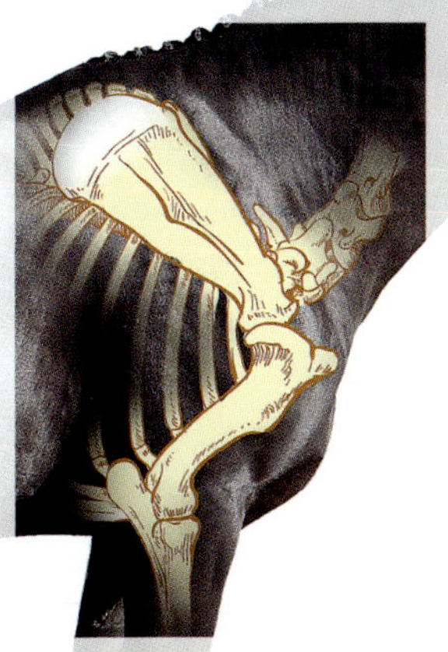

During both the standing and suspended phases of movement, the shoulder blade must be able to glide in every direction. It must be able to glide and turn downward, upward, diagonally toward the front and diagonally toward the back. Therefore, it's important that all the muscles that bind the shoulder blade to the trunk must be strong but also elastic, in order to allow this movement.

When the leg touches down, the energy generated should travel upward. If the shoulder blade doesn't glide optimally along the trunk, then the energy cannot be moved along completely. In my practice, I often encounter limited mobility of the shoulder blade. Some good news: because the shoulder and trunk are connected by soft tissue (ligaments, muscles), you can make this area more mobile through massage and stretching exercises, even without being a medical professional.

● Shoulder Joint

The shoulder blade and the strong humerus bone form the shoulder joint. The horse cannot bring his humerus forward without there being a movement in his shoulder blade. This joint is responsible for the sideways movement of the forehand, which isn't large because the sideways movements are limited by the shoulder blade. Unusually, the shoulder joint does not have any stabilizing ligaments. The stability is realized through the muscles. This leads to the fact that this joint is sensitive and often prone to pain.

Fact: Through muscle groups and fascia, the shoulder joint is connected with the jaw and hip joints. This is the reason that a block in the shoulder joint, for example, can also affect the hip and/or jaw joints.

• Elbow Joint

The elbow joint is formed from three bones, the humerus and two radius bones, the ulna and radius. In people, the two radius bones are separated. This allows us to turn our lower arms. In horses, these two bones are fused together, which prevents it from turning.

A further distinction between horse and human anatomy is that the horse cannot completely extend his elbow joint. The reason can be found above the joint in form of an extension of the radius bone. This bone limits the extension. Through this special construction, the elbow joint is a solid joint and an optimal shock absorber in the region of the foreleg.

Fact: In jumpers and event horses, painful bruises can occur on the elbow when the horse hits a jump with his forehand. Because of the concussion from the pole/jump, the hoof can get out of control and be catapulted against the elbow.

• Muscles of the Upper Forehand

As already mentioned, the musculature of the forehand has a shock absorption function; it absorbs the forward movement generated by the hindquarters and is, therefore, less directly responsible for forward movement. During acceleration and braking, the role of this muscle group increases.

Fact: If the goal is to build up the muscles of the forehand, include transitions, gymnastic lines, and small jumps in the training program. Traveling at a consistent tempo requires little from the forehand muscles.

Because of the form, function, and central position of the forehand, there are many muscles in this area. I'm only going to describe those muscles that most commonly trigger a biomechanical disorder. In order to clarify their tasks and to which groups these muscles belong, I've divided them as follows:

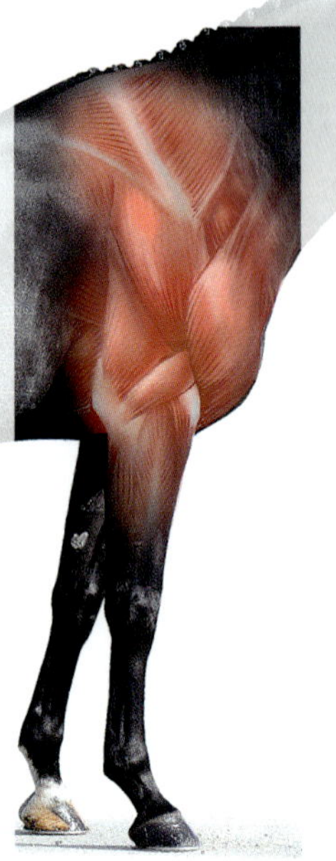

- Muscles that suspend the trunk.
- Chest muscles (pectorals).
- Muscles that suspend the limbs.
- Muscles that move the limb forward.
- Muscles that move the front limb backward.

■ Muscles That Suspend the Trunk

As the heading implies, these muscles carry the trunk. The "trunk-bearing muscles" include the chest muscles (*mm. pectorales*) and the ventral serratus muscles (*m. serratus ventralis thoracis*).

There are four chest muscles that connect the limbs with the lower part of the trunk. As connector muscles between the trunk and the forehand, the chest muscles catch/cradle the trunk. In addition, they help move the limbs forward, backward, and inward. Horses that tend to travel on the forehand or that are ridden with draw reins have lots of tension in this muscle group. Apart from short, dull gaits, triggered by this tension, lateral movements can also be a problem as they require so much elasticity here.

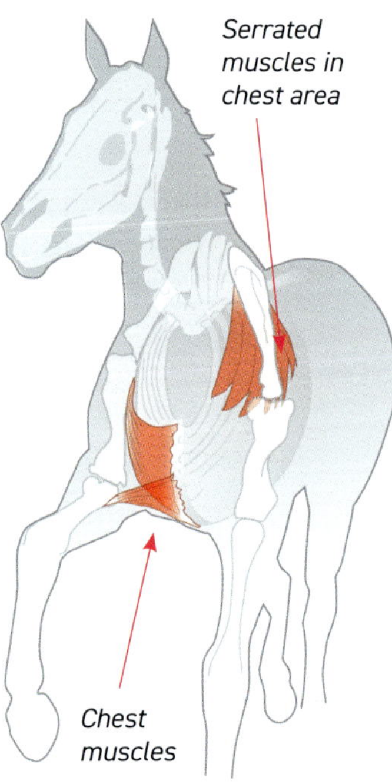

On the superficial chest muscles, there can be lots of swelling in the girth area, which is at the height of the elbows. This tension can even cause "girthy"

behavior. When a horse has muscular tension in the muscles that suspend the trunk, his way of going will be dull and his strides won't cover ground.

However, of the muscles that suspend the trunk, the most important, is the serrated muscle (*m. serratus ventralis thoracis*), which spreads like a fan along the trunk and neck. It's this muscle that allows your horse to have a beautiful, flowing way of going.

You can easily see the neck section of the serrated muscles in front of the shoulder blade. It should fill up the triangle between the shoulder blade, lower cervical vertebrae, and the withers. Its job is to lift and carry the neck when the leg is in the standing phase, and together with the wide back muscles, this muscle brings the shoulder blade forward.

When your horse has a dip in front of his shoulder blade, this muscle is too weak and underdeveloped (unfortunately, many horses are this way). A reason for this can be a block in the lower cervical vertebrae, but most often, the problem can be found in the hindquarters. These horses don't engage their hindquarters correctly (whether because of a functional impairment or rider error). What follows is that this muscle is not able to carry the neck. You'll notice that your horse either lies on the bit or curls back behind it. Thereby, it can be difficult to bring the neck to a long-and-low stretch and, at the same time, maintain a springy, loose gait from the shoulder.

The chest section of the *ventralis serratus* also begins at trunk and rises farther upward between the shoulder blades. When landing after a jump, the trunk glides between the "poles" (the forelimbs) toward the ground. As this takes place, the *ventralis serratus* muscle is stretched. (Consequently, it works eccentrically.) With horses that have tension in the chest section of the *serratus* muscles, this wonderful shock absorption doesn't take place. In this case, the energy from below can't be delivered and channeled upward again. The burden remains "caught" in the lower extremities, creating circumstances ripe for injury and wear and tear on the joints.

The *serratus* muscle is most stressed by jumping. When the muscle is tense, the trunk will not be lifted back upward after the jump. The effect is as if the horse stays standing a second longer because the trunk doesn't spring upward and the forehand can't get out of the way. A strong (but unfortunately also tense muscle) can position the shoulder more steeply, so that the horse will end up standing with his forelegs too far behind as he lands.

Often, these horses won't want to be touched in the girth area. During grooming and girthing, they appear unhappy because they don't like any pressure on this muscle.

The sources of tension in the *serratus* muscle are often avoidable. Most often, tack is the source of the problem. With long girths, I often see that the buckles bore through the leather (saddle flap) and apply pressure directly on the muscle. With short girths, the buckles are often not well padded enough. In addition, a girth that is too thin or over-tightened can bring too much pressure on the trunk muscles, which causes pain here (see chapter 12, "Preventive Measures," p. 200).

■ Muscles That Suspend the Limbs

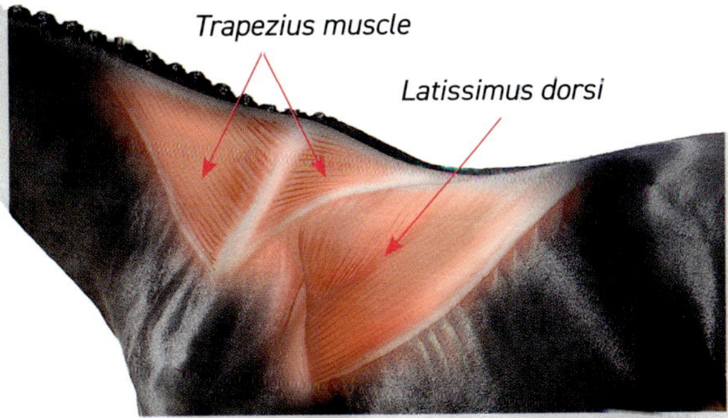

The muscles that hold up the limbs originate from the cervical vertebrae, as well as the nuchal ligament, and run almost all over the entire back. They attach again at either the shoulder blade or the upper arm (humerus). They fulfill various functions such as bringing the limb forward and backward, stabilizing and bringing the limb outward—to name just a few of their functions.

There are two muscles that I want to call your attention to. The first is the wide back muscle (*m. latissimus*). It contracts the shoulder joint and moves the leg toward the back. In addition, the *latissimus dorsi* muscle pushes the trunk forward between the shoulder blades. It tips the shoulder blades toward the front and plays an important role in the spring mechanism of the forelegs. Many mechanical problems can originate in this broad muscle: if there's a blockage in the saddle area, the resulting limitations of movement can compromise the shoulder freedom in the forelimbs. This leads to unevenness. Eventually, the tension in this muscle can even cause lameness in the forelimbs (shoulders).

Fact: The wide back muscle is the counterpart of the brachiocephalicus muscle. When the wide back muscle has tension, the brachiocephalicus muscle will eventually be affected, and vice versa.

Many riders will be familiar with the second muscle, the *trapezius* muscle. It looks like the fin of a fish, as it also stretches from the middle of the nuchal ligament back to the T10 vertebra. The wide point of insertion is found on the outside of the shoulder blade. Because its extension stretches in both directions, this muscle is involved in both bringing the forelimbs forward and bringing them back. When the shoulder blades pull upward, this muscle also guides the leg away from the center of the body and is, therefore, an important muscle for all lateral movements. It's common for the *trapezius* muscle to be diagnosed with muscular atrophy when, for example, a too-tight saddle gullet causes a dip beside the withers. But, because this muscle is actually very thin and wide to begin with, it's really not possible for it to lose too much substance. More likely, these dips beside the withers are actually a sign of weakness in the muscles that suspend the trunk. Instead of the trunk being properly suspended, the thoracic vertebrae "hang" between the shoulder blades and are the source of these dips.

In addition, you can't underestimate the possibility that the musculature is actually suffering from too

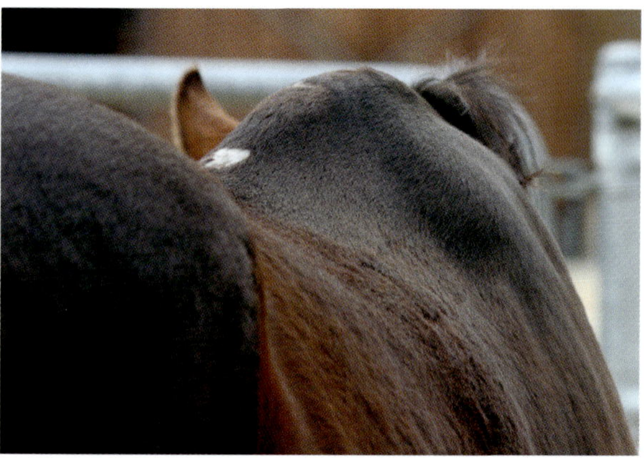

The dips at the withers can either be from muscular atrophy in the deep layers of the back muscles or they are a sign of trunk instability.

much pressure from the saddle. The muscles more likely to lose mass as a result are the *longissimus dorsi* and/or the spinous processes muscles (*m. spinalis*) and not, as is so often assumed, the *trapezius*.

Fact: When a horse has dips to the right and/or left of the withers, it's not due to atrophy of the trapezius muscle. Rather, the source of the problem lies in the deeper muscle layers or an unstable forehand.

■ Muscles That Move the Limbs Forward

Among the muscles that move the limbs forward, you see muscles that originate at the shoulder blade or upper arm (humerus) and insert at the neck or head. Their function is to bring the foreleg forward or to contract the neck and head as well as to stretch or execute a longitudinal bend.

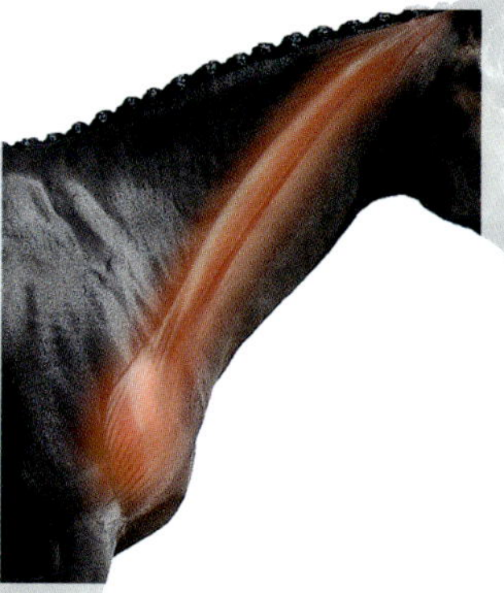

A muscle that should often be massaged and stretched is the *brachiocephalicus* muscle. The literal translation from German is the "head-arm-muscle." As the German term implies, this muscle binds the head to the forelegs. It's one of the forelimbs' most

Physical Therapy for Horses

important connectors and helps to execute longitudinal bend during the leg's standing phase.

It's interesting to know that the *brachiocephalicus* muscle, along with the position of the neck, influences the movement of the forelegs.

> Example: A horse at a full gallop doesn't have any "knee action," which allows him to bring his forelegs much farther forward. A gallop is flat. When the neck is elevated, like a canter for dressage, it's much more difficult for the horse to bring his forelegs forward, but it leads to a higher front leg action because the muscles can pull upward more.

In daily life, many horses have overly tense *brachiocephalicus* muscles and unfortunately, the muscle is also overly developed. They are responsible for the built-up, lower side of the neck. Horses that don't step off from behind use this muscle in order to "get into gear." In order to transition to a higher gait, they must always "lift up" with their head and neck in order to be able to move forward. When the horse is, for example, too tight in his neck—meaning behind the vertical—this muscle loses length in its contraction and the forward stride will be shortened. Because of the tightened position of the neck, these horses are then able to bring their forelegs even higher. This looks spectacular, but it's not ground-covering—or correct. In order to be able to use this muscle optimally, and so maintain ground-covering activity of the forelegs, the neck must be carried in front of the vertical and with elevation.

My Tip

Pay special attention to the *brachiocephalicus* muscle. The way it develops will reveal how you work with your horse. Through correct dressage work, this muscle will develop so that the horse achieves a gait that is both ground-covering and fully expressive. But this can only be achieved when combined with thrust from the hindquarters.

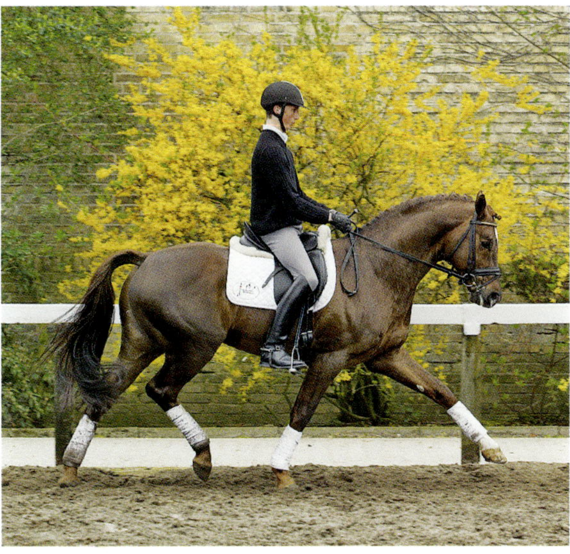

The position of the neck is vitally important to the forward movement of the front legs. When the horse is both carrying his own neck and moving toward the bit, the forelegs extend well from the shoulder, but not too high.

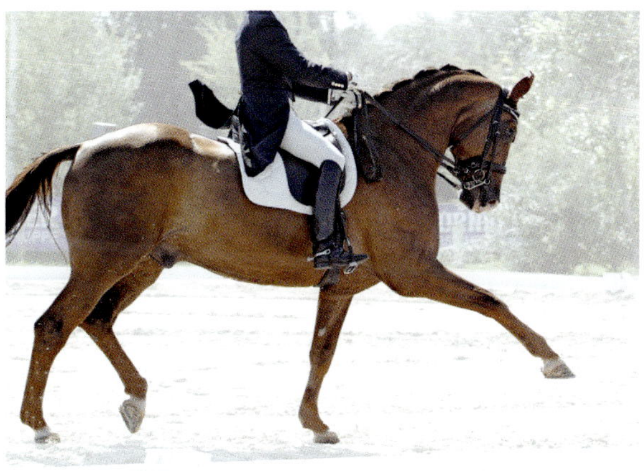

When the horse is behind the vertical, the forelegs travel higher, but they are not moving loosely forward from the shoulder.

■ Muscles That Move the Limbs Backward

The neck section of the *trapezius* muscle and the diamond-shaped *rhomboids* belong among the muscles that move the limbs backward. They tip the shoulder blade forward and, in this way, they help to execute the backward movement of the limb. The two muscles lie on top of one another, originate in the shoulder blade, and attach to the nuchal ligament.

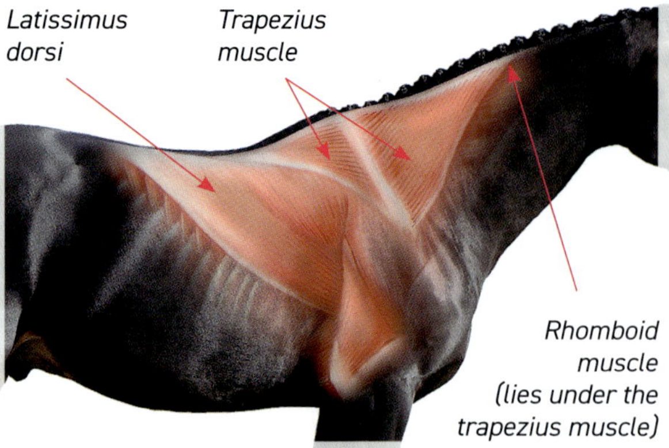

Therefore, the nuchal ligament is also indirectly involved with the attachment of the shoulder blade to the trunk. When the nuchal ligament is being pulled too tightly, as, for example, with the use of draw reins or when the horse is ridden behind the vertical, the movement of the shoulder blade is also automatically limited. Here's what follows: tension in the shoulder-girdle muscles that can lead to an altered angle of the shoulder blades.

Fact: The shoulder-girdle muscles include all muscles that have their origin in the neck or trunk and their point of attachment in the front limbs. For example, the muscles that hold up the trunk, chest muscles, trapezius, rhomboids, and even the brachiocephalicus muscle.

I've already mentioned an important muscle that moves the forelimbs back, which is the *latissimus dorsi* (wide muscle of the back—see "Muscles that Suspend the Trunk," p. 78). The most important muscle that works with it is the triceps (*m. triceps brachii*). This is the large, fleshy muscle directly in front of the girth area. It originates on the shoulder blade and gets smaller as it travels toward the elbow, where it attaches. This upper arm muscle contracts the shoulder joint, extends the elbow joint, and in this way, brings the legs back.

When there's tension in the neck and back, you often find tension in this three-headed muscle. Because the *triceps* muscle is large, accessible, and fleshy, it's easy to massage here. To relieve

tension is usually relatively easy and the horses enjoy having this muscle treated.

Fact: Tension in the shoulder-girdle muscles affects the position of the withers and breastbone in relation to the forehand. These horses may stand ahead of or behind with their forelimbs.

■ The Lower Forehand

● Knee Joint

The knee joint is comparable to your wrist joint. It consists of eight bones of various sizes, in two rows, plus an accessory carpel bone, which is found on the backside of the joint. Contraction and extension are its strength. Movement toward the center of the body (adduction) or away from the body (abduction) mostly happens in this joint.

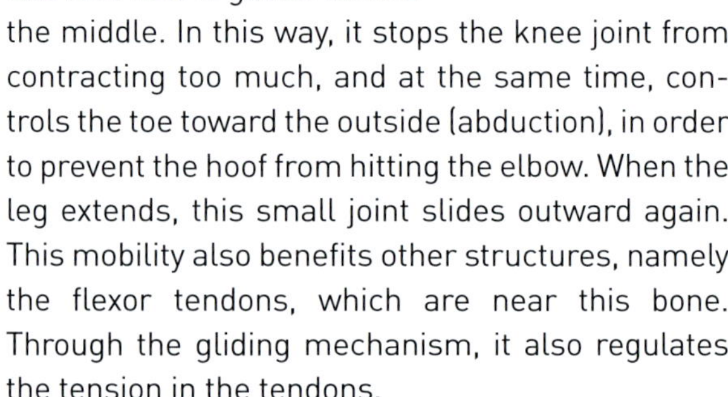

Just a short note about the accessory carpel bone: This small-sized bone plays an important role in the mechanics of the forelimbs. Without it, you would have many more injuries to the elbow.

You can easily feel the accessory carpel bone on the outer, backside of the knee joint. When this joint contracts, you can feel how it glides toward the middle. In this way, it stops the knee joint from contracting too much, and at the same time, controls the toe toward the outside (abduction), in order to prevent the hoof from hitting the elbow. When the leg extends, this small joint slides outward again. This mobility also benefits other structures, namely the flexor tendons, which are near this bone. Through the gliding mechanism, it also regulates the tension in the tendons.

Time after time, I find that this bone is blocked; this means, the gliding toward the inside and outside has been reduced. Over time, what follows can lead

Physical Therapy for Horses

to injury of the flexor tendon. In addition, blood vessels and nerves that are important to the lower limbs also run near the sesamoid bone. Due to blockages, they can be compromised, which can cause circulation problems and loss of sensitivity in the tendons. This can be compared to carpal tunnel syndrome in people.

■ Joints of the Lower Limb

Whether I'm talking about the forelegs or hind legs, the lower bones form the horse's toes. At the end of the cannon bone, you find the fetlock joint, then the pastern, and coffin joints. The construction of this part of the horse's body can be compared with your hands and feet. The coffin bone is the middle of your hand or foot. The splint bones are two bones that are "remnants" from the time when the horse had more toes. The fetlock joint can be compared to the first joint of your finger/toe, then comes the pastern joint. The tip of your finger/toe with the nail is comparable to the coffin bone of the hoof (see illustration at the top of p. 84).

In the toe, you also find the basic movements of flexion and extension. There are also small turning movements and a slight guiding toward the inside or outside. In turn, the fetlock joint is quite different. Due to a rise in the middle of the joint, it's not able to turn, and you only find a little splaying (abduction) and pull (adduction) in the fetlock joint. However, the range of flexion and extension is larger.

The genius of the horse's musculoskeletal system is easily recognizable in the lower limbs. Evolution has developed the horse from a small, compact animal that hid in the woods to a prairie-dwelling prey animal with long, thin, and light limbs. This allows him to run fast and far when it's necessary to his survival. It's notable in the large, voluminous muscles that belong to the middle of his body. The farther you get from them, the lighter the structure of his limbs. The entire ligament and tendon system is laid out so that the horse, with the help of his sesamoid bones, can absorb and let loose a lot of energy without using up a lot of his power.

Imagine the following: the entire system of tendons and ligaments in the lower limb functions like a spring. When the horse lands on a leg, the fetlock moves toward the ground. Thereby, the ligaments and tendons are stretched. Afterward, the leg and trunk are brought upward again, as if by a spring: this means, the leg lifts from the ground without requiring much muscle power.

Combined with the rather more stable trunk, this mechanism enables the horse to be able to be able to run long distances at a maximum tempo. The same construction allows the horse to jump: by loading the hindquarters, the horse catapults himself high in the air. To do so, the horse needs less power than you would imagine.

When you observe the mechanics of these joints, it's actually astounding that the fetlock joint is not injured more frequently when the horse gallops or jumps, for example. Let's imagine the horse at a gallop. In one phase of this gait, a single foreleg carries the weight of the entire horse, during which the fetlock joint takes the most concussion and receives the heaviest burden. Under this burden, it may compress all the way to the ground during its standing phase.

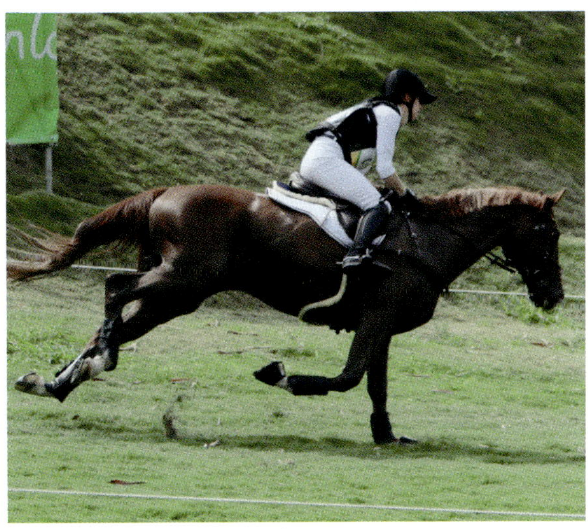

You can recognize how low the fetlock is toward the ground when this leg must carry the horse's entire weight.

A comparison of the hand/ foreleg and foot/ hind leg of human and horse.

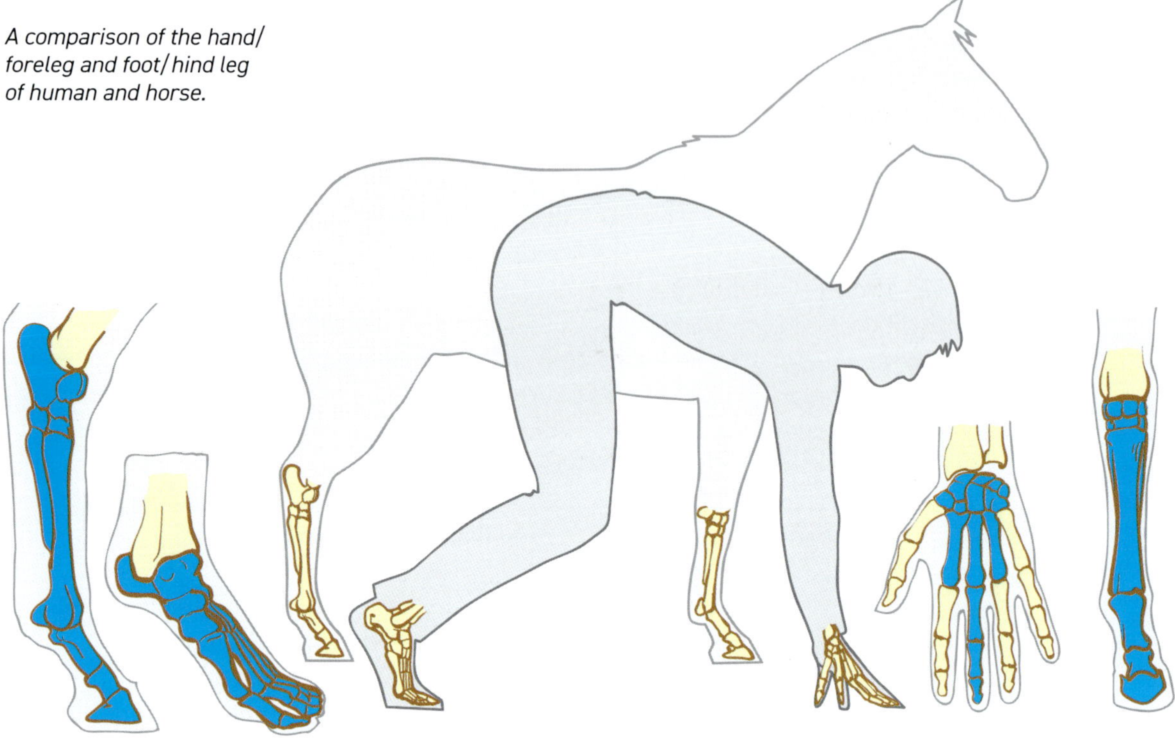

■ Musculature of the Lower Limb

When it comes to the musculature of the lower forelimbs, or the lower hind limbs for that matter, we distinguish between two muscle groups:

- Flexors of the lower limb.
- Extensors of the lower limb.

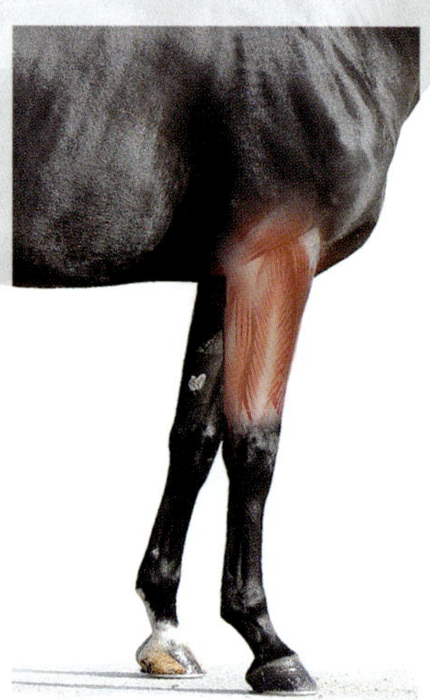

The flexors and extensors are comprised of multiple muscles. Their job is to bend the lower limbs or to stretch them, respectively. It's interesting to note that the muscle bellies are all located above the knee joint; below the knee, you only find the tendons that belong to them.

● Flexors of the Lower Limb

The *flexor* muscles are found on the backside of the lower arms and legs, as shown in the example. They work like a spiral, are extremely elastic and, therefore, can take on eerily heavy burdens.

Example: Imagine the following: a horse lands after a jump. He must take his entire weight and that of the rider with his two front legs. The fetlock joints, with their distinct ability to flex and stretch, partially touch the ground. This means the flexor muscles must be able to get longer by 10 to 15 centimeters and withstand the weight. That's quite a lot!

The *flexor* muscles work eccentrically as this takes place, which means the muscles must get longer as they accept the weight—the hardest type of work for the muscles. The stretch is found only in the muscle belly, which is found between the elbow and knee joint.

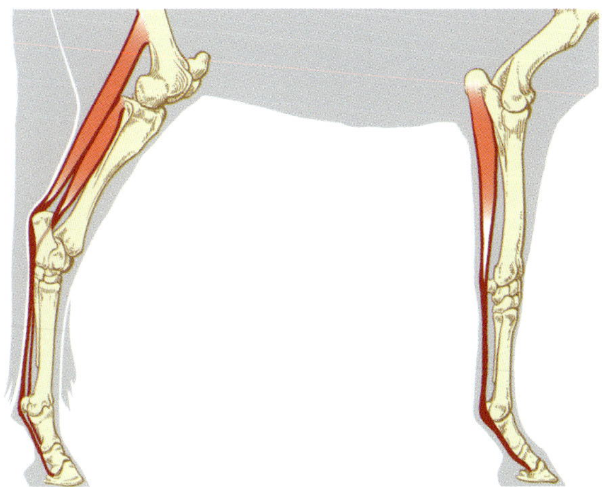

Flexors, front and rear

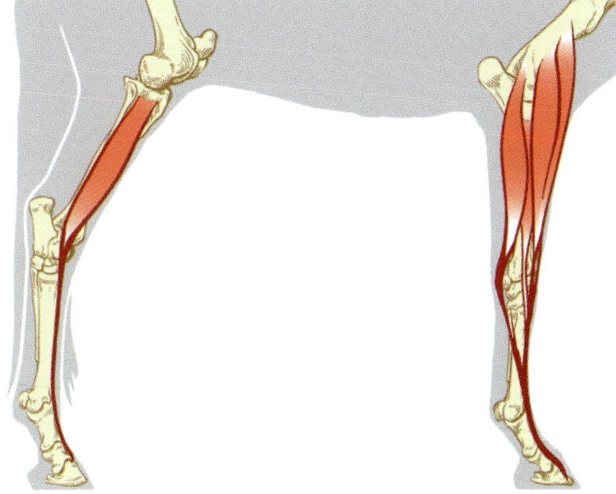

Extensors, front and rear

Because the muscles are marbled and sinewy, there are rarely injuries to the *flexor* muscle bellies. However, the tendon system is the weak spot of this construction. An important consideration for a tendon injury is that you have the ability to support the healing process. Generally, when there's a tendon injury, there's also a negative tension in the corresponding muscles. What follows is that there's a major pull on the tendons. This disrupts the healing process. Therefore, it's advisable to treat the muscle bellies that belong to the tendons with massage.

■ Extensors of the Lower Limb

The extensors of the lower limbs originate at the elbow up front and around the stifle joint behind and insert at the toes. They consist of multiple muscles, and here, too, there are no muscular fibers below the knee joint (or hock joint in the hind legs). This muscle group has the job of stretching the knee and hock joints as well as the toes.

In this photo, you can clearly see how elastic the flexor muscles are. With this horse, the trunk is hanging low, the body has little stability, and the soft tissue (the tendons) are clearly too weak. The spring mechanism isn't working optimally, which means the horse has to use more energy to move himself forward. If a horse with these conditions is not worked correctly, but rather asked for too much, it can later lead to health problems involving the tendon and muscle structures.

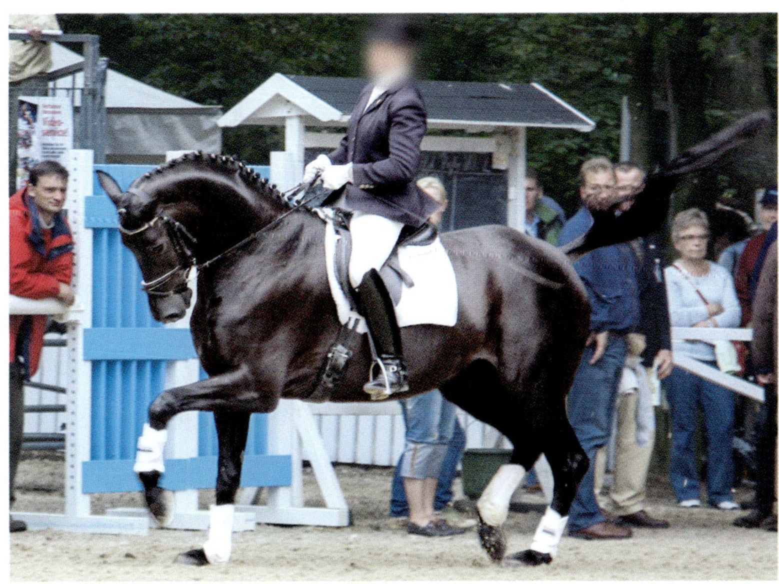

The Nervous System

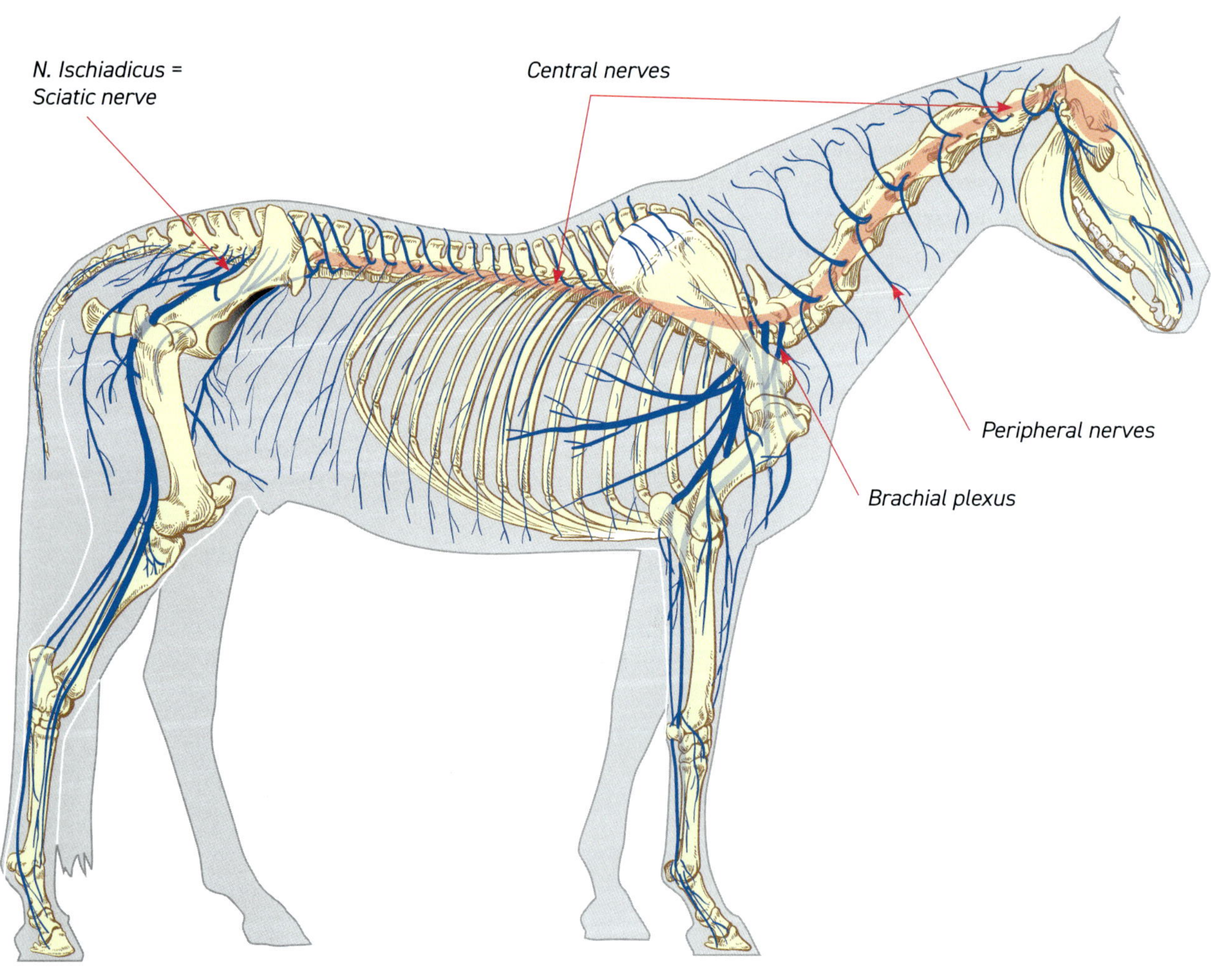

You're galloping through a corner, seeing the jump, riding directly toward it and you need to make decisions and react. In a split second, you judge the distance and decide whether you should ride more forward, hold back or just "passively" sit as you approach the jump. Your decision must be recognizable to your horse, be processed by his nervous system, and activated with the desired movement.

We can wonder at the unbelievable complexity of how this all works. We're talking about millions of pieces of information, which precede each individual event at unbelievable speed.

The nervous system is the management and control center for all living creatures. Horses, as flight animals, must have fast and efficient communication inside their body in order to survive. The horse's strong flight reflex is initiated by the nervous system, just like all other functions of the horse's body such as muscle contractions, digestion, blood circulation, and heartbeat.

With physical therapy, you have a big influence over the nervous system and can even affect metabolism, release of tension, and pain relief.

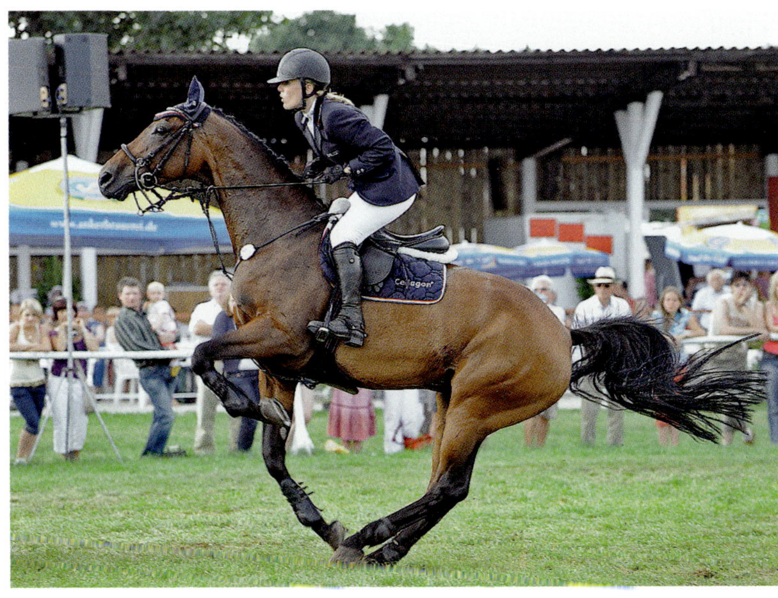

In order to correctly approach the jump, it's necessary to have good "body language" between rider and horse.

The Anatomy of the Nervous System

The nervous system can be divided into two parts:

- The central nervous system.
- The peripheral nervous system.

The Central Nervous System

The central nervous system consists of the brain and spinal cord and can be seen as the center from which the horse receives the signal to move and the motivation to see the movement through. The information travels from the brain into the spinal cord,

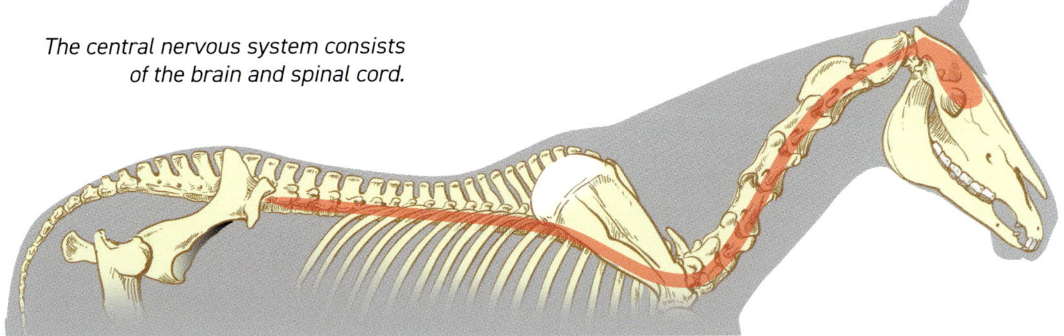

The central nervous system consists of the brain and spinal cord.

where the signal is coordinated and conveyed further by nerve pathways (the peripheral nervous system). The brain is well protected in the middle of the skull and the spinal cord is pulled/continues like a cable through the vertebral canal. Through the vertebral foramina (holes), which are found between the individual vertebrae, a part of the nerves branches out and travels to the different areas of the body. Roughly stated, the nerves that exit between the cervical vertebrae supply the neck and forehand extremities. From the thoracic vertebrae, nerves extend that lead to the organs, while the hindquarters are supplied by nerves in the lumbar region.

Figuratively speaking, the nervous system can be compared to a telephone wire. The main wire, which runs under the street in the ground, is like a mammal's central nervous system. It then divides into individual households using many cables, which is like the peripheral nervous system.

The peripheral nervous system is responsible for communication inside the body.

The Peripheral Nervous System

As soon as a nerve cord leaves the spinal cord, it's categorized as part of the peripheral nervous system. The nerve cord will divide many times. Neurons and cords possess contact points, called synapses. They pass the signal along to other neurons.

Over the entire body, you find sensory neurons, which constantly receive stimuli and also communicate with one another. This complex data is sent back to the central nervous system and processed here, then the central nervous system sends it back out to the executing organ via motor-nerve fibers (see illustration below).

In the peripheral nervous system, you find neurons that fulfill various tasks in the body.

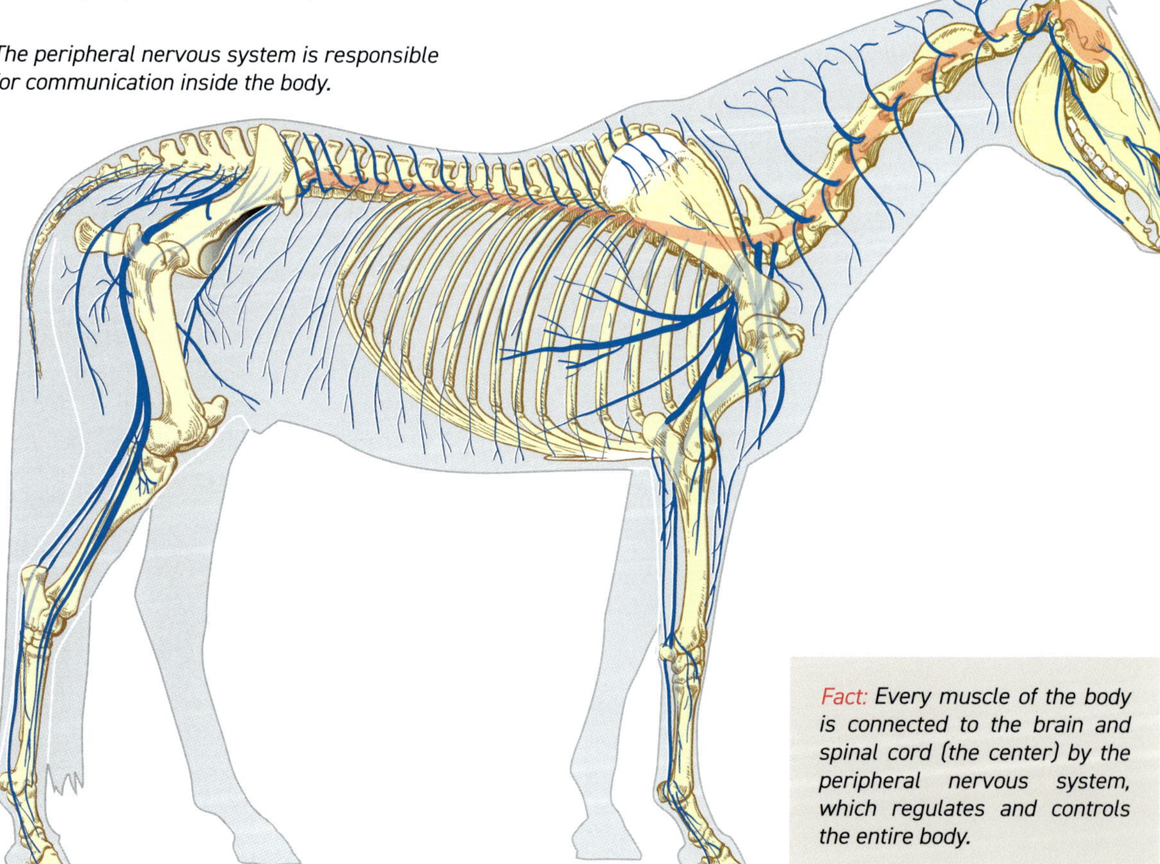

Fact: Every muscle of the body is connected to the brain and spinal cord (the center) by the peripheral nervous system, which regulates and controls the entire body.

Physical Therapy for Horses

■ The Sensory Neurons

Sensory neurons, which belong to the peripheral nervous system, can be found all over the body. These nerves register environmental influences. When the horse sees something unknown, senses pain, or loses his balance (see photo), this information travels via sensory nerve fibers back to the spinal cord and brain, where it is processed. As a reaction to potential imminent danger, signals travel to the muscular cells and trigger movement and/or a flight reflex. When giving a massage, you also have direct influence on these nerves. These nerves register your reassuring touch, which does the body good and in this way reduces muscular tension (tone).

■ The Motor Neurons

Motor neurons control the muscles. During movement, information flows constantly between the central nervous system and the muscles. Through this interaction, the power and degree of movement is regulated.

■ Proprioceptive Receptors (Positional Reflexes)

The proprioceptors (positional reflex neurons) are receptors available to the muscles, tendons, and joint capsules. They regulate how various body parts are positioned in relation to one another. The receptors respond to strain and compression. For example, they're responsible for posture or for avoiding injury to the musculoskeletal system.

When the horse steps funny on a stone, for example, it's these receptor neurons that are elongated and stimulated. The information "we're being over-extended" will immediately be conveyed to the central nervous system; from here, directions will immediately be given to the muscles to prevent a twisted foot.

For riders, these receptors are like an insurance that make the horse more sure-footed. The body learns to react quickly to unevenness and, thereby, maintain balance. By riding only on one even surface (such as in your riding arena), these receptors will not become optimally trained. Therefore, I

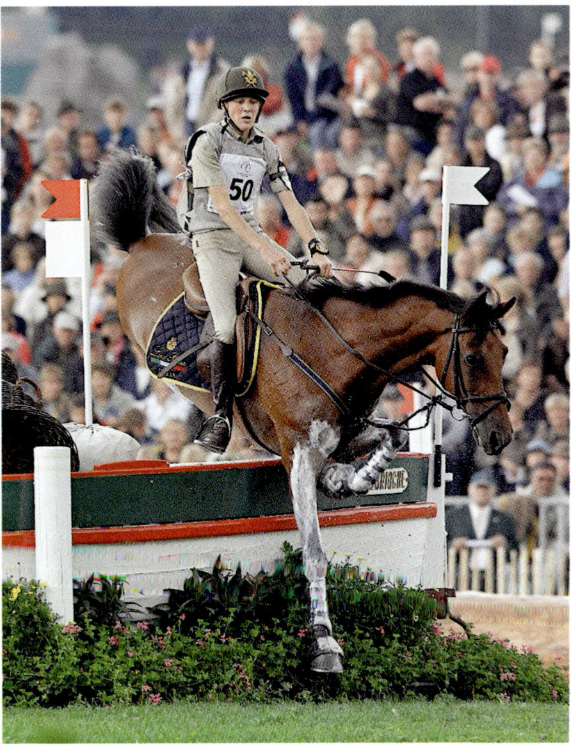

In order for the horse to rescue himself from such a situation and find his balance again, the nervous system must react quickly.

believe that no matter what discipline a horse is intended for or what career he may go on to have later in life, all horses should be ridden out in the open at all three gaits. They should also jump small jumps and be ridden over cavalletti. It's only in this way that he'll develop his positional reflexes and sure-footedness.

When a horse has been injured, the proprioceptive receptors can be affected and suffer. When injured, the musculoskeletal system can no longer protect itself optimally. The healing of these receptors can last longer than the actual injury. Please don't forget this when your horse is recovering.

But how can you best restore these receptors?

These proprioceptive receptors must relearn everything. This means they need lots of varying stimuli in order to come back to full performance and protection. When your horse has had a ligament or tendon injury, it's not enough to lead him around an arena for four weeks. These horses need to move on various types of footing during their rehabilitation (indoor and outdoor arena, grass, paved roads) in order to recover fully. Otherwise, it can happen that the horse will re-injure himself the first time he encounters uneven footing, as the receptors can't respond to the larger strain and compression. The tissue will over-stretch once more and incur injury.

You'll encounter these proprioceptive receptors again in chapter 8, "Stretching Exercises" (p. 144), as they take on an important role in stretching.

The Autonomic Nervous System

The autonomic nervous system is yet another nervous system that I'd like to briefly describe. Formerly, it was referred to as the "vegetative" nervous system. This nervous system controls important organs, which normally work involuntarily and without our awareness, such as for digestion, breathing, and heartbeat. In addition, it regulates the expansion of the blood vessels, metabolism, water supply, and gland secretion.

The sympathetic and parasympathetic nervous systems are part of the autonomic nervous system. These two systems work antagonistically, which means against one another.

■ The Sympathetic Nervous System

The sympathetic nervous system is active during training or danger: the heart pumps harder, respiratory and heart rates climb. The blood vessels widen and both sweat production and adrenaline levels rise. At the same time, digestion slows in order to allow the muscles to be fully supplied.

■ The Parasympathetic Nervous System

The opponent of the sympathetic nervous system is the parasympathetic nervous system. It reduces respiration and heart rate. Blood vessels contract, sweating is reduced, adrenaline production stops. The circulation to the internal organs increases again and the horse becomes calmer.

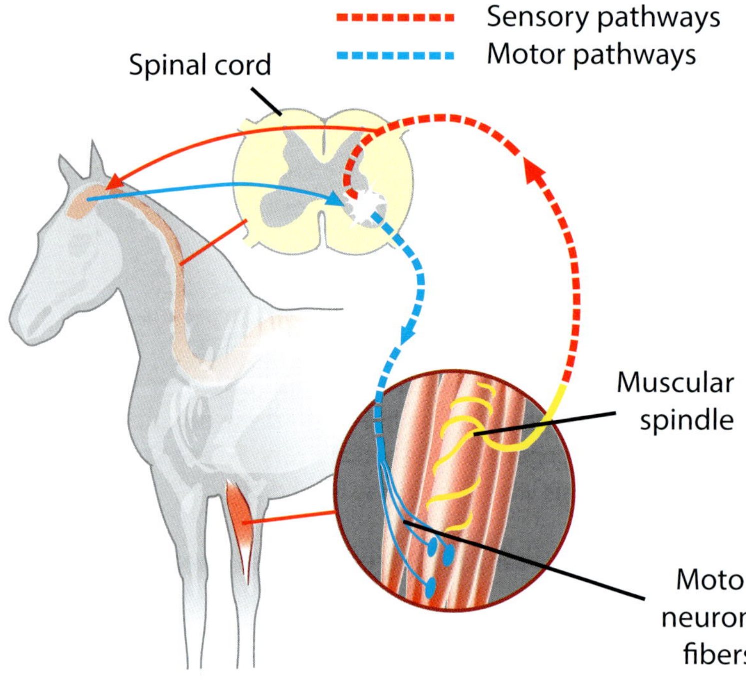

Pathways of the sensory and motor neurons.

The Nervous System and Movement

One of the nervous system's important tasks is to coordinate movement. The first step that a horse (or a person) takes is initiated by the nervous system. In the beginning, it doesn't work so well: both human and animal babies fall down frequently. But soon one doesn't even have to think about it. Walking has been made automatic by the nervous system. Thereby, the body economizes its brain capacity and the brain can occupy itself with new exercises until these are ready to become automatic. That's why we practice! In order to make a movement automatic, movement patterns are repeated. This is why you can't only learn to ride by

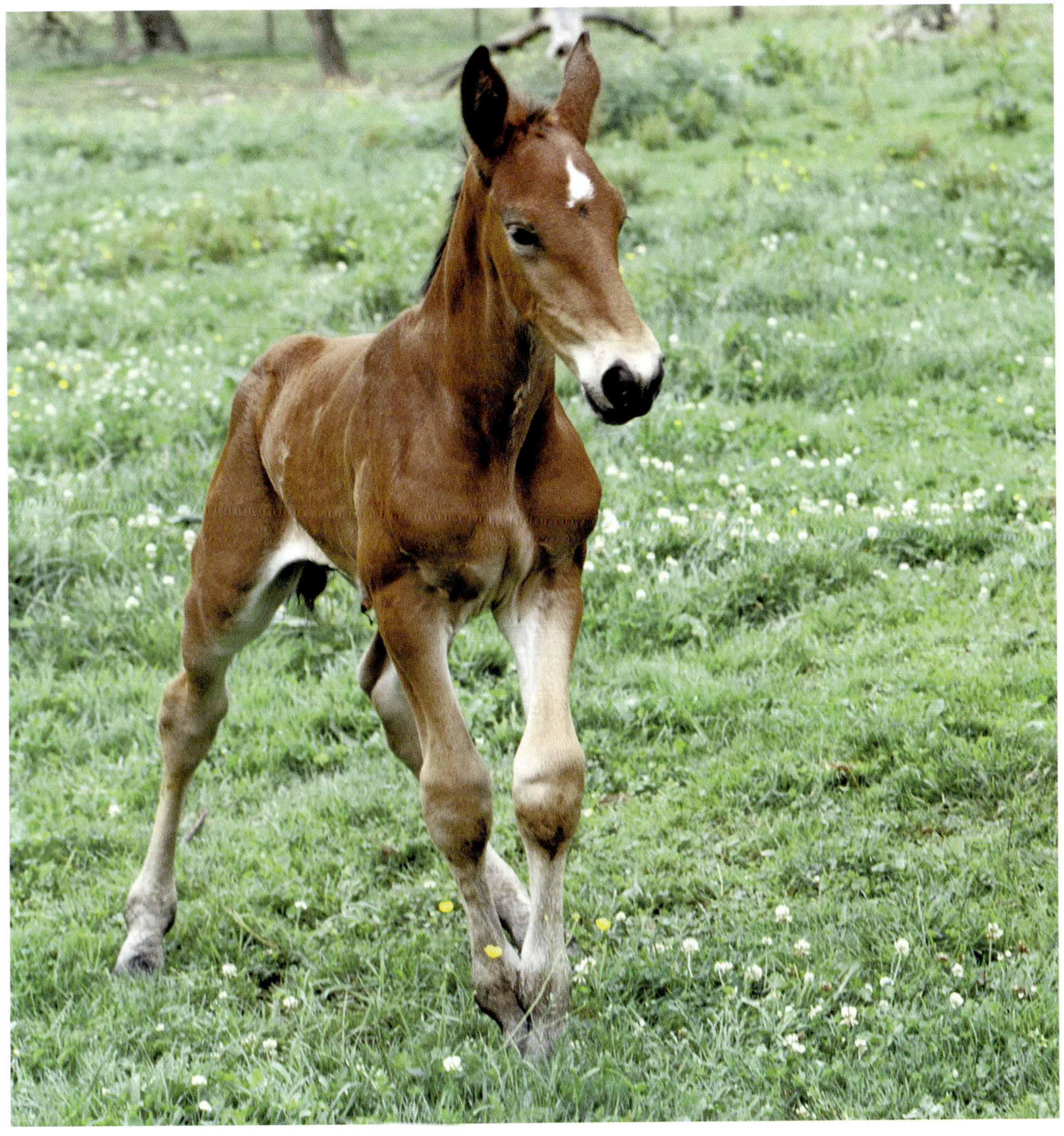

Movement is trained and becomes automatic thanks to the nervous system.

reading books. You must feel and process the movement. Here's an example from a rider's daily life. You want the horse to learn a new movement, for example, a canter departure. Your body gives the horse the aids (very clearly) and after a few successes the horse has learned: increased weight on the inside seat bone, forward-driving inside leg, and an outside leg placed in the "guarding" position means "Canter." Over time, these aids will become lighter and more refined. Your goal is to become so refined with your aids and for the horse to become so sensitive that he can respond to just a light, practically invisible aid. You can thank the nervous system for this accomplishment.

Observation

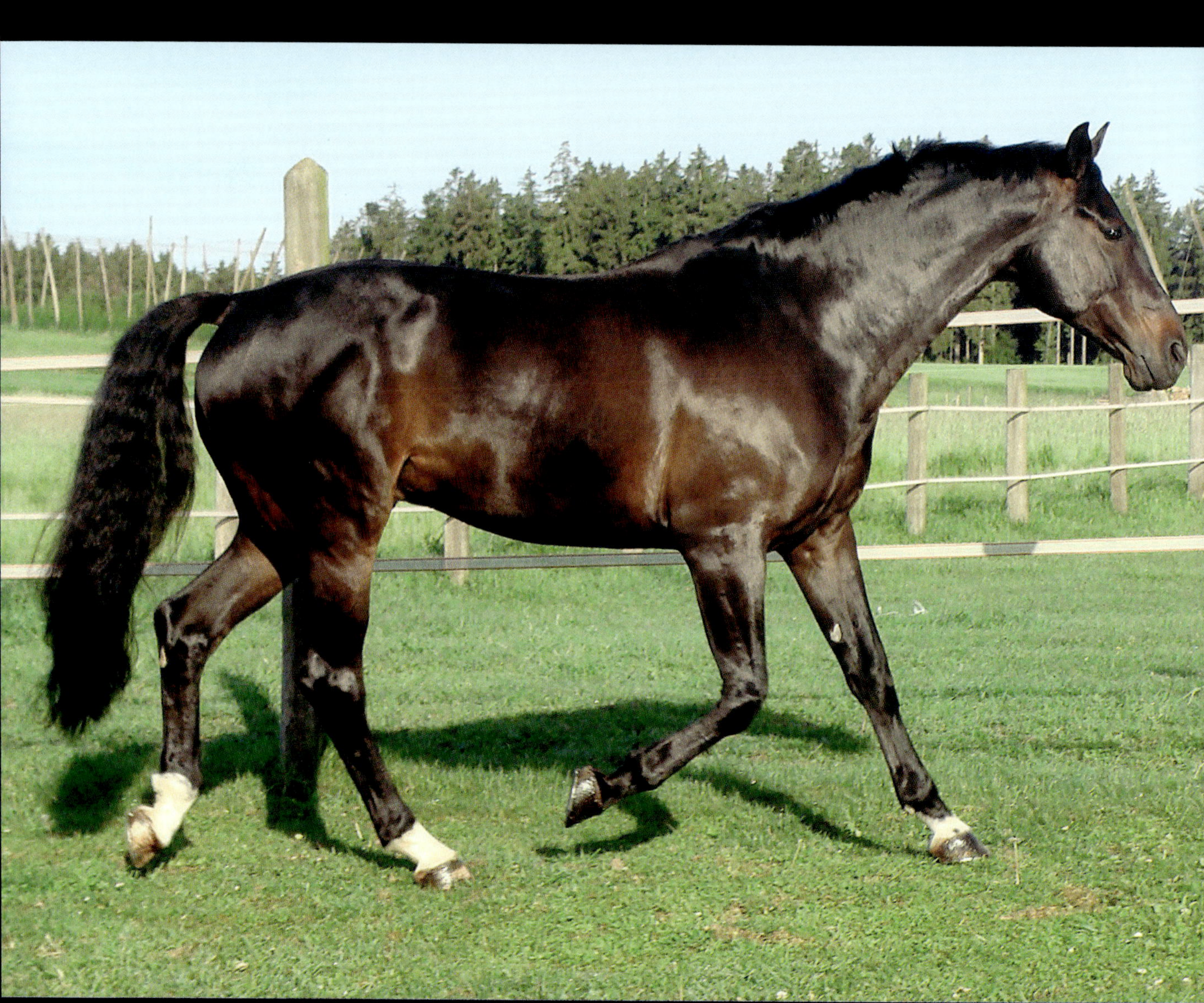

Like me, you probably enjoy standing in a pasture and looking at your horse. You notice his coat, how he keeps his surroundings in his gaze, how he can move his head, and how his body flows when in movement. Some of your fellow boarders may laugh when you appear just a little bit "in love" with your horse. However, what you're observing so closely when you stand by the pasture fence, longe your horse, or work at liberty is actually really important for the horse owner. Why? You're getting a ton of important information that will help you get to know your horse better and be able to react sooner when something isn't right.

When "observing," the point is to recognize your horse's current state of well-being. You get a sharp look at his posture when he's healthy. The best thing about observation is that it's fun and you don't need any expensive equipment to do it. You already have the necessary equipment with you. A steady gaze, the necessary interest and—most import-ant—a plan in your head about what exactly you need to pay attention to. The goal of observation is to get to know your horse's distinct characteristics. Only then will it be possible to notice changes to the musculoskeletal system in a timely manner. Observe your horse regularly and keep his "normal" in your memory. This baseline observation makes it possible for you to discover early on changes such as muscular development, muscular atrophy, blockages, subluxations, and compensatory move-ment patterns. It's possible that even naturally occurring weaknesses in your horse's conforma-tion don't have to inevitably become the sources for joint or muscular problems. You should recognize these weak spots and keep an eye on them, and if changes occur, you can be an important partner to your physical therapist or vet in that you can describe them correctly and in detail.

In this chapter, you'll receive "tools of the trade" for effective observation. For each specified anomaly (deviation from normal), a possible source of the problem will be named as an example. This can't possibly be a complete reference, as the sources of

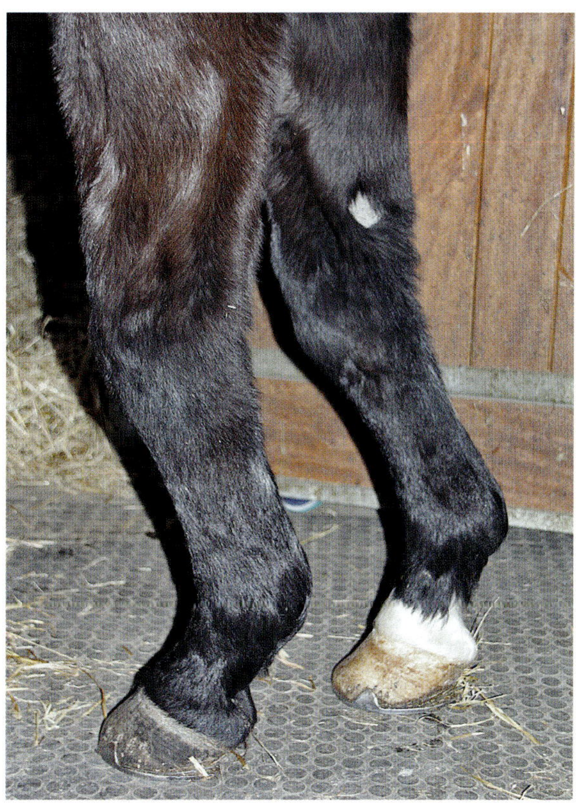

This horse is over at the knee. Conformational faults do not necessarily have to affect the horse's movement: this horse, who is 31 years old, has had this flaw since birth. Yet, in his dressage training, he reached Fourth Level.

anomalies are highly complex and would go beyond the scope of this book. Therefore, I've included those anomalies that I encounter most frequently in my practice. If your horse should have multiple or more serious changes to his musculoskeletal sys-tem, I would advise you to seek professional advice.

On the following pages, there are many factors that you should pay attention to. Because there are so many points, it's perhaps best that you take this book with you to the stable and compare on the spot! Soon you'll see your horse with new eyes.

I personally observe my horse almost daily in order to monitor that his training is on the correct path. In my dressage work, I was riding in too much collection for some time and within two weeks, I could determine that my horse's croup muscles were becoming too dominant and tight. This was a sign that my training program could not continue as it had been, as my horse did not have the strength for it. I immediately changed my work, incorporating more forward riding, and the tension in the hindquarters went away. What I'm trying to say is that it can happen—tensions emerge. However, you need to keep a daily eye on the horse to ensure the musculoskeletal system is handling everything well. This is the only way to avoid injury and ensure the horse can develop soundly.

General Inspection While Standing

You're now going to systematically observe your horse, train your powers of observation, and learn to "palpate" your horse with your eyes.

When you do the inspection, it's advisable to be in a place where the horse feels secure. Here, you'll be able to observe his normal muscular engagement and way of going.

Step One is to keep in mind a picture of your horse's general condition:

- How is his weight?
  Is he overweight or too thin?
- How is his coat?
  It should be smooth and shiny.
- Is he alert?
  He should be taking in his surroundings, not shut down.
- How are his eyes?
  Alert and without fear? (The eye is a window to the soul.)
- How is he breathing?
  With relaxed nostrils and regular breaths (12 to 18 breaths per minute)?
- How is he standing?
  Evenly on his limbs? Leaning forward or backward?

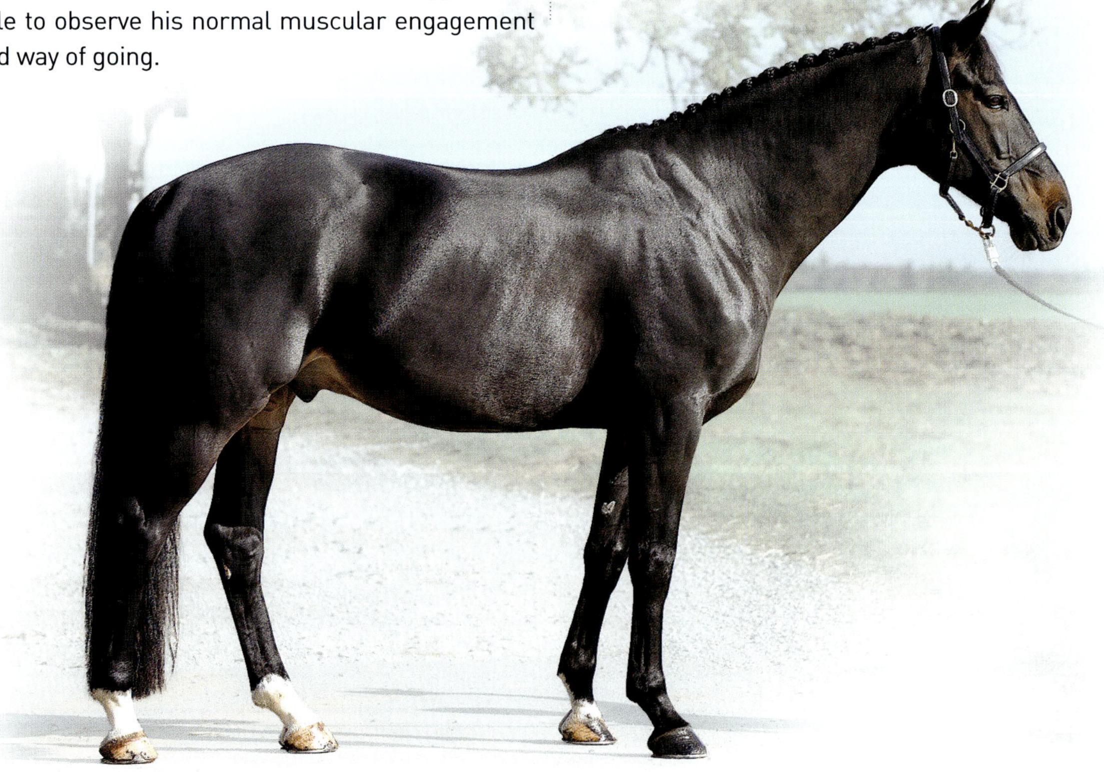

Physical Therapy for Horses

Detailed Inspection While Standing

Position yourself at a distance of three to four meters from your horse. In order to be able to inspect him in detail, he must now be standing square on an even, hard surface. His neck must be straight.

As a physical therapist, I look over every horse that comes to me for treatment from various perspectives and observe him based on the following criteria.

Observing from the Front

1 In the normal position, the eyes and nostrils are parallel and even with one another.
2 The jaw muscles are equally developed on both sides and relaxed.
3 The muscling of the neck (*brachiocephalic*), shoulder (*triceps*), chest (*pectorals*) and lower arm (extensors and flexors of the leg) are developed evenly and powerfully.
4 Both forelegs bear even weight.
5 The forelegs form a vertical (plumb) line and the hooves point to the front.
6 The hooves must be evenly formed. One hoof should not be flatter or steeper than the others.

The following examples illustrate the most common sources for the misalignments that I see in my practice (see illustration right):

Anomalies

1 **The eyes and nostrils are not even horizontally.**
   A blockage or muscular tension in the upper cervical vertebrae can be the source of a crooked head. This misalignment can be caused by an especially big effort involving a lot of strength (for example, the horse panics when tied or is cast in a stall), so that the upper cervical vertebrae become blocked due to the intense pressure in this area. A misaligned jaw joint can also be the source of the problem.

Another source, which is actually located far from the poll, is a twist or blockage in the sacroiliac joint. Such blockages often result in symptoms at the poll.

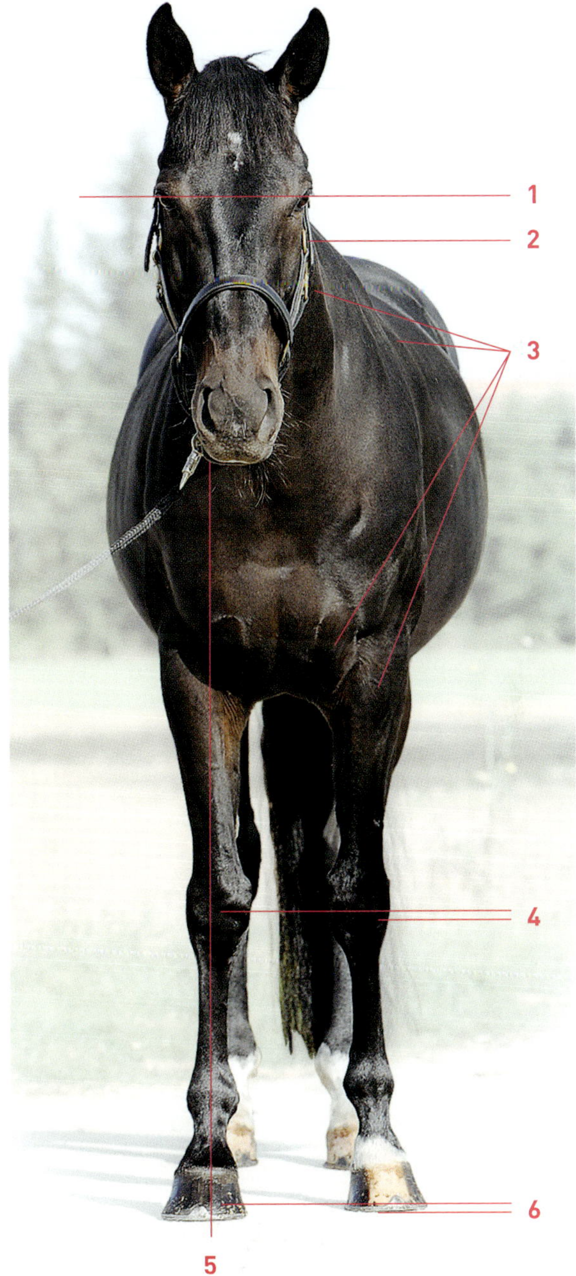

2 Irregular Jaw Muscles

An irregular jaw muscle on the right or left side, or a permanent strain in the masticatory muscle can be the result of tongue ailments, such as hooks on the teeth. Another source can be a reduction of mobility in the jaw joint, which is triggered by a blocked cervical vertebra. Other possible reasons are harsh riding hands, an inappropriate bit, or an overly tightened noseband. But a crooked pelvis can also be the source of the problem, although it lies far from here.

3 Irregular Muscular Development in Neck, Shoulder, Chest, and Arm

In these muscle parts, it can be that irregular muscular development (atrophy or hypertrophy) is a sign of a compensatory movement pattern, which has been established due to injury, arthritis, blockages, lameness, etc.

4 Bearing Weight Unevenly on the Forelimbs

Uneven weight-bearing is common when there are, for example, underlying lamenesses. When you notice this, alarm bells should be going off. The horse needs a veterinary examination without delay, because through the horse's effort to relieve one leg, he can quickly develop secondary tension and injury throughout his entire musculoskeletal system.

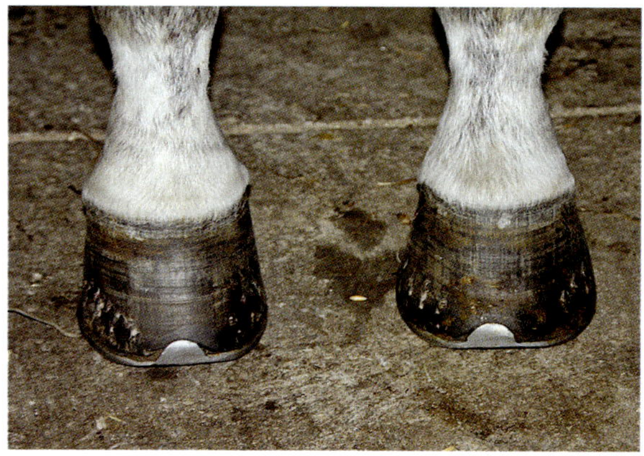

Unevenly formed hooves can hint that the horse is bearing weight unevenly.

5 Uneven Positioning of the Legs

When the horse has a base-wide stance with his forelegs, he'll have less carrying ability. If he stands narrow, it's a sign that he's experiencing tension in his neck or shoulder girdle.

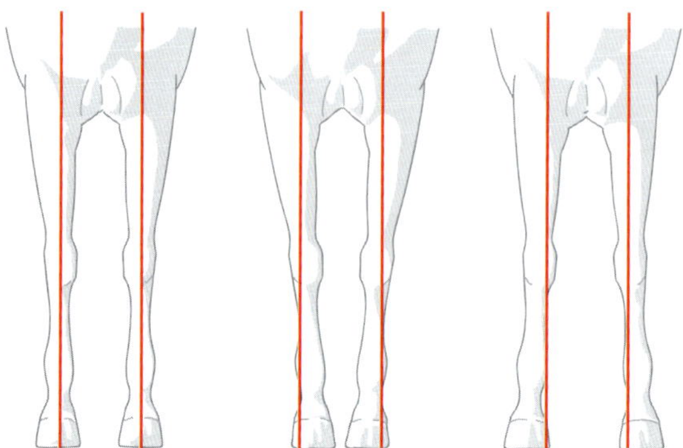

Horses can have misaligned limbs from birth (turned toward the inside or the outside). Later in life, this can only be corrected with difficulty, if at all. Over time, these misalignments lead to stress on the affected limbs, which also triggers tension in the shoulder/neck/chest areas.

It can also happen that these misalignments occur during the course of a horse's life; for example, due to a faulty trim or from tension in the shoulder/elbow area. When possible, you should correct these changes.

6 Hoof

At the hoof, you can recognize whether the horse is bearing weight evenly on his forelegs over a long period of time. When the horse favors a side, the hoof on the affected side will get higher and smaller over time due to bearing less of a burden. In contrast, the other side will get broader and flatter because of bearing more burden.

My Tip

Always check the hooves when purchasing a horse. They can give you a hint about how evenly the horse has utilized his forelimbs over a longer period of time.

Physical Therapy for Horses

From the Side at a Standstill

When you observe from the side, begin at the front (see illustration below):

1 The angle between head and neck should be about 90 degrees. The head is carried in a relaxed manner.

2 The muscular development of the neck should be even. The space between the nuchal ligament and the cervical spine should be filled with muscle mass (this means no dip in front of the shoulder blade).

3 The angle of the shoulder blade: a 90- to 100-degree angle between the shoulder blade and upper arm is good here.

4 The forelegs are perpendicular. This means you can draw a plumb line from the middle of the shoulder blade through the elbow joint, to the middle of the knee joint to the backside of the bulbs of the heel. The legs are not positioned in front of or behind this line.

5 The topline musculature is relaxed and evenly formed all the way to the hind end.

6 The abdominal muscles are naturally taut, not hanging low and not pulled up tightly. The horse breathes into his belly.

7 The croup muscles are also even and strong. They form round hindquarters.

8 The hind legs are perpendicular. From the seat bone points (*ischial tuberosity*), you should be able to draw a straight line down to the ground, over the rear edge of the hock and fetlock joints.[5]

9 The tail should be held loosely and close to the body.

Obviously, it's important to do this observation on both sides of the body.

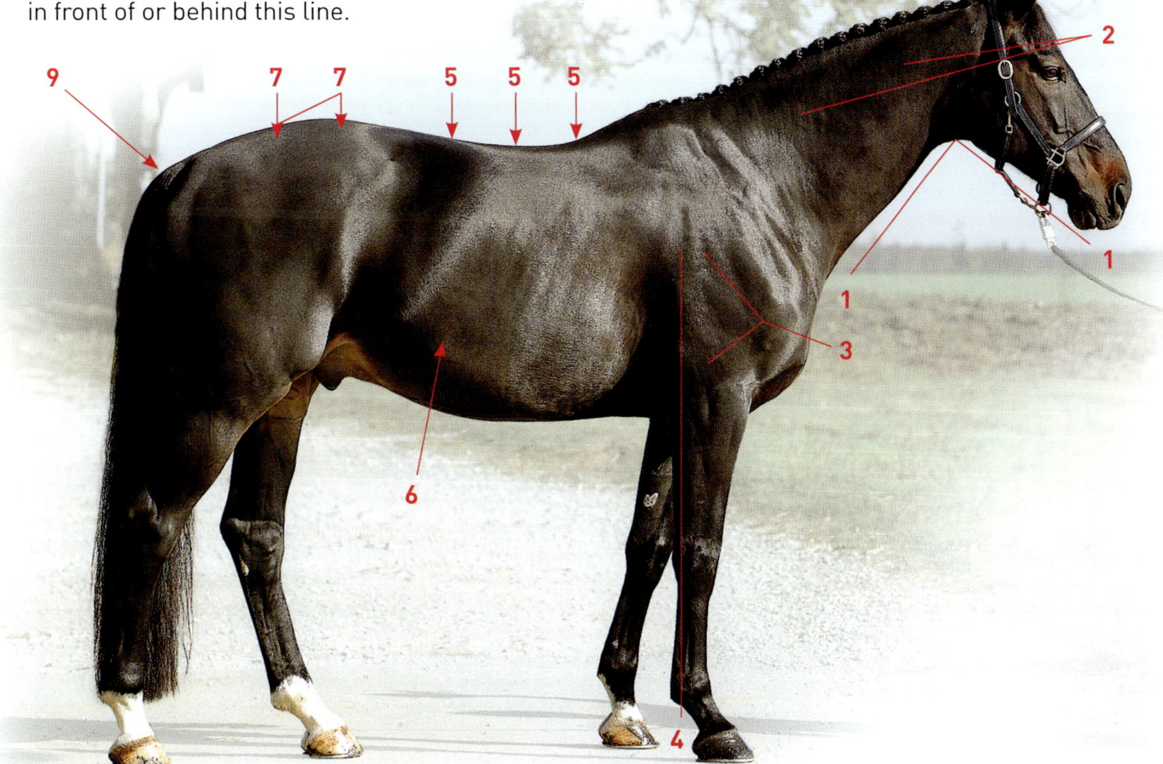

5 Because the horse is not standing square, I did not draw the plumb line for the hind legs.

Anomalies

1 The Poll

From the side, you can easily recognize changes in the poll. The sources of the issue can be the same as those described when observed from the front (see "Observing from the Front," p. 95). However, from the side, it's usually easier to discover whether the contraction and extension of the neck has been altered. You already know how important the joints of the poll area are, how quickly changes can occur here and what effects this can have.

One source of a poll-area blockage is a fall forward. The horse hits his nose falling forward and the head can then be shoved slightly upward, above the first cervical vertebrae. The blockage is often recognizable by a change to the angle between head and neck, a posture adopted to avoid pain.

Another source for a change of the head and neck angle is uneven engagement in the surrounding musculature. When the poll and neck extensor muscles are experiencing pull and tension, the horse will stand with a lightly outstretched head. If the head is more "rolled inward," it's the contracting muscles of the neck that have too much tension.

There are two bursae (sacs of synovial fluid) located at the poll, which ensure the tendons can glide over the bones there. These bursae can become inflamed and swell up if they are under too much pressure due to muscular tension or a concussion (for example, from a door or window). There will then be noticeable swelling behind the ears.

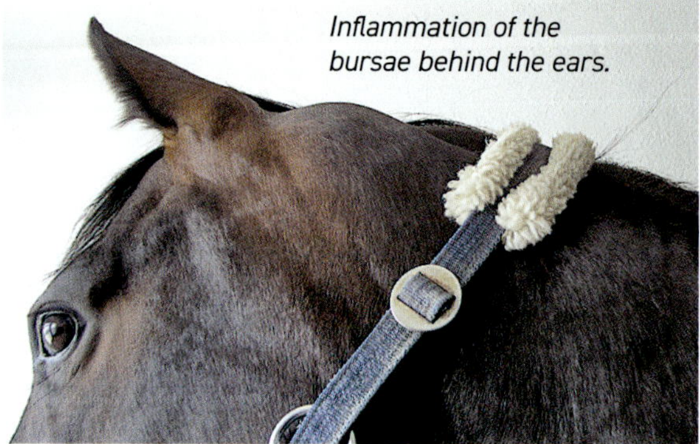

2 The Neck

The neck should have a beautiful, full, even muscling from poll to shoulder blade and between the nuchal ligament and cervical vertebrae.

When a horse is not able to take enough weight onto his hindquarters, for example, then he won't be able to carry his neck himself, and the carrying muscles of the neck will appear underdeveloped. You can recognize this by a dip in the neck, directly in front of the shoulder blade. In turn, there will be increased muscular build up around the poll and the large *brachiocephalicus* muscle will be tensed. If the neck muscles are underdeveloped, the horse's ability to lift through the back is also restricted.

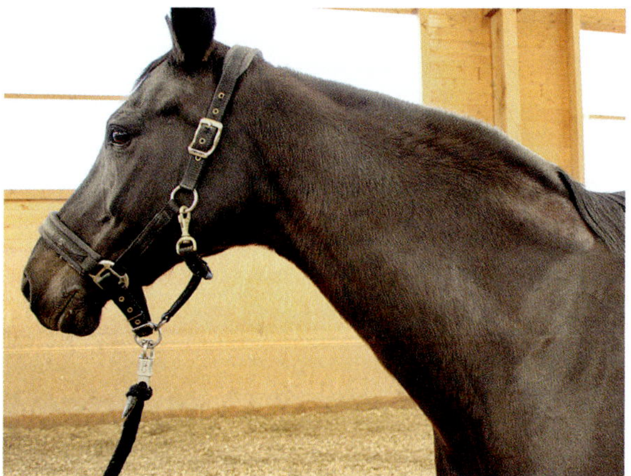

This neck is unevenly muscled. There's too little muscle in the poll and shoulder-blade areas, while the underside of the neck is too strongly pronounced. The nuchal ligament has an uneven bulge and the semispinalis capitis *muscle is too pronounced as well.*

3 The Angle of the Shoulder Blade

As you know, the shoulder blade and trunk are connected only by muscles. This provides the forehand with excellent shock-absorbing ability. However, when there's accumulated tension in the shoulder-girdle muscles, the shock-absorbing ability is impaired. You can recognize this because the shoulder blade will be positioned higher in the direction of the withers, which can also cause the angle of the shoulder blade to alter along with a leg-positioning that is in front of or behind the vertical plumb line.

4 Legs That Are Not Straight

When the forelimbs are no longer standing perpendicularly, it can be a hint of various problems. If the forelegs are too far forward, this can be a sign the horse is trying to take weight off his lower limbs or, as described in the last section, the horse is tense in the shoulder-girdle muscles.

If the limbs stand behind the vertical plumb line, this can indicate a blockage in the lower cervical vertebrae.

If the hindquarters are too far under the body, this indicates restriction in the stretch of the lumbar region and that the horse may have back pain.

If the hind legs are too far back, this indicates he's having difficulty lifting his back. It's also a position the horse may adapt to relieve pain/stress, which would be welcomed by the back and pelvis when there's pain in these areas.

Fact: When your horse is always resting the same hind leg, this can be a sign of nerve compression in the lumbar region on this side. This position relieves the area by taking weight off the leg.

5 Muscling of the Back

Please always keep it in the back of your mind that the horse's trunk is his center of movement. One of the most important muscles in this area is the *longissimus dorsi* (long muscle of the back). The muscling should be evenly formed from the withers to the lumbosacral junction. Often, you see a bulge in the muscles behind the saddle area. This buildup of muscle (muscular hypertrophy) is negative. It means that the small, deep muscles are overtaxed and, therefore, the *longissimus* and the *gluteus medius* must act as stabilizers. However, this is not their job—both these muscles are intended for movement, not

stability! When ridden, these horses can't get loose, and the impulsion of the hindquarters will not make it past the lumbar region.

In addition, over the long term, a poor saddle fit can also limit muscular development if it is

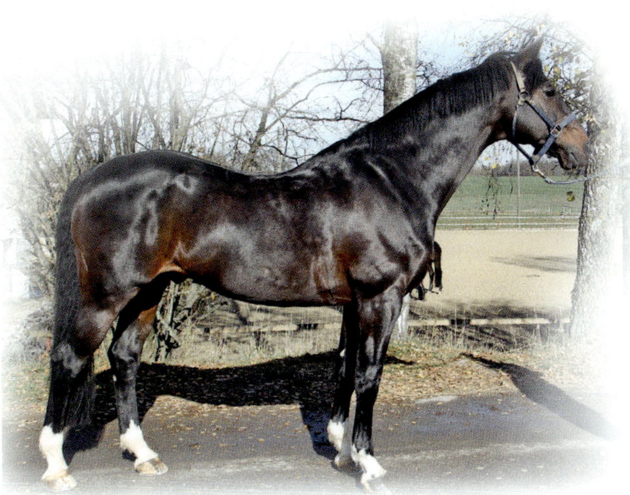

This horse has an extreme swayback, but likely no back pain thanks to his very strong abdominal muscles. He's 19 years old and has competed successfully in show jumping in the past (up to 4'6"). There are many horses that can become solid, long-term partners for both pleasure and competitive riding, despite physical defects.

putting uncomfortable pressure on the muscles. The result is muscular atrophy in the saddle area with a restricted lift in this area. Also, a gullet that's too tight puts pressure on the muscles around the withers and the *trapezius* will recede. This can lead to a movement dysfunction where the swing of the front limbs forward and backward in both the stance phase and swing phase suspension is visibly disrupted.

6 Muscling of the Abdomen

The abdominal muscles are the "opponent" (antagonist) of the back muscles. The abdominal muscles stabilize the trunk from below, straighten the pelvis and lift the back. When the abdominal muscles are too weak, the back is not stabilized from below and it "hangs down."

As a result, the horse's ability to step up under his body is restricted and the trunk lacks stability. With this as a weak point and with a rider on his back, the mechanics of movement can't function.

Further, the abdominal muscles encounter problems when the belly is sucked up high. Your horse then breaths superficially (not deeply in his belly). This can be a sign that the diaphragm (the largest respiratory muscle) is accumulating tension. This will inevitably affect the horse's performance.

7 Uneven Muscling of the Hindquarters

Often, muscles of the hindquarters develop unevenly. The *gluteal* muscles are too strong while the *biceps femoris* are too weak, and the *hamstring muscles* are again too strongly pronounced (see photo, at right). This is a sign that the horse is compensating at work and not engaging enough with his hindquarters. Thrust and impulsion are not developing sufficiently in the hindquarters.

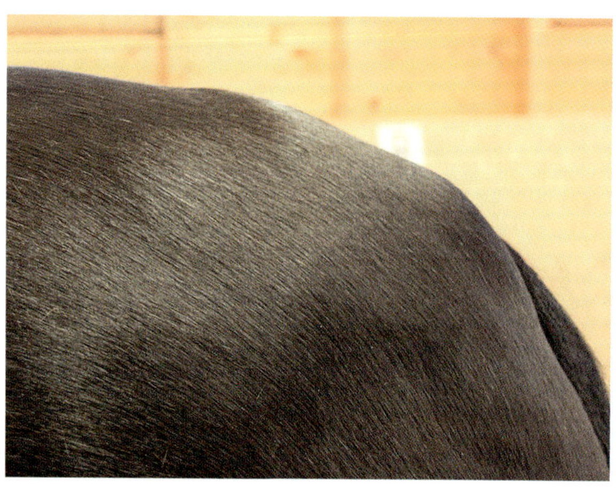

8 The Tail

The tail should hang close to the body. When it's crooked, as in the photo, tucked in tightly, or held overly far from the body, there's a definite dysfunction in the back or sacroiliac joint. Causes might include muscular tension, accumulated

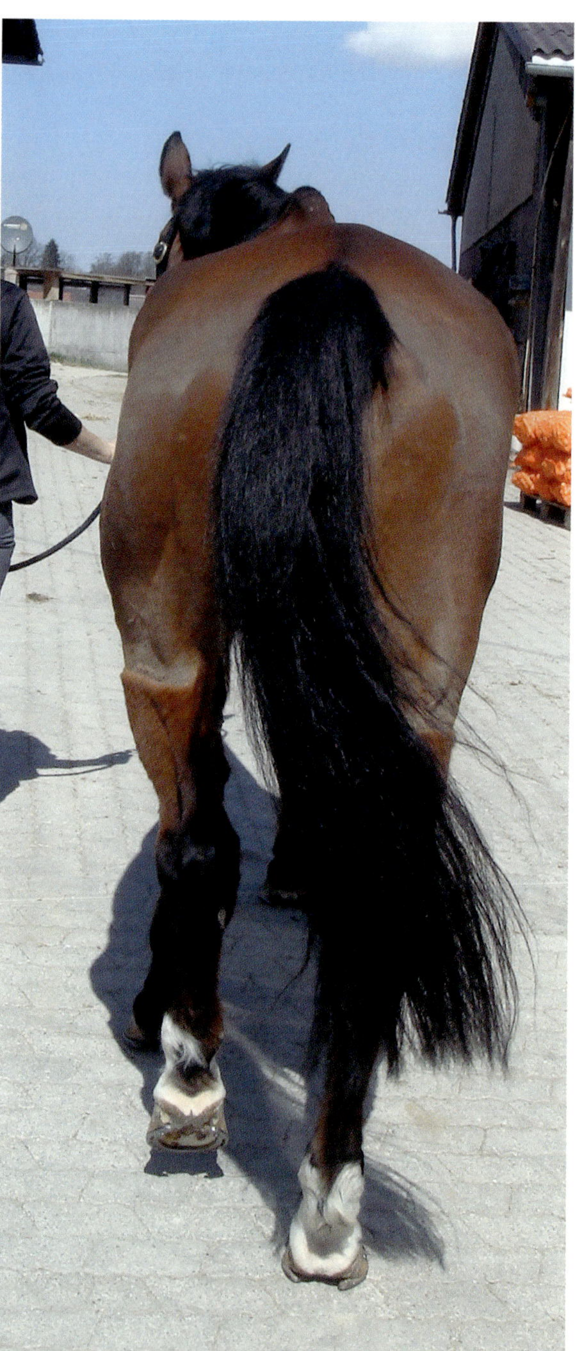

It's obvious here that the horse's pelvis is twisted and he's carrying his tail off to one side. The whole horse is shortened on the left side.

tension in the tendons between the pelvis and sacrum, or a twisted sacrum (see photo above).

From the Back at a Standstill

The horse must stand square with his hind legs parallel.

1 The two iliac tips (*tuber sacrales*) must be at the same height and clearly recognizable.
2 Both hip bones are even.
3 The croup musculature has developed evenly on both sides.
4 The tail hangs in the middle, relaxed.
5 Pull the tail to one side. The inner muscles (the adductors) should be even and form a consistent angle.

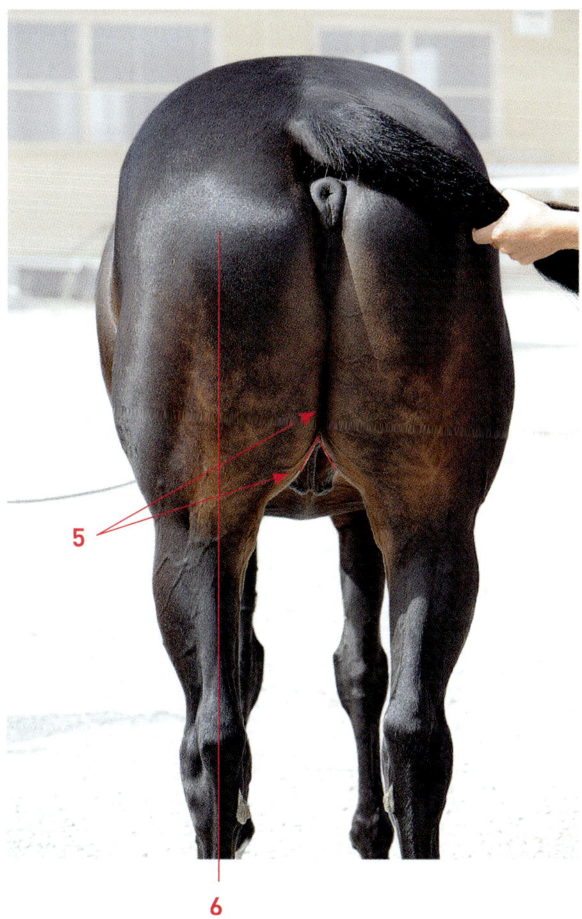

6 From the ischial tuberosity down, you can draw a plumb line through the middle of the hock and fetlock joints to the middle of the hoof.
7 The hooves should point forward.

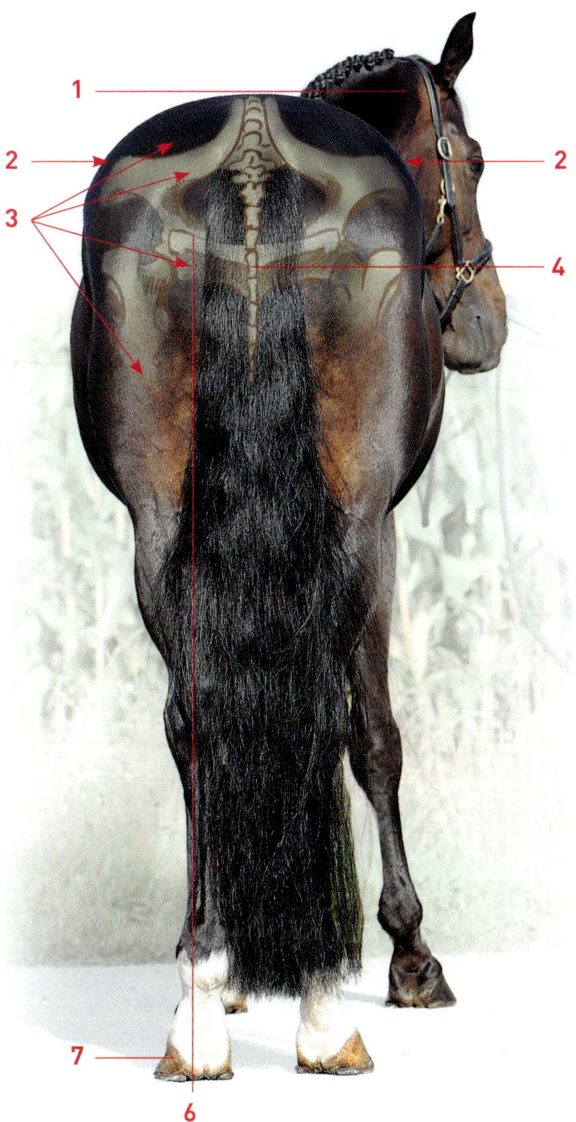

6 Possibly stands slightly to the outside.
7 The hoof tends slightly outward.

Anomalies

1 Crooked Pelvis

As you know, the sacroiliac joint (SI) is a relatively small, flat joint. Symptoms in the SI joint can occur as a result of subluxations. When observed from behind, you'll recognize that the left and right points of the sacrum (*tuber sacrales*) are at different heights. In addition, you'll recognize muscular atrophy of the hindquarters on the same side.

Upon examination, I often find a pelvic misalignment and I then ask whether this has been a long-term condition. Most of the time, the owner and rider haven't recognized it at all. In addition, a swelling above the ilium is a sign that the joint is not functioning optimally or is being overly taxed.

Fact: My experience shows that the SI joint often shows symptoms that don't always have a primary cause there. But you'll often discover anomalies in this joint that have enormous influence on the horse's performance.

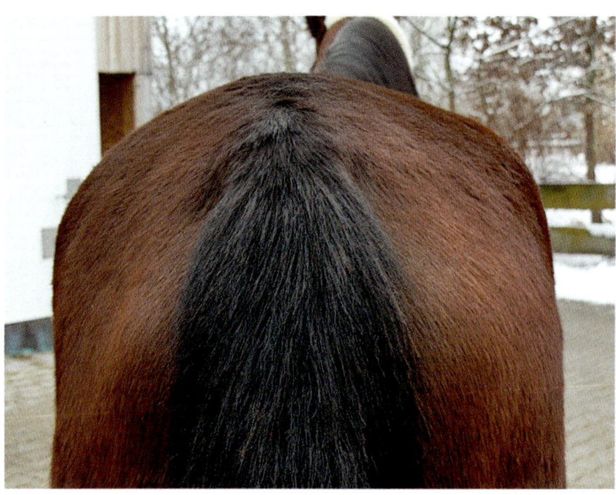

This horse has a crooked pelvis. In addition, it's easy to recognize a tilt in his longitudinal axis. The muscling of his hindquarters could be better.

2 A Twisted Pelvis

Keep a close eye on your horse's hip bones. Don't underestimate the force of accumulated tension in the muscles (often the loin musculature). As you know, the bone is not fixed. And, if one side of the hip flexor is tense, this muscle can pull the pelvic bones forward or down, so that you can see a height difference of the hip bones. The affected side will be lower.

3 Uneven Muscular Development

The musculature around the pelvis is the horse's motor and it will quickly build up or waste away

when a horse has a mechanical disorder. The muscles of the hindquarters must be developed so that they form a "beautiful, round bottom." No muscle group can be allowed to be over- or underdeveloped (see photo, p. 100, left).

4 The Tail

The tail forms an extension of the spinal column. It very precisely reveals the present condition of a horse's back. If it's tight and cramped or hangs sideways, this can indicate joint or muscular problems in the back and/or in the SI joint.

5 The Adductors

When the inner leg muscles are unevenly developed, this can hint at problems with the pelvis.

6 Perpendicular Hind Legs

As with the forelegs, you can also find horses that stand wide or narrow with the hind legs. When a horse stands narrow behind, it can be that his adductor muscles are too strong or a dysfunction of the pelvis or hip joints can be the source of the problem. If the horse stands wide, his croup muscles are too tight.

Fact: Be careful! This false positioning of the hind legs can develop during training when the hindquarters are put under too much strain.

7 Leg Position

Especially with the hind legs, it's important that you monitor where your horse's toes are pointing. For example, muscular tension in the loin muscles (*iliopsoas*) can cause the toes to turn outward.

From Above at a Standstill[6]

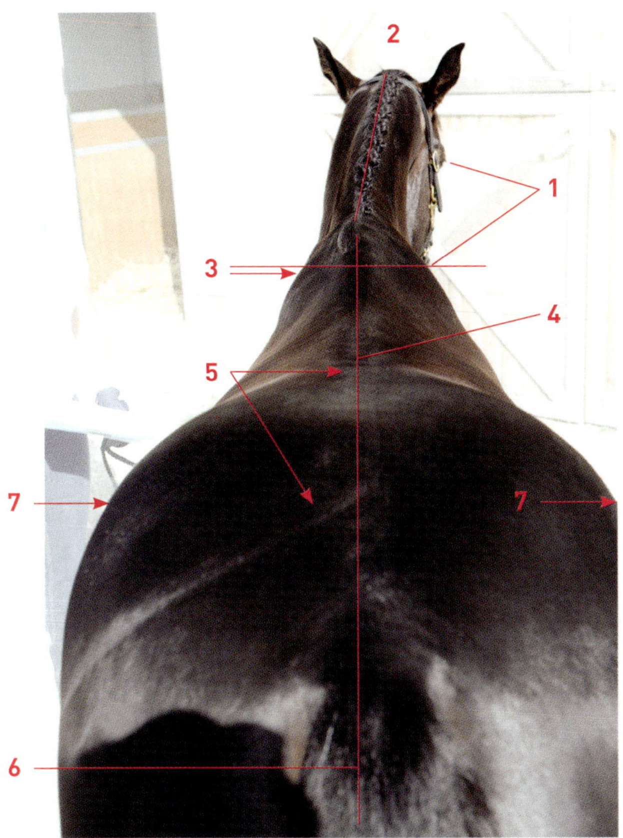

Looking from above you can get the impression as to whether the horse has uniform diagonal development. Stand behind your horse on a stepstool or grooming box. As you do so, make sure your horse is standing square on all four limbs.

1 The head position. You can see the same amount of eye and nostril on both sides.
2 The crest runs straight.
3 The shoulder blades are evenly wide and stand at the same height.
4 The spinous processes form a straight line.
5 The back and croup musculature are evenly built.
6 The middle of the pelvis is an extension of the back.
7 The hip bones are of the same height and in a parallel line with the shoulders.

---

6 Note: The horse in the photo is not standing completely straight and his right shoulder blade is somewhat wider.

Anomalies

1 Crooked Head Position

A blockage in the upper cervical vertebrae can cause a twist to the head, which means you'll see more nostril on one side than the other. It's also good to recognize the ears' position. If the head is crooked, they will not be the same height.

2 The Crest

The crest can give you a hint about the mobility of the cervical vertebrae. If you discover an irregular drop in the crest (for example, in the middle of the neck), you can take this as a hint that there's a blockage in the cervical vertebrae.

3 The Shoulder Blades

There are many causes for anomalies in the shoulder-blade area.

One cause is heightened compression from the saddle on the right side, which is caused by always mounting your horse from the same (left) side. In this case, you'll recognize that the horse's right shoulder is farther forward.

A further possibility is uneven weight distribution on the legs, which is not only recognizable on the hooves, but also at the shoulder blades. The shoulder blade is higher and wider on the side where the leg is bearing more weight. There can be numerous causes for this: generally speaking, I often find this in connection with a blockage in the lower cervical vertebrae and the 1st thoracic vertebra.

4 A Crooked Spinal Column

When the spinal column isn't forming a straight line, your horse has scoliosis. This can greatly reduce the horse's flexibility. He may have been born with scoliosis, but inappropriate workload during his training can also be the cause.

5 Unevenly Developed Muscles

Here again, you want to compare the evenness of the spinal column from left to right. Due to blockages, changes in muscular volume can happen quickly. For example, if there's a blockage in the lumbar/loin area, you will see flatter muscular development there.

6 The Pelvis

A shift of the longitudinal axis can hint at a twisted pelvis, which in turn can be traced back to blockages in the lumbar vertebrae or shortened muscles in the lumbar and pelvic regions (see photo, p. 102).

7 The Hip Bones

Observing from above, you'd best be able to recognize when the pelvis is twisted. You should find both hip bones on a single line. As I've already described, the most common reason for this twist is accumulated tension in the loin muscles (*iliopsoas*), which tilt the pelvis forward and down.

In Movement

Again, you'll observe your horse from all three angles (front, side, and back) while he moves. Watch as he walks and trots on a straight line, and trots and canters on the longe line.

To do this, have an assistant lead your horse away from you, about 20 meters, on a hard, even surface. The leader travels near the horse's left shoulder and looks straight ahead. The leader should hold on lightly—so lightly that she does not inhibit the movement of the head, but firmly enough that she can control the horse.

It's easiest to recognize movement anomalies at the walk because the horse has less muscular engagement and problems become visible.

Fact: The horse's movement should be balanced, loose, have even rhythm, and be full of swing and power.

The Hindquarters at the Walk

Fact: You can best identify weak, tense, injured muscles at the walk. Because many muscles work together at the trot, they can "cover up" for one another. At trot, it's easier to recognize joint problems.

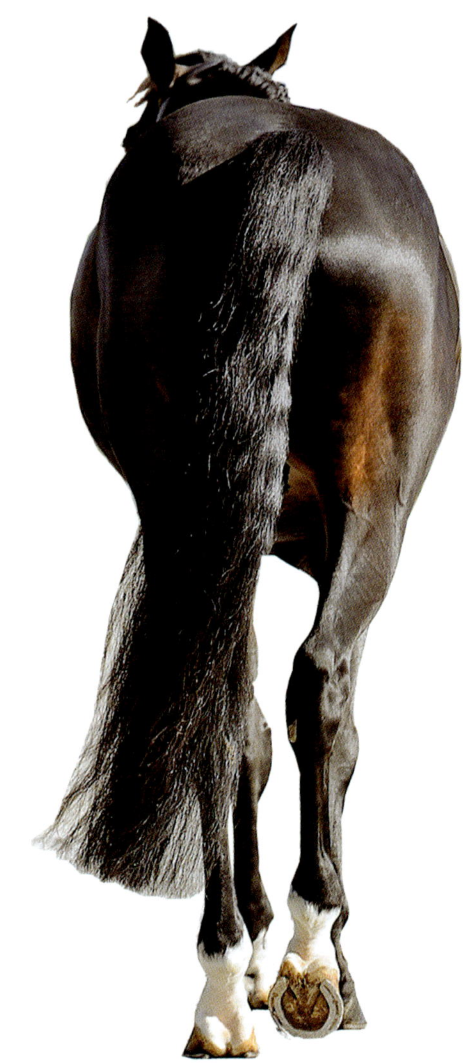

The horse walks away from you.

The Horse Walking Away from You

In all gaits, movement should come from the hindquarters, the motor. How can you best assess the condition of the hindquarters?

1 The Pelvis

- Left and right iliac tips (*tuber sacrales*) should rise and fall independently from one another (see illustrations on pp. 67 right and 101).
- The same goes for the two hip bones (see illustrations on pp. 67 and 101).
- Through this movement, the entire pelvis makes a rotating/rolling-forward movement (see illustration below). Figuratively speaking, imagine a combination of a duck's movement with that of a lizard's. This combination of movement is found in both sides of the pelvis.

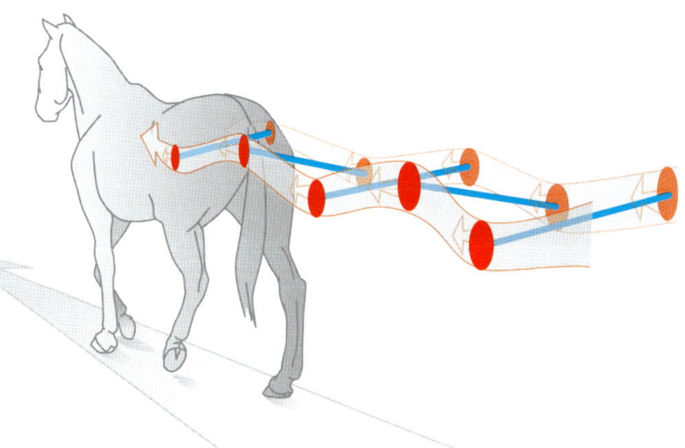

2 The tail swings loosely back and forth.
3 As they move forward, the legs are evenly lifted and rise to the same height.
4 During the standing phase of the gait, there can't be any inner rotation of the hind legs.
5 The hind feet descend vertically downward from the hips.
6 The hindquarters follow straight back from the forehand.

Anomalies

1 The Pelvis

The pelvis is one of the most important areas of the horse's body. Unfortunately, I frequently find disorders here. The causes can be primary or secondary.

Through trauma, subluxations or acute blockages in the SI joint can occur in the pelvic area. Then the horse goes lame, can bear only a little weight on the affected side as the ligaments and muscles are overstretched or tensed.

With chronic blockages, you could see that the affected leg moves forward more slowly. The desired pelvic movement (a mix of duck and lizard) is no longer there; this can affect one or both sides.

Lameness can trigger the same symptoms as the muscles recede prematurely. As already discussed, movement dysfunction in the poll or forelegs can also manifest as secondary symptoms in the pelvis.

2 The Tail

The tail is an extension of the spine and is always an indicator for the condition of the back. Tension in the back muscles or a twisted sacrum automatically cause a tense and crooked tail. This shows up when the horse clamps his tail, carries it crooked, or too high.

Exceptions are horses of certain breeds, such as the Arabian, that like to carry their tail to the left. This is genetic and is not an anomaly.

3 Differences in How the Limbs Lift or Move

All forms of uneven movement can be caused by lameness or muscular tension. I would advise taking these signs seriously and enlisting professional help as a first step.

4 Turning of the Hind Legs in Standing Phase

Blockages or instability around the hip joint or lumbar vertebrae can be the source of this rotation. As the hind leg moves back, the shifting of weight and/or longitudinal bend in the lumbar region is not happening and, therefore, the hind leg executes an evasive movement (see chapter 3, "Biomechanics," p. 34). This puts more stress on the stifle and hock joints as the horse, due to the evasive/turning movement, has put extra weight on the standing leg.

5 The Hind Feet Are Not Set Vertically

When your horse sets down his hind legs too far to the inside or outside, this evasive movement can mean a blockage in the upper area of the limb. Likewise, a low-grade lameness and muscular tension can trigger these symptoms.

6 A Crooked Horse

From the back and front, you can easily see if your horse is straight. If he's very crooked, you'll recognize it in his extremities. The hindquarters come down to the side of the forehand. He walks "half-pass like"; the legs stagger slightly.

A helpful trick is to shut your eyes and listen; this will help you recognize when there are clear differences in the weight affecting the rhythm of the extremities.

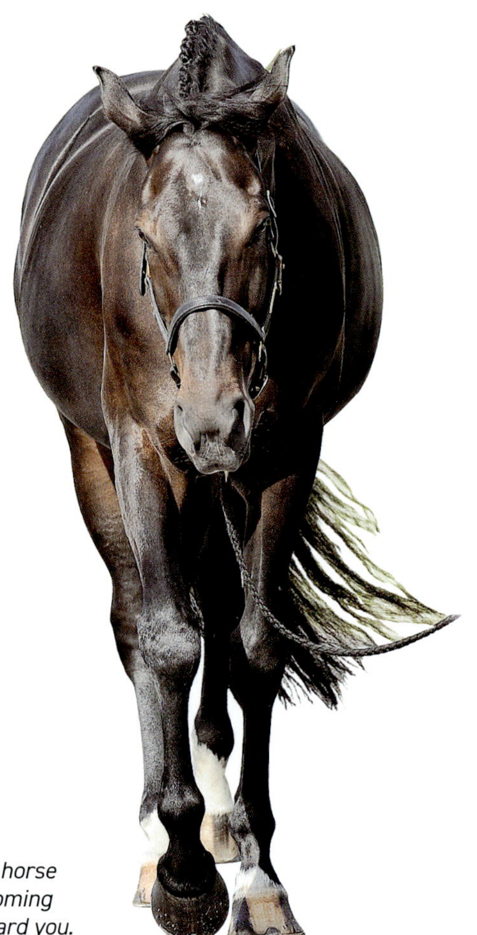

The horse is coming toward you.

The Forehand at the Walk

1 The horse's head is relaxed and slightly down.
2 The head swings back and forth like a pendulum and moves with a slight nod.
3 The shoulder blades glide out from the trunk, up and down.
4 Both shoulder joints move evenly toward the front.
5 During the moment of suspension, both legs reach the same height. The hooves land flat.
6 The trunk swings evenly out to the sides, back and forth.
7 A straight horse should be recognizable. The hindquarters follow the forehand, as if in a single lane.

Anomalies

1 Head Carriage

When the horse travels with his head really low, it may be that he's trying to shift his weight to the front in order to take weight off his hindquarters. When it's reversed and he's carrying his head too high, he's trying to shift more weight to his hindquarters in order to relieve the forehand. An uneven nodding/bobbing of the head means that he is not fully weighting one of his limbs, but rather making an evasive movement. The horse is lame.

2 The Head Doesn't Swing

Viewed from the front, the head should move in a small "eight" pattern: swinging up and down and lightly to each side. I often observe that the head can only swing up and down. If the horse can't swing his head to the side, a blockage in the poll is likely.

3 The Shoulder Blades Don't Glide

When one or both shoulder blades can't optimally glide from the trunk, there are tensions and adhesions present in the shoulder-girdle muscles. The horse moves dully on the forehand and "stamps" his feet onto the ground.

4 The Shoulder Joints Come Forward Unevenly

There can be various reasons that the shoulders do not move forward evenly (see Number 3): a muscular injury (acute or chronic) or muscular tension. In addition, a blockage at the C1 or T1 vertebrae with involvement of the first rib can trigger this same symptom.

5 The Hooves Don't Land Evenly

It's common to see horses step sideways with their forelegs. When you lift the leg up, stretch it forward and try to turn it, the turn on the longitudinal axis is restricted, usually toward the inside. The reason may be a blockage in the shoulder— or elbow joint.

When a hoof is not set down flat, it brings about a biomechanical imbalance in the hoof area, which can manifest as painful dysfunction all the way to the back.

Irreparable damage to the joints and ligaments of the lower limbs can follow.

Fact: Close your eyes. Often, you can hear an unevenness in the landing phase (and rhythm) more easily than you can see it.

6 The Trunk Doesn't Swing Enough

Because the trunk is suspended between the shoulder blades (the posts), it's able to swing back and forth like a pendulum (the ship). You should be able to see the following: an even, outwardly swinging trunk, which hangs between the shoulder blades like a "hammock," moving back and forth. However, if there's an accumulation of tension or restriction of movement in one of the shoulder blades, it may indicate a blocked rib or problem with an internal organ, which will reduce the swing.

7 A Crooked Horse

As with the observation from behind, you must periodically observe and monitor your horse's position from the front view. The source of the problems will be the same.

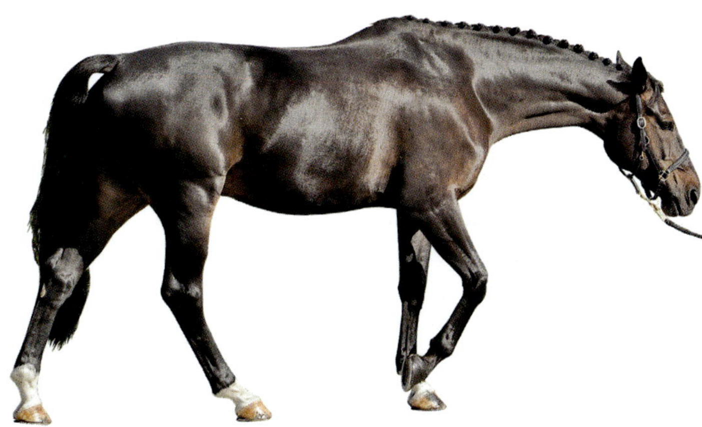

You position yourself beside the horse so that you can easily follow the movement pattern from back to front—through the entire body. From the side, you can also best observe the flow of movement throughout the whole body. Obviously, you need to observe both sides and compare them.

1 As the horse puts his foot down, the nose is pushed forward slightly. A slight lowering of the head and neck as the front feet are set down will be visible.
2 The up-and-down glide of the shoulder blade is recognizable.
3 The foreleg moves forward evenly, the "hanging" phase, and doesn't require much effort. There's an even striking off at the end of the standing phase.
4 Engagement and releasing of the back and abdominal muscles. The back swings lightly with the movement.
5 The thrust comes from behind and comes forward over the back.
6 The contraction of the stifle and hock joints happen without much visible effort and delay.
7 The hind hooves track in the same lane as the front hooves (= tracking up).
8 The forehand comes away from the ground quickly. The hind hooves shouldn't touch the front hooves.
9 No dragging toes.
10 The tail is held lightly away from the body.

Anomalies

1 Abnormal Head and Neck Movement

When the head is pushed forward too much (the horse's head movements resemble a chicken when he walks), the poll is suffering from restricted movement.

2 Too Little Glide in the Shoulder Blades

There are accumulated tension and movement restrictions in the shoulder-girdle musculature, as already described (see p. 98).

3 Shortened Movement of the Forelegs (Forward or Backward)

When the muscles that move the legs forward or backward are tensed, or there are blockages in the cervical vertebrae, and/or blockages in the thoracic spine area, it can lead to a shortening of the standing or hanging phases of the front legs.

4 No "Relaxation Phase" in the Abdominal and Back Muscles

The reasons for this (see Number 6 on p. 99).

5 Hindquarters Lack Impulsion

See Numbers 1 and 2 on p. 105.

6 The Mechanics of the Hind Legs Are Restricted

The movements of the stifle and hock joints belong together. This means that if the horse has a problem with his hock, it will also affect the biomechanics of the stifle. The horse will have a stiff gait. If he doesn't care to bend one of his hind legs, it can hint toward a dysfunction in these joints. Another reason can simply be muscular tension in the hamstrings, which always coexists with tension in the back muscles.

7 Tracking Up Unevenly

The horse should track up evenly. This means, his hind hoof should come past the print of his front hoof on the same side. In addition, he should lift both hooves to the same height.

8 The Hind Hoof Makes Contact with the Front Hoof

When the horse's hind hoof makes contact with his front hoof, he may constantly pull off a front shoe. Or worse, he may repeatedly injure himself. On the one hand, this can mean that the horse has tension in his shoulder-girdle muscles and isn't moving his forelegs out of the way quickly enough. On the other hand, the overreaching can go back to a coordination problem, which means, the horse lacks control of his hindquarters. He doesn't know exactly where the leg is, and just sets it down.

9 The Horse Drags a Hind Toe

This symptom can occur for many reasons, but often the source is either a blockage in the poll, tension in the hamstrings, or inactive hind quarters.

10 The Tail Isn't Loose

The causes have already been described, such as accumulated tension in the back (see Number 2 on p. 105).

Through Tight Turns at Walk

The point of this exercise is to test your horse's longitudinal bend and coordination. The horse turns tightly around you, at a distance of one to two meters.

In the turn, it should be possible to see a bend through the whole horse, from the jaw to the tail, and more so in the cervical, thoracic, and lumbar regions. The inside hind leg should cross over the midline without any difficulty. The outside leg travels in a sequence from the midline (inside) outward and forward and is not just moving out.

Blockages in the poll become very clear in tight turns. With this diagnosis, the horse will either position his head to the outside, stretch his nose too far forward, or tilt/turn the head (bringing the nose either to the inside or outside).
Compare both sides with one another.

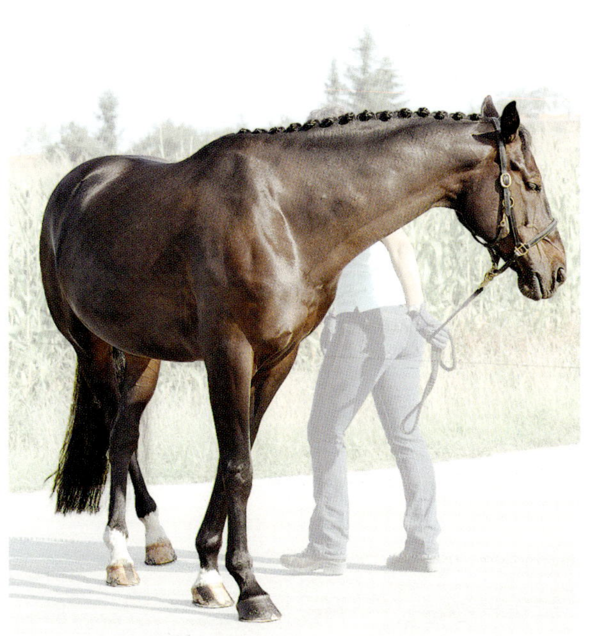 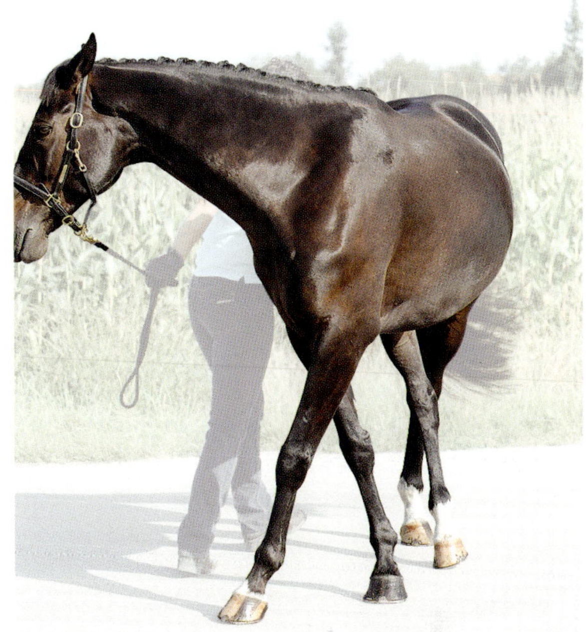

Note: This horse could position himself a bit more to the inside at the poll.

Anomalies

The following symptoms are possibilities: as the horse turns around you, he either falls in toward you or he doesn't want to—or cannot—bend. The most common causes are blockages and/or pain in the spine.

When the horse has difficulty crossing his legs, the problem comes from the upper hind end, the sacroiliac joint, and even the lumbar/loin area.

While Backing Up

Your horse should be able to back up effortlessly. When he does, you can see an even, diagonal movement of the legs with a slight lift to the back and a lowered croup. The hindquarters lower slightly and the hind legs are lifted to an even height, brought back and set down again.

Anomalies

When there are blockages in the lumbar vertebrae or sacroiliac joint, or there is low-grade lameness, the horse will not back up willingly. Pay attention to his back—it should not be too strongly arched—and also make sure that as he begins to back up, the body doesn't push back too far over the hind legs without them moving.

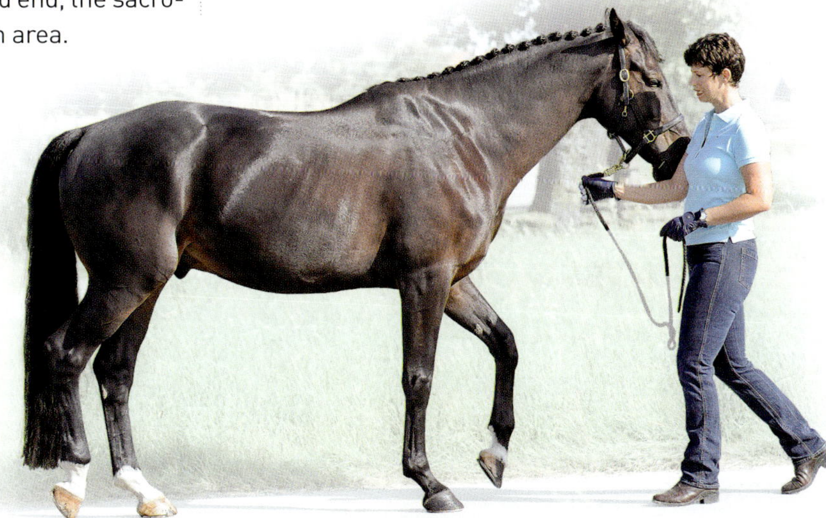

Observing at Trot

Pay attention to the same criteria at the trot as you did at the walk, except for the tight turns, which should only be executed at walk.

At the trot, muscular engagement is heightened, which can cover up many compensatory biomechanical processes. Chronic blockages will not be as visible as at the walk, but lameness will be more visible at trot.

1 You should see an even, two-beat rhythm with the horse carrying his head at a consistent height.
2 The transition from walk to trot comes from behind, without the head/neck lifting higher.

Anomalies

1 **A Definite Head-Bobbing**

When you can see an uneven head bob at the trot, there's a lameness present.
If you've discovered that the horse is lame, ask an assistant to lead him at a trot on hard ground on a circle of 8 to 10 meters in diameter. Here, lameness is often much more recognizable.

2 **No Push from Behind and the Horse Raises His Head**

In the upward transition to trot or canter, the movement must originate from the hindquarters. Horses that always come above the contact at the first stride, are using their *brachiocephalicus* muscle to get into gear and the hindquarters follow without thrust. These horses always have pain in their back or hindquarters.

At Trot on the Longe

When your horse is trotting on the longe line, you can easily observe the use of his back and mobility of his pelvis. The *longissimus dorsi* should alternately engage and relax, and his inner croup should lower when the leg is lifted.

If you determine there is a movement dysfunction, the causes will be almost identical as "at the walk."

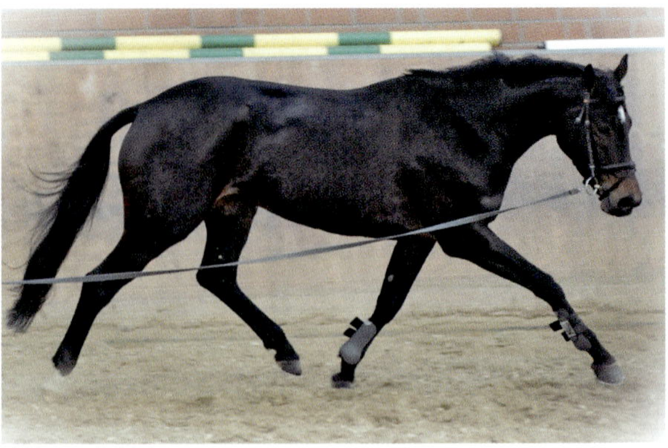

Horse on the longe at a trot.

At Canter on the Longe

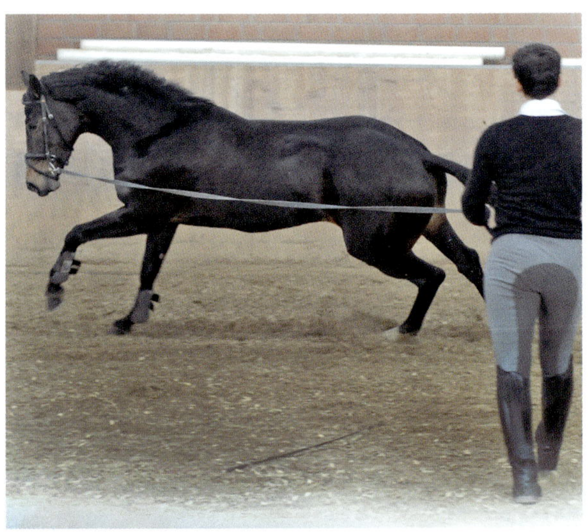

Horse on the longe at a canter. As the horse canters, he's positioned to the outside and tense. Tension in the horse must be considered in an overall observation.

When I watch the transition from trot to canter, I want to see the hindquarters push from below, which they should continue to do at the canter. Because of the engagement on both sides of the *longissimus dorsi*, the forehand will lift up. At the canter, there should be a clear stretch and lift in the back. A definite three-beat rhythm should be recognizable, too. In the moment of suspension, there must also be a contraction of the abdominal muscles.

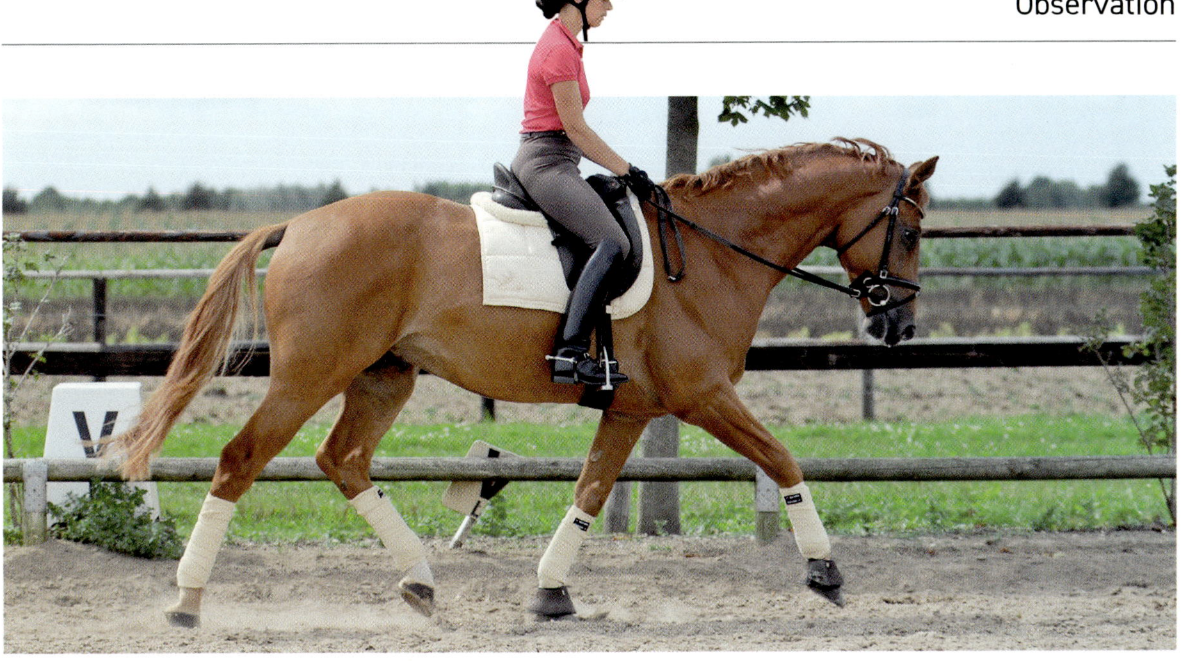

The horse's way of going should also be observed under saddle.

Anomalies

Most of the anomalies that are recognizable at canter have causes in the hindquarters. It's common to see a horse that always falls into a cross-canter or tries to run away. This points to dysfunction in the lumbar and pelvic area, or to balance problems.

When longeing, you have a connection with the horse through the longe line. You can reference this to determine whether the horse is bending well and evenly on both sides. It's also interesting to observe the bend in his neck, if the horse is positioned to the inside or outside, whether the horse's hindquarters are staying "in lane" or falling to the outside.

When the horse has difficulty with coordination with stopping, turning, stepping sideways, or backing, you should investigate the source of the problem as it could be a disorder of the spine.

Hint: If you notice symptoms and changes, please consult a professional before you get started with massage and stretching.

Observing Under Saddle

You should also observe your horse's movement patterns when he's being ridden.

You can already learn a lot about your horse's condition when tacking him up. A demonstration of aggressive or fearful behavior when being saddled or bridled means the horse isn't feeling well.

When mounting, there are signs such as:

- Evading as the rider sits.
- Dropping through the back or "humping" the back when the rider sits in the saddle.
- During the first steps, the horse "crouches," won't move forward, runs away, or bucks.
- Tossing the head.
- Posture and movement flow are different with a rider than without.

With these signs, alarm bells should be going off. Your horse is in pain and you must find the cause of his behavior (see chapter 1, p. 1).

Of course, the end of this chapter does not mean the end of observing! Remain attentive—constantly and in all situations. If symptoms and changes occur, your first response should always be to consult an expert.

Palpation

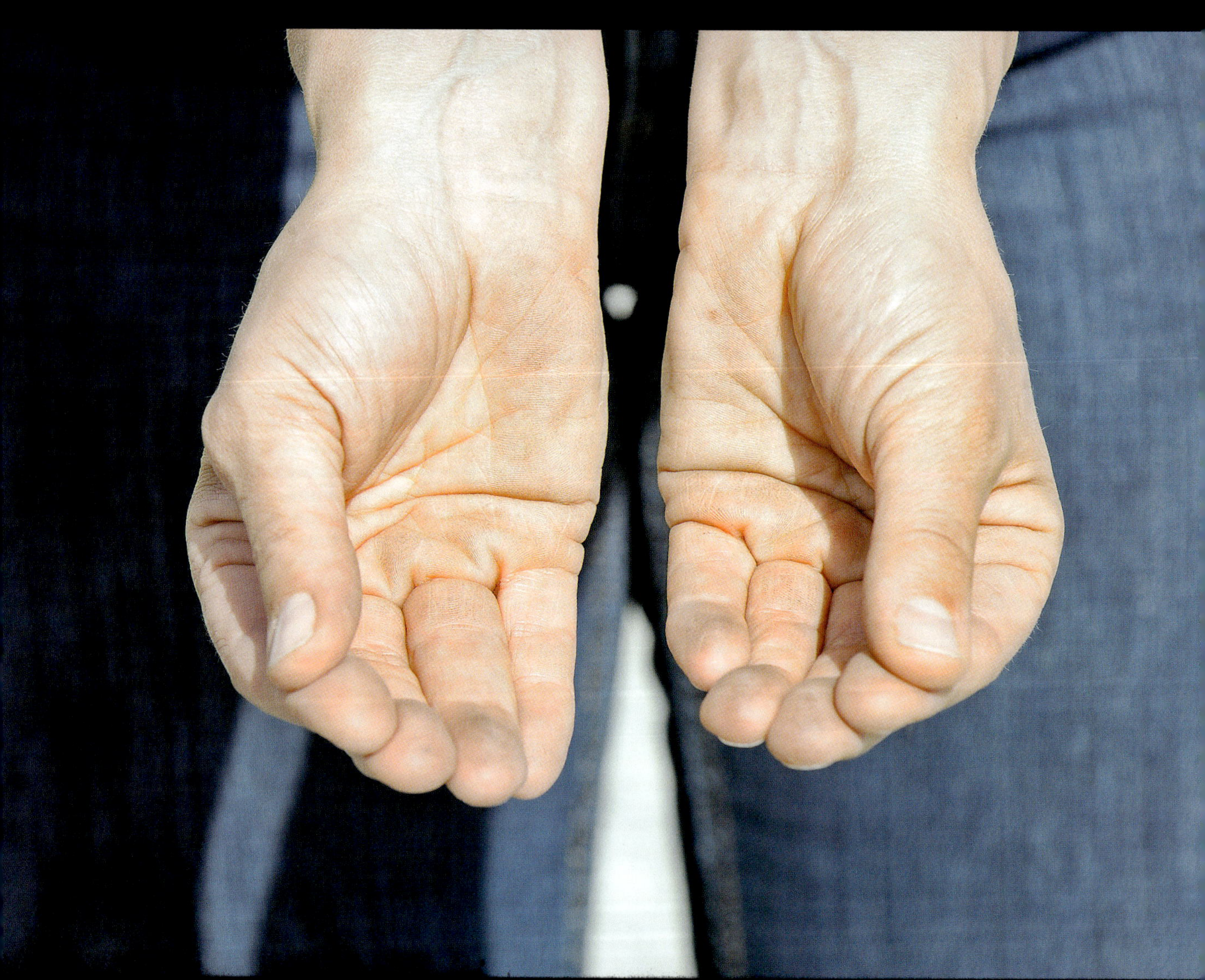

I'm finally getting to the *hands-on* part of this book! Now, you'll use your sense of touch to explore. Your hands are a wonderful instrument—nearly indispensable in daily life. And how sensitive they are! Your fingertips have a huge number of nerves and are just waiting to get to work now. To learn to employ their sensitivity, you must practice and continuously learn.

The term "palpation" means examining the body through touch. With this method, you can determine the body's consistency, elasticity, mobility, and sensitivity to pain at the surface. You're looking for areas of tension, adhesions, growths, muscle knots, swellings, and differences in temperature—all of which are anomalies that can hint at illness.

My Tip

To monitor temperature, use the back of your hand. You have a better ability to feel hot and cold there, so it will be easier for you to feel the differences.

Palpation should always be done before, during, and after a treatment. In this way, you can locate and monitor any points of pain or tension. As a "beginner," you may have difficulty remembering the exact location of pain points. It will help to simply mark them with chalk, finger paint, saddle soap, or with streaks in the horse's coat. During treatment, these marks will make it easier to monitor whether the point of pain is feeling better. Often, pain is already reduced during a treatment.

As with any examination, you should find a quiet workplace. It's imperative to remove any jewelry that could get caught and/or hurt your horse. It's best to have short fingernails, which makes the examination easier and is more comfortable for your horse. Don't apply any fly spray as it makes the coat slippery and you won't have the necessary resistance from the coat that you need for palpation and further treatment.

Before you begin, please look your horse over for any wounds or injuries.

If you're massaging multiple horses—for example, first a mare and then a stallion—you will have the first horse's scent on your body. This can lead to complications. In this case, it's better to change your clothes so that the stallion doesn't become excited.

In addition, please don't wear any perfume or after-shave. These scents make horses uncomfortable.

Practice on the Horse

Always keep an eye on your horse and his reactions. It's important to notice how he reacts to various levels of pressure. Pay attention to your own safety as horses can react very strongly to pain or a bad feeling. Please don't tie your horse the first time you palpate, massage, or stretch him. You may trigger pain points that can cause the horse to react strongly and possibly spook. In this case, he needs the option to move in order to communicate to you how he's feeling. When you have a "helper" hold your horse, this person should always stay on the *same side* as you're working, but otherwise not interact with the horse too much.

My Tip

If you're not sure what a tense muscle feels like, palpate several different horses in order to learn the difference between tense and relaxed muscles.

Unless you have a lot of experience, I advise you to palpate the same body part on both sides. To be more specific: first, palpate the head on both sides, then the neck on both sides, then the shoulder, and so forth. Later, with experience, you can palpate a single side in one go, before moving to the other side.

Hint: Begin with light pressure when palpating!

Position yourself near your horse. Always work with both hands. This means you should position the hand you're not using somewhere on the horse's body. This will be calming for your horse. In addition, when you employ techniques that only require use of your thumb or fingertips, I advise you still try to allow your whole hand to have contact with the horse and follow along. You may know this from your own experiences with massage—a small, direct point of pressure is uncomfortable, but when the massage therapist uses a flat hand, it's more comfortable and easier to relax.

How Hard Should You Press?

When it comes to deciding how much pressure to use, your best bet is practicing on yourself first. There are three different levels of pressure. All three should feel comfortable to you, as long as you yourself aren't suffering from accumulated tension.

Light Pressure 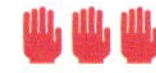

Bring one or two fingertips or the palm of your hand to your forehead and make small, round movements. Try out the difference between using the tips of your fingers or the fingers' fleshy pads. Can you feel the difference? Please keep in mind the most comfortable application and level of pressure.

Medium Pressure

To experience medium pressure, use the fleshy pads of your fingertips or your thumb directly on the inner half of your clavicle. In the same spot, press with both your thumb and fingers at once. Here, too, please try out various positions with your fingers.

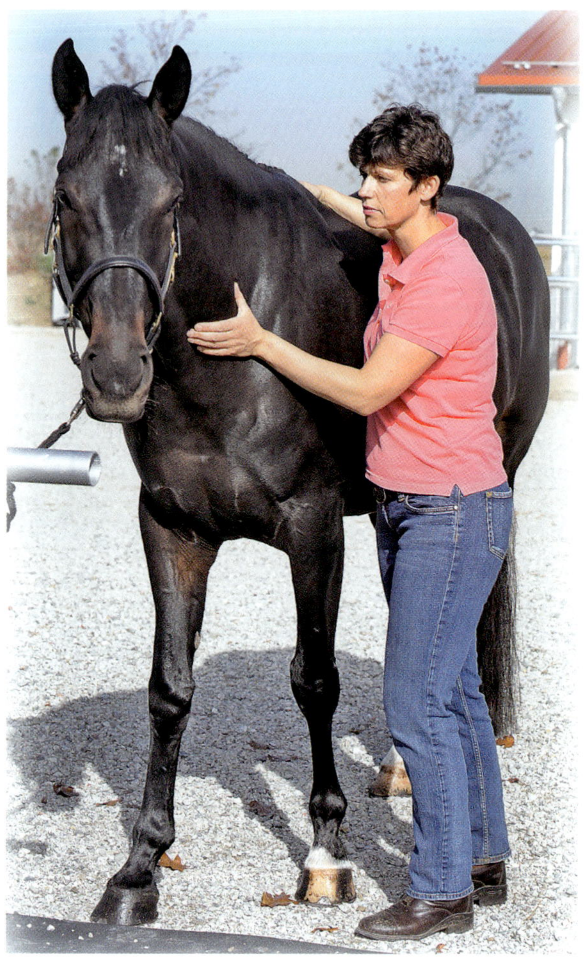

When palpating or massaging your horse, keep your body in connection with his. This will have a calming effect.

Hard Pressure

Using the palm of your hand, massage your thigh or practice applying direct pressure to your elbow. As you can certainly feel, you can really apply your strength here, without causing pain.

Fact: Eventually, you should be able to apply pressure all over your horse without him having a reaction. Of course, the less muscular places/bones that are not covered with much soft tissue will remain more sensitive.

Techniques to Palpate the Horse

Depending on the shape of the muscle or the body part/area, you'll utilize one of the following to palpate: your thumb, pads (tips) of your fingers or palm. As I come to various muscle groups in the book, I'll give hints based on what level of pressure I use to palpate these muscles.

- Use your fingertips or thumb for small areas, such as at a tendon's point of insertion and the small muscles of the head and poll. Make small, circling movements directly on the tendon or muscle; the skin slides/moves with you.

Fact: Studies have shown that the pointer and middle finger have the most receptors. These are located in the pads of the fingertips.

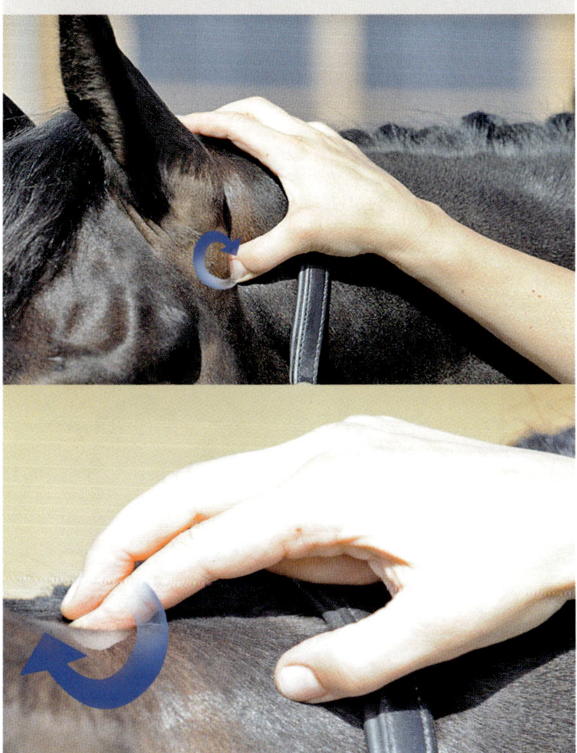

- Palpating with your palm, while applying more pressure with the fingertips. This touch is for the larger, flatter muscles, such as along the neck, shoulder blades, back, and flank. You press and glide the palm of your hand down the whole muscle. When you've done this two or three times without the horse reacting, you can up the pressure by using your fingertips. Now, you can either just glide your fingertips down the muscle or use them to push into points along the muscle, every 2 to 3 centimeters.

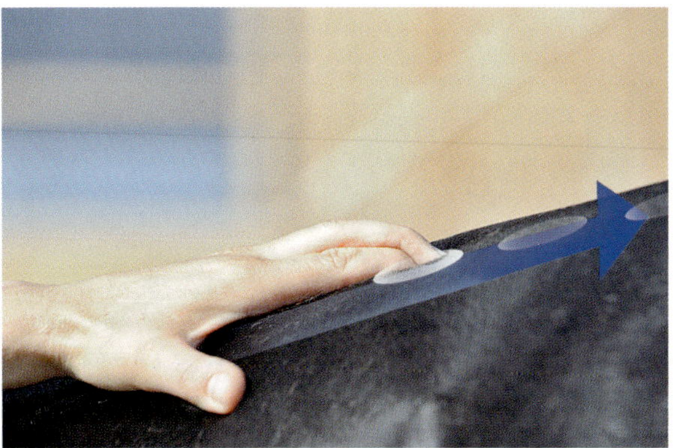

- With large, round muscles, you can really wrap your hands around them and use your fingers to just rock them and apply pressure at points. This is a good technique for palpating the large *brachiocephalic* and *hamstring* muscles.

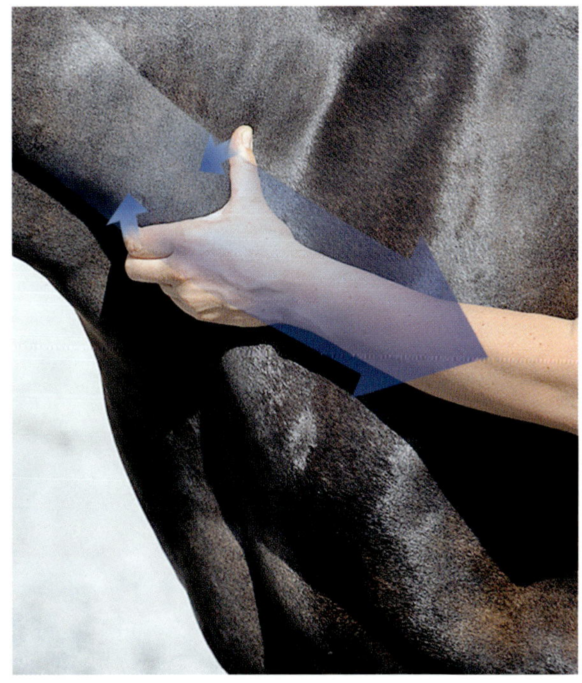

Triggering Pain

Of course, it's possible that you'll trigger pain in your horse during palpation if he has a problem at a certain point. Once you've found a pain point, try to feel what the tissue is like there. This is the only way your fingers and hands can get trained.

Your horse is your "teacher": he'll show you when he doesn't feel good.

Possible signs of pain:
- The skin shakes when touched lightly.
- The muscles feel tight. The muscles tense up, get hard, when you palpate.
- The horse moves away from a light pressure.
- He pins his ears.
- He pinches his nostrils.
- He shakes his head.
- The horse has an excited gaze and his eyes widen.
- He switches his tail.
- He tries to push away with his body.
- He kicks or bites.
- His breathing is quick and shallow.

How Should a Relaxed Muscle Feel?

Even when you're just palpating the muscle, the horse can like and enjoy your touch.

Signs of well-being:
- The muscles are pliable.
- The head lowers.
- The ears hang relaxed to the outside or are directed back in concentration.
- The lower lip hangs down and away from the gums.
- The eyes get smaller and softer.
- The horse dozes off.
- Breathing slower and deeper.
- The horse snorts. (The mucous membranes in his sinuses relax and there's a clear discharge from his nostrils.)

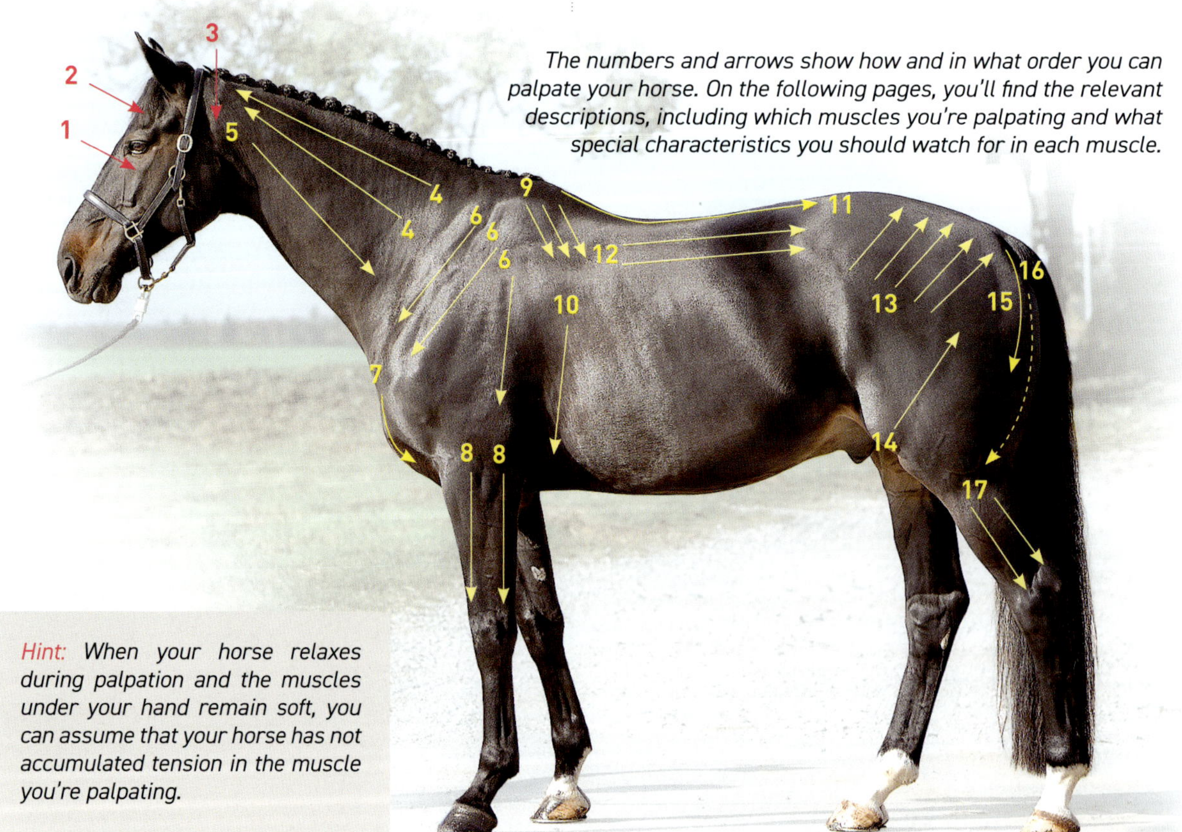

The numbers and arrows show how and in what order you can palpate your horse. On the following pages, you'll find the relevant descriptions, including which muscles you're palpating and what special characteristics you should watch for in each muscle.

Hint: When your horse relaxes during palpation and the muscles under your hand remain soft, you can assume that your horse has not accumulated tension in the muscle you're palpating.

- Every now and then, he chews lightly, shakes his head gently, or yawns.
- He rests/shifts a hind leg.

Now, I'm getting to the various regions of a horse's body. In the following section, I've listed and described the most important muscles that you can feel (and which are most often suffering from tension).

When you begin each muscle group, always start with light pressure. If the horse doesn't react, you can increase the pressure. If you've had a massage, you know how this goes. You don't know what's coming, so you tense up at first until you realize that it doesn't hurt. Horses are the same way. I always palpate each muscle group two or three times. In the process, the horse gets used to my hands and I can better assess the pressure and the consistency of his muscular tissue.

I also recommend that you start up front at his head and work your way back, as described in this book. It's helpful to have the palpation diagram in your head.

Let's Get Started!

1 The Outer Masticatory Muscle
(*M. masseter*)
This area frequently suffers from tension. The muscles tense up because of dental problems or when there are disorders elsewhere in the body (for example, with the pelvis).

> **My Tip**
>
> Take the crest and shake it back and forth. If it's tight, this is an indication that the neck muscles that you've just palpated are also tight. Compare both sides of the neck.

Please be careful: when horses have tension and pain in this area, they can react strongly by quickly bringing their head up high or trying to run away from the pressure.

2 The Temples 
(*M. temporalis*)
Looking at the horse from the front, you'll see two "bulges" directly under the spot where the forelock attaches. You can palpate them easily with your thumbs.

Horses that are frantic and nervous have lots of tension here. But, strangely, this muscle is not that sensitive—it will just feel hard when it should feel soft.

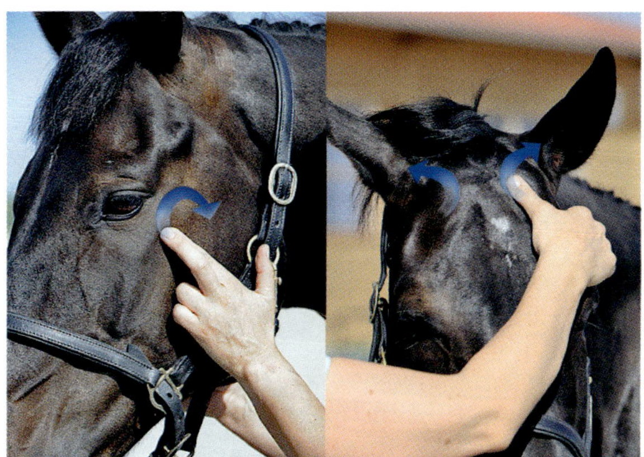

3 The Poll 
This area can be palpated with light to medium pressure. Horses that tend toward nervousness have lots of tension here. In my experience, if you find tension in the poll when you palpate, you'll also find tension toward the tail. In this case, please only apply light pressure when you palpate!

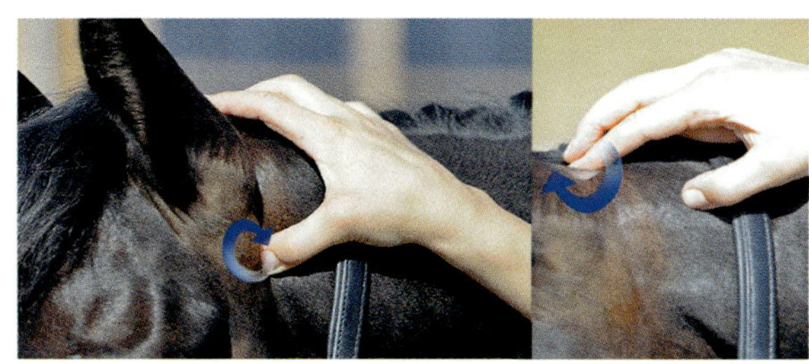

4 Neck Area 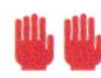

In this area, palpate the muscle below the crest, between poll and shoulder, with a flat hand and heightened pressure on the fingertips. I glide my hand from the shoulder blade toward the poll (against the direction the hair grows) and press points along the way.

As you palpate, the muscles should give slightly. Generally, there are few pain points here, but there can often be increased muscle tension, especially in the *trapezius* muscle.

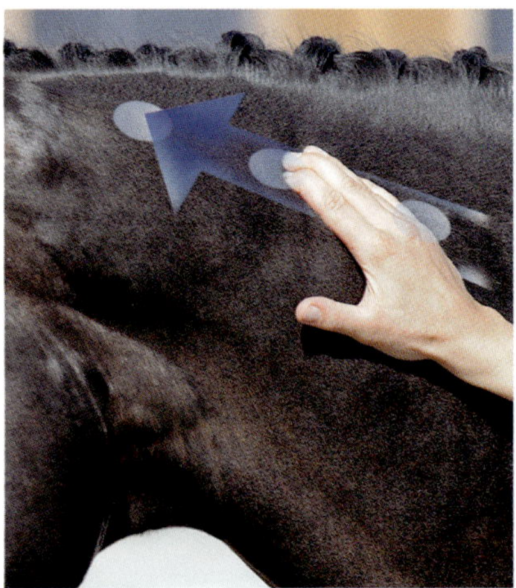

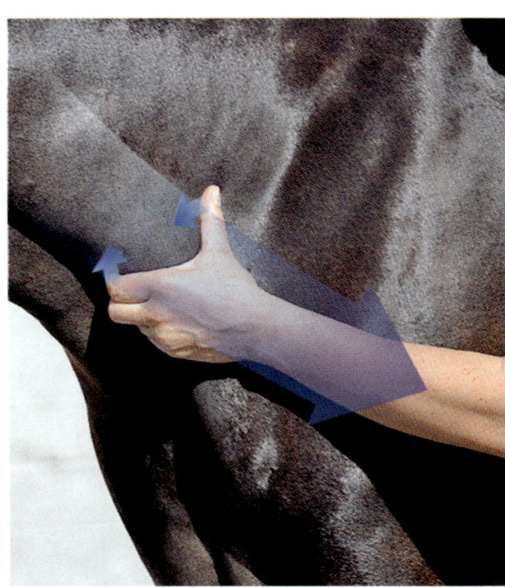

5 Brachiocephalicus Muscle

(*M. brachiocephalicus*)

You should find this muscle supple and that you can shake it lightly. Unfortunately, it is often tight and painful.

6a Shoulder Blades

You'll palpate the muscles that lie on and beneath the shoulder blades. The muscles on the shoulder blade are thin and, therefore, feel tauter. So, don't press too hard. In between these muscles, you can feel the fishbone-like "bulge" of the scapula, a bony ridge on the shoulder blade.

6b Triceps

(*M. triceps*)

This is a large, loose muscle below the shoulder blade. Here, you can press harder. It's frequently affected when the *brachiocephalicus* muscle is tense. When tension accumulates, both muscles shorten and this restricts the horse's length of stride.

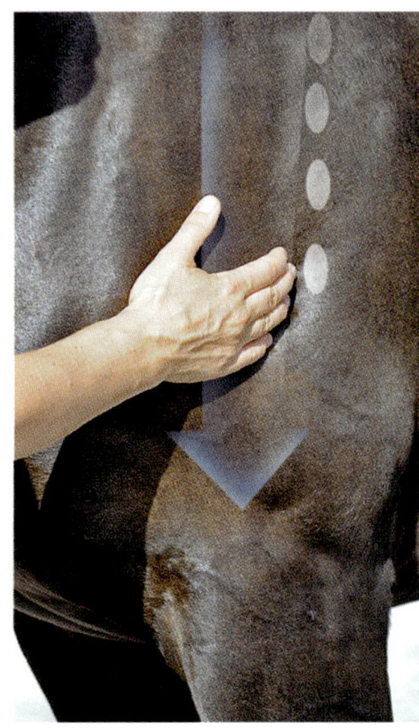

7 Pectorals

(*Mm. pectorales*)

To palpate the *pectoral* muscles, grasp in between the forelegs. Normally, this muscle group is soft. However, horses that travel too much on the forehand or are ridden with draw reins will have tension in these muscles.

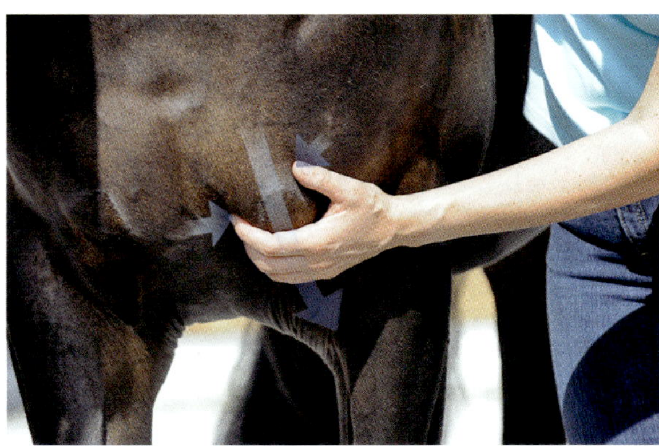

8 The Forearm 

The muscles of the forearm are always relatively taut, although the extensors on the front side are somewhat softer than the contractors/flexors on the backside of the leg. After a hard training session or a tendon injury, you'll find both groups of muscles are tighter and will be grateful for a massage.

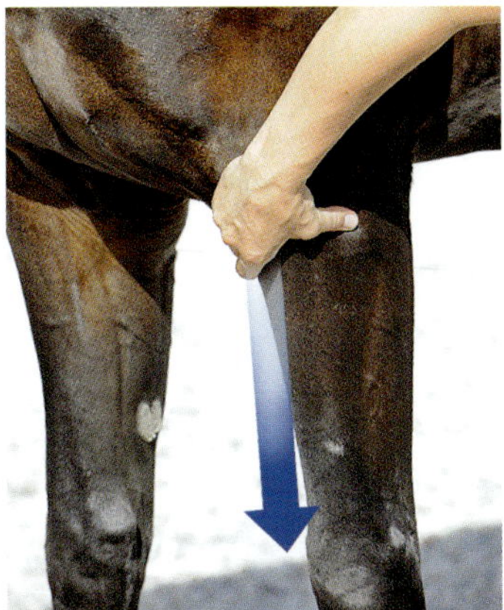

9 The Withers 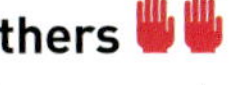

At the withers, you're palpating the *trapezius* muscle. This muscle will frequently be painful when there's lameness or poor saddle fit.

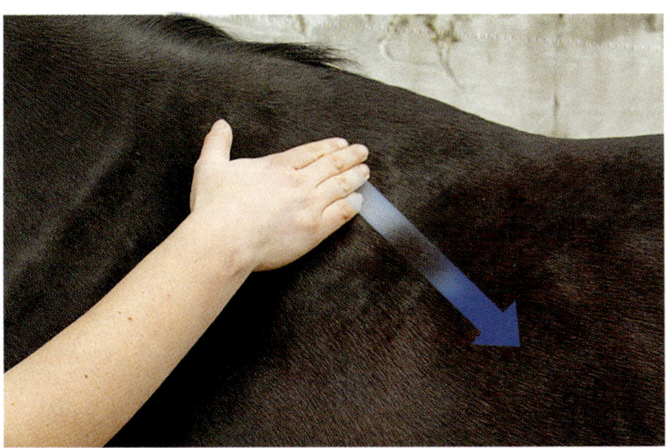

10 The Girth Area 

In the girth area, the skin has a reflex that should not be mistaken for pain. This reflex causes the skin to shake/tremble and should disappear if you run your hand over this spot multiple times. If this shaking remains, however, it can be interpreted to mean there's pain in the ventral serratus (*m. serratus ventralis thoracis*). Unfortunately, I also often find a swelling in the girth area. If you encounter these symptoms, you should inspect your girth (see chapter 12, "Preventive Measures," p. 200).

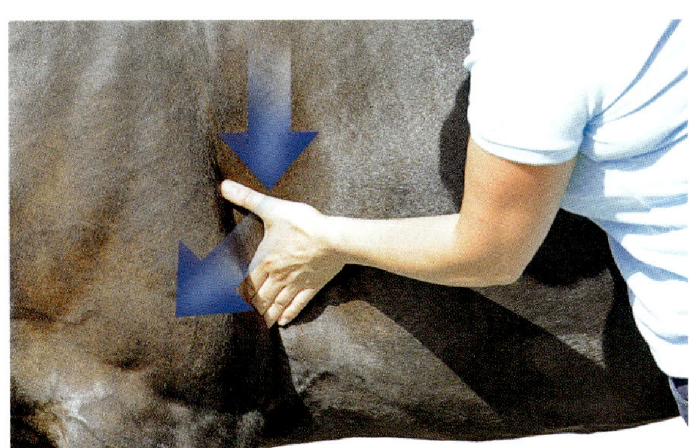

11 The Spinous Processes and Supraspinal Ligament
(*Ligamentum supraspinale*)

Here, use only the soft pads of your fingertips, as you're palpating around bone. Stroke from withers to sacrum along the spinous processes. When your horse has a reaction, it can indicate inflammation along the back or pain in the spinous processes, which you find with kissing spine, for example.

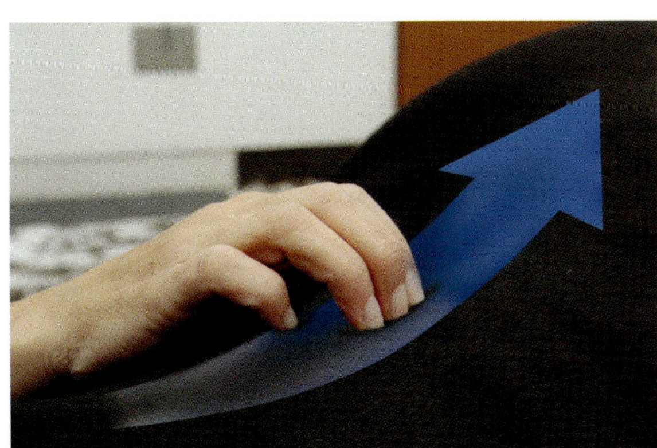

12 Back Muscles 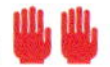

These muscles lie directly along the spinous processes and run to the costal arch, approximately one to two hand-widths toward the ribs.

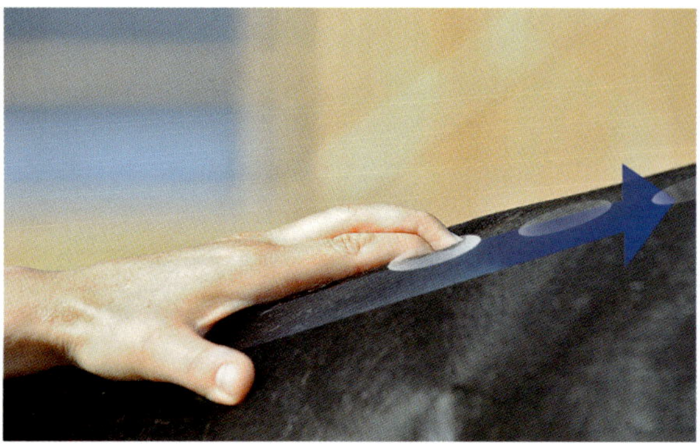

When you palpate the back muscles with a consistent pressure, they'll give slightly. With light pressure at various points, you can check for sensitivity/pain. Simply stroke your flat hand and slightly bent fingertips over the back. There shouldn't be any reaction when you're palpating with a flat hand. You should feel the muscles give to your touch. Having said that, this musculature is often painful. You'll notice it because the muscles beneath your fingers will get hard, the horse avoids the pressure or clearly shows you that he's uncomfortable with the pressure.

13 Croup Muscles and Biceps Femoris 

Begin with the muscles around the hip bones and palpate toward the croup. When you apply hard

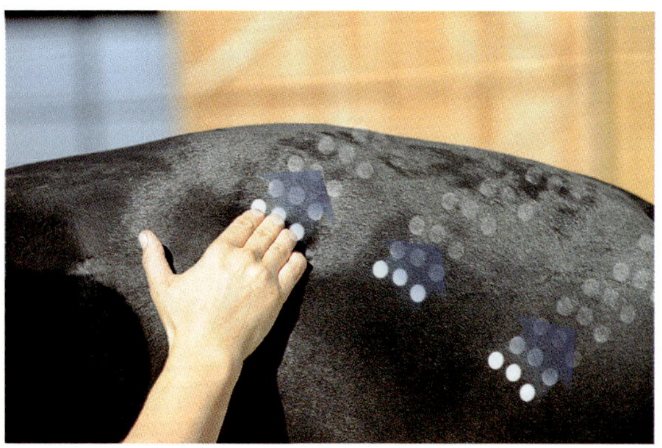

pressure, the muscles should give. If the horse tips his pelvis or buckles at his stifle, it's a sign of pain in the *gluteal* muscles or, as often proves the case, tension in the broad pelvic ligaments. When there's accumulated tension in the back muscles, you can expect to also find increased muscular tension and pain in this area.

14 Quadriceps 

(*M. quadriceps femoris*)

This should be very relaxed and soft. When there are stifle problems, these muscles can be very sensitive. Please be careful in this area as horses can be ticklish here.

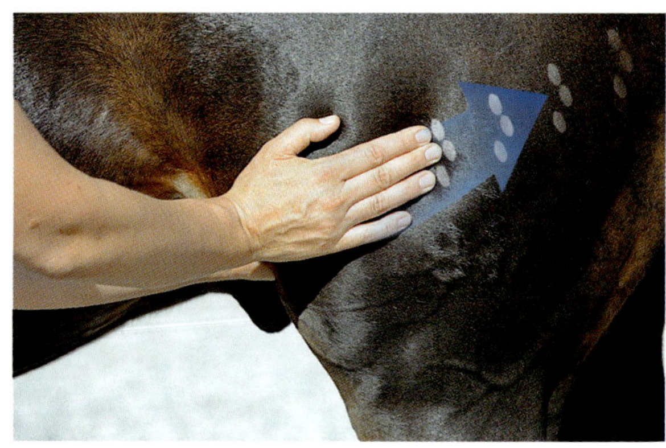

Hint: When you palpate the muscles of the hindquarters, they must and should be about the same in terms of softness and should feel flat and supple. A separation between the various muscles shouldn't be easy to feel. You'll recognize large muscle knots or adhesions of the muscular tissue, as you'll find spots that are really hard and other spots that are really soft. Knots/adhesions are fatal to the development of strength, as part of the muscle isn't functioning. Then, circulation in this area is also compromised. It's painful. This is a clear sign that the horse is compensating as he moves, does not have enough strength and is not getting enough recovery time during training.

15 The Hamstrings 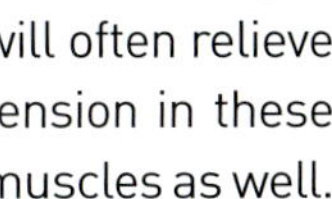

The hamstring muscles (*M. semimembranosus and M. semitendinosus*) should also be relaxed and soft. But, please be careful when you palpate! These muscles may be so painful that the horse will kick out. They have a close relationship with the back muscles and can be affected as a result of back tension. If you can relieve the tension in the back, you will often relieve tension in these muscles as well.

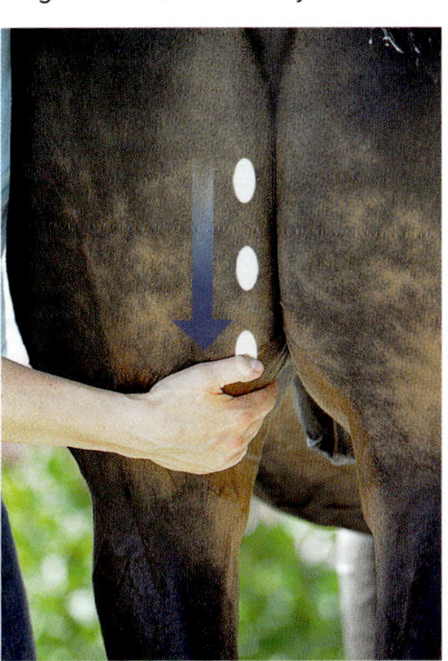

16 The Adductors

These muscles lie on the inside of the upper thigh. They should be soft. You can palpate them from the front or the back, along the inside of the upper thigh. Because many horses are tense here or simply ticklish, please palpate with caution.

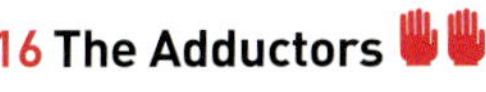

17 The Lower Leg Muscles

Just like the forelegs, this part of the hind legs is relatively taut.

Generally speaking, when palpating, horses should not have pain, not show signs of being unwell, and not try to move away from the pressure. If they do, there is accumulated tension or injury at hand, which must be treated.

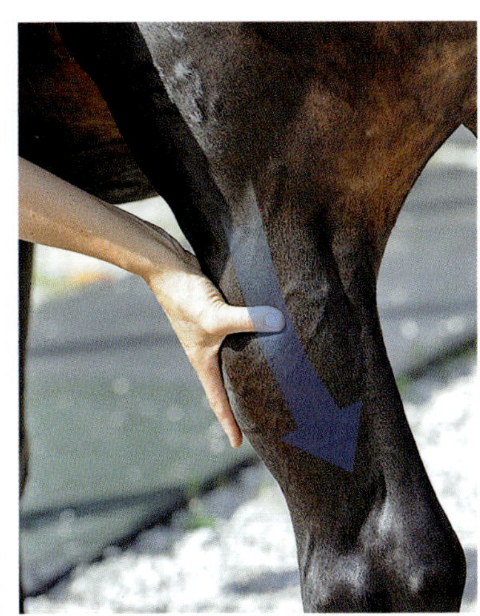

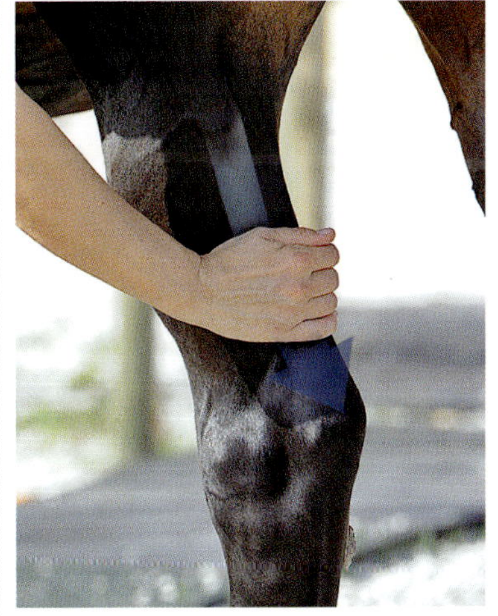

My Tip

Palpate the tendons and joints of the lower limbs on a daily basis, feeling for increased temperature or swelling—even when you're not planning a treatment.

Massage—The Art of Healing with Your Hands

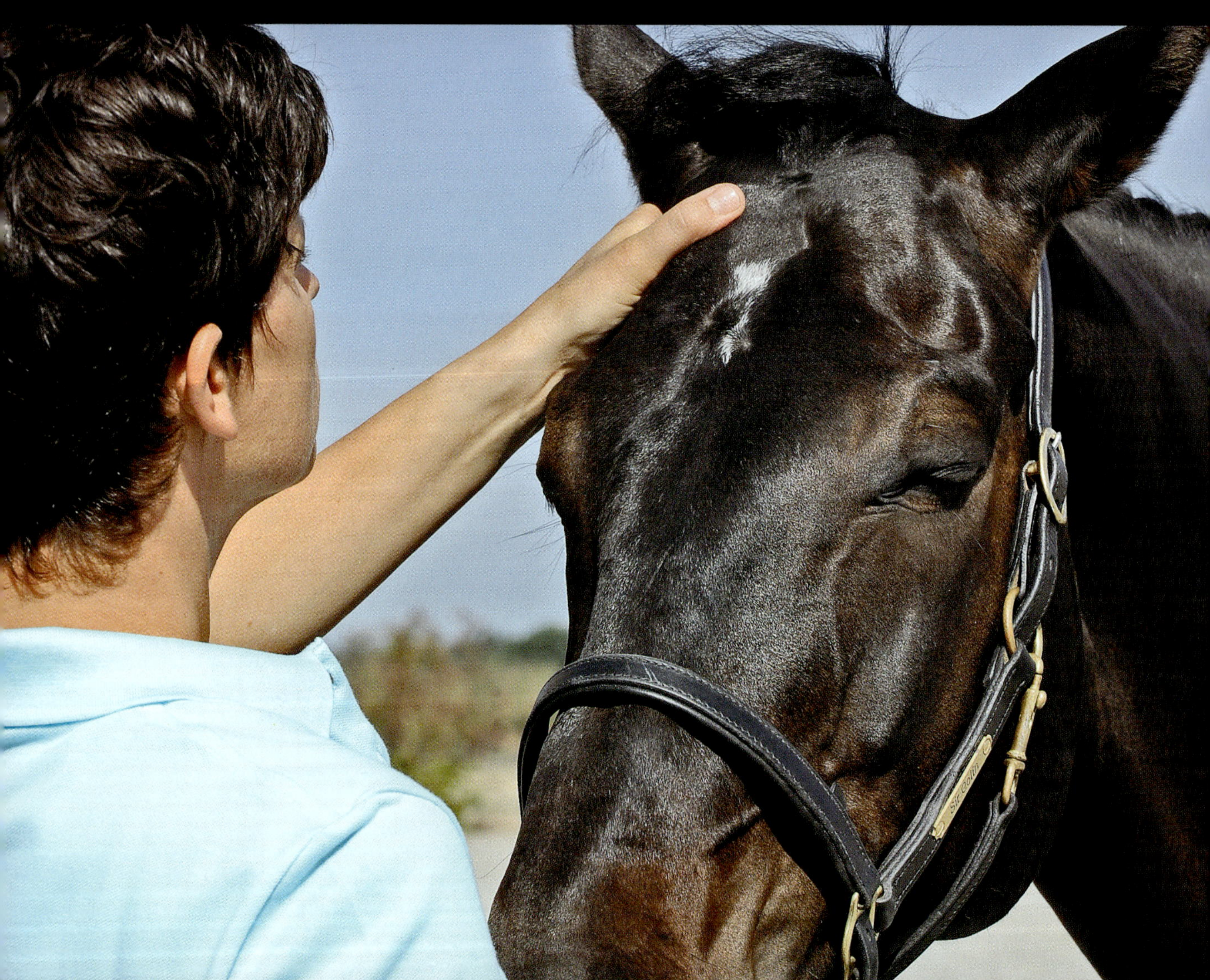

I'm sure you've enjoyed a massage at least once in your life, so you know how wonderful and good this is. On the other hand, you also know how much a massage can hurt if you have tension in your muscles, and how good it can feel when the pain lets go. Perhaps, while grooming your horse, you've experienced that he becomes unsettled, moves away from the brush and even turns with his body, as if to say, "That hurts!" In contrast, you've probably experienced a horse leaning into your brush and communicating with his body language when he likes something, and that he's enjoying the pressure and massage you've provided by brushing him.

The word "massage" is Arabic in origin and means "to touch or feel." Massage is among the oldest healing methods in existence. Yet, incredibly, every culture on earth still considers massage "cutting-edge." To me, this shows what enormous effects this form of treatment is having today and will continue to have in the future. Even in the animal world, massage is a part of wellness. Think about animal films in which you've watched elephants, apes, and deer as they scratch one another. Horses in a herd will also often stand and massage each other with their lips and teeth.

Of course, massage methods have evolved over time. There is sports massage, fitness massage, fascia-release techniques, trigger point massage, and more. From these original healing methods, other manual therapies such as osteopathy and chiropractic have developed. These treatment methods are very specialized and should only be administered by professionals. All these techniques have shown that they are highly applicable and can be wonderfully incorporated for animals as well as people. I have colleagues who have successfully treated dogs, cats, hamsters/guinea pigs and birds as well as zoo animals such as elephants.

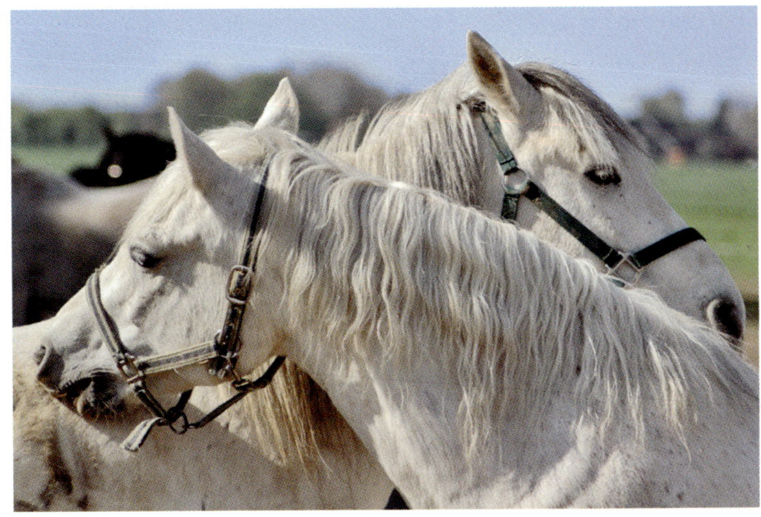

Scratching a friend's back is also a form of massage.

In this book, I'd like to introduce you to classical massage, techniques that you can apply to your horse without worrying that you'll hurt him or cause him to be unwell (provided that you observe your horse's body language and pay attention to any contraindications—see p. 128). In classical massage, the therapist uses her hands to give the massage. The different types of touch and pressure bring the desired result—relaxation or stimulation. It's a treatment of the soft tissue; this means, you'll be influencing muscles, tendons, ligaments, and fascia. In the application sections, I'll elaborate on different techniques in the practical/hands-on part of this chapter. A prerequisite for giving a massage is that you have basic knowledge of your horse's anatomy (see chapter 2, p. 18). Only then will you be able to distinguish between different structures and apply the described techniques. I'll guide you through how to give both preventive and preparatory massages.

The Effects of Massage

Almost every day, you experience how good the effects of massage can be. When you have pain somewhere, such as tension in your neck, back, or shoulders thanks to working at your computer for a long time, you automatically touch the painful spot. By putting your hands on and rubbing the painful spot, hormones (endorphins) are let loose in your body, which alleviate the pain and increase circulation.

Further effects of massage include:
- Regulates muscular tension.
- Loosens scars and soft-tissue adhesions that have been there for a year or less.
- Dissolves blockages in the veins and lymph system.
- Has a supportive influence on the internal organs via reflex arcs (neural pathways), such as when a horse is suffering from colic.
- Provides mental relaxation, which means reduction of stress hormones and slowing of the respiratory system.
- Restores full mobility.
- Improves performance.
- Improves the relationship between rider and horse.

As you've just read, the effects of massage are both amazing and multi-faceted because it can have an influence on the horse's entire body. During a massage, you'll notice your horse relax quickly, as the massage is influencing the autonomic nervous system. Because many muscles are directly and indirectly connected to one another, it is possible that tension in the neck area will also lead to tension in the musculature of the hindquarters. When you give a massage that relieves problems in the neck, you've often also treated and brought relief to secondary problems in the hindquarters.

Where Should You Massage?

Just as when you palpate the horse, you want to be in a familiar, quiet space when you give him a massage. In addition, you want somewhere with a wall for the horse to lean on. Make sure it's a place where you won't be distracted. For example, a barn aisle where other horses are constantly going to be led past just isn't appropriate.

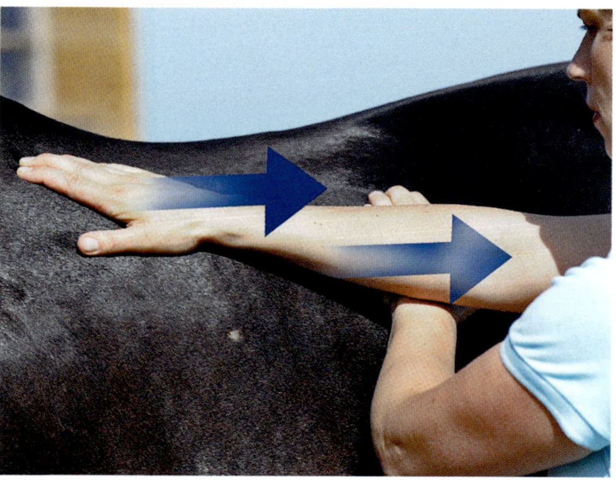

It's best to massage with your hands. Thanks to their warmth and energy, your horse will relax more.

In the beginning, it's helpful if you can have a helper hold the horse. Otherwise, tie him loosely with a lead rope. Personally, I then like to tie the horse's lead rope to a thin piece of baling twine, so that if the horse gets startled and pulls back, the baling twine will rip (see "Tying," p. 201).

What Tools Should You Use?

Mainly, you'll use your hands. In time, your fingertips will get more sensitive. You'll learn to differentiate between various structures and how a possible place of tension feels.

By working with your hands, you'll exude warmth and improved stimulation. You personally are brought closer to your horse. You can feel how the body tissue responds to your treatment, and adjust the level of pressure accordingly. Therefore, working with your hands is preferable to using a tool.

Hint: Massage is also an opportunity to clean your horse! If you have little time for grooming and massage, you can use your hand instead of the brush. You'll see how clean and shiny his coat will become—and how dirty your hands get!

There are also tools to support your massage available on the market, such as rollers, massage balls, vibrating devices. For you as a beginner masseuse, it may make the work easier at first, but you won't be able to feel your horse's most delicate responses. The sensitivity of your hands, the warmth and energy that they bring, are the "icing on the cake" of massage. You can quickly develop the sensitivity of your hands and, thereby, discover the necessary flexibility within your technique.

> **My Tip**
>
> If you've never given a massage before, it may be that you can't feel the difference between various phenomena in the body; for example, whether the muscle is hard or not. Don't doubt yourself. When you concentrate on this work and always keep this guidebook nearby, you'll learn quickly.

How Hard Should You Press?

The amount of pressure that you should (or can) use depends completely on your horse. Getting a massage should always be comfortable for him. Although a massage with light pressure will be superficial, the effects of the massage will "domino" to the deeper tissue as well. Therefore, strength is not necessarily required in order to give an effective massage. Pressure that's too hard is always bad. You're not accomplishing anything when the muscles get even more tense or you have to "fight" with your horse because the massage is hurting him.

Fact: Massage is not rocket science. Anyone can learn it.

After your horse has become used to the massage and has released tension in his superficial muscles, you can slowly increase the pressure. But, keep in mind that the muscles on the shoulder blade are thinner than the muscles of the hindquarters, for example. For you, this means you'll need to use less pressure where there are thinner muscles. In contrast, you can press harder on the thickly muscled hindquarters if you find there's no pain there.

You can review how hard to press on various body parts in chapter 6, "Palpation." There, the amount of pressure is spelled out.

Hint:
As hard as necessary and as softly as possible.

Please remember that horses have varying levels of sensitivity and tolerance for pain and pressure. Therefore, a Thoroughbred with much more sensitive nerves might react to gentle palpating, more so than a Appaloosa.

> **My Tip**
>
> In the beginning, you're still developing a comfortable routine and learning how to touch the horse. You should proceed with caution and care. You must both get used to this new experience.

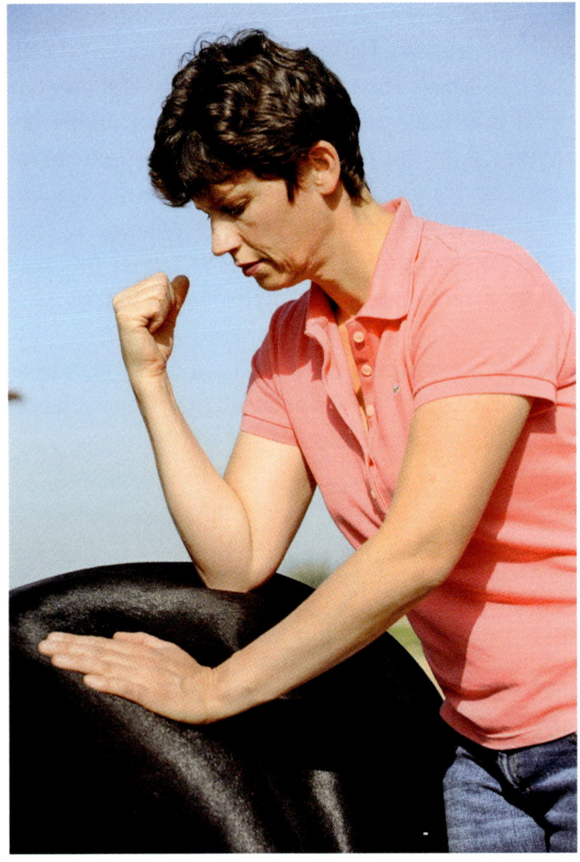

Use direct pressure to loosen tension in the croup muscles.

these horses will also benefit from your massage. Once or twice a week will suffice here.

On the other hand, there are "hot" horses, such a Thoroughbreds, who tend to get agitated, are spooky and consequently get tense easily when ridden. These horses should be massaged as often as possible, even daily, in order to lower tension in the body. You'll notice that your horse will become calmer and more relaxed to work with. In the case that you find it difficult to massage daily, keep in mind that even 10 minutes a day after riding is very helpful.

A second reason for massage is when there's chronic pain, tension, and/or injury in the muscles. As long as there's tension and pain, a daily massage is advisable. How much time you need to spend depends on the degree and severity of the problem. You'll see how your commitment pays off. Within a few days, you'll see that your horse has more mobility and less pain.

With an injury, you first need the advice of your veterinarian and/or physical therapist in order to determine a treatment plan and to learn which massage techniques are appropriate for the horse at this time.

> *Fact: Massages will do your horse good, regardless of how long or how frequently they happen.*

How Often Should You Massage?

Theoretically, you could give your horse a massage every day—he'd love it. But, being a realist, I know this is impossible! However, there are two different reasons to give a treatment.

The first reason is preventive, a massage that doesn't need to be given daily. Therefore, the frequency of treatment depends on what type of horse you have. There are horses that innately tend to be more relaxed. They're not easily agitated and don't spook or react too quickly. These horses do not tend to develop muscular tension. Therefore, they don't need preventive massage on a regular basis. Having said that, every massage does some good and

How Long Should a Massage Last?

The length of treatment depends on your horse's reaction. If he's nervous and uneasy, you should begin with no longer than about 10 minutes per day. After he gets used to it, when you notice that he's enjoying the massage, you can lengthen the time to between 20 and 30 minutes. Once you and your horse have become accustomed to it, after five or six treatments, there is no longer a time limit as long as your horse remains patient. Your horse will show you when he's had enough. He'll become uneasy and distracted.

With horses that enjoy the treatment and relax into it right away, you can begin with about 20 to 30 minutes of massage.

If your horse has pain points, you should massage them for no longer than three to four minutes, and at most just every other day. When you massage a pain point, you are causing an "inflammation," which can be very painful the next day.

Of course, with the first treatment, your horse may have a reaction such as stiffness or not wanting to move. If your horse reacts this way, just longe him for the next two days, turn him out to pasture, or just work him very lightly. But don't be afraid—it's simply a reaction that will lead to the body healing itself. Because of the possibility of an initial reaction of this kind, I don't recommend giving the first massage right before a big event, such as a show you must attend, clinic or long trail ride. Once your horse knows and loves massage, you won't need to give this a second thought. Massage will do your horse good, even before an important performance.

When to Massage— Before or After Work?

I'm often asked whether it's better to massage before or after work. As a preventive measure, I recommend massaging after work. Your horse has used energy at work and will, therefore, be calmer, as long as he doesn't have any major pain while working that will cause him to be frantic and tense after work.

If your horse does have accumulated tension, however, I advise you to massage the tense area before exercising him. Why? To prepare the muscles and get them ready to work: through massage (and stretching) muscular tension is alleviated,

circulation is increased, and the affected muscles can both contract and stretch more optimally during work. The horse's muscles will become more supple, which contributes to a more ground-covering stride and more powerful movement that's full of impulsion. Finally, the pre-work massage stimulates muscle growth and stretch. Consider this: when your horse has a tense muscle or chronically tense muscle group, circulation to this area is reduced and the muscles lose their ability to stretch and contract. Over either a short or long period of time, your horse will lose muscular strength and elasticity.

> *Fact: During a British study, muscles of the hindquarters were massaged for 30 minutes and afterward there was a measurably larger range of movement (Hill & Crooks, 2012).*

An Important Tip for Treating Muscular Tension

In order to achieve optimal, lasting muscle relaxation, it is wise to also treat the affected muscles with massage and stretching after the horse has worked.

> *Fact: When a muscle is tight, it will not be able to get stronger!*

My Tip

With a really tense horse, I recommend leading him around for 10 to 20 minutes after the massage. This allows his body to perceive its new mobility and relaxed state.

The First Time!

The first time you massage your horse, he'll be curious, but perhaps also confused. Some horses respond by becoming nervous, impatient, or even defensive. Don't be discouraged by a defensive reaction. Stay calm, breathe deep, and remain relaxed throughout. Check in with how you are touching the horse. In these cases, it's advisable to stick with "long strokes." Your first goal should be for your horse to relax and get used to massage.

If you have a large horse, have a block available to stand on. This also allows you to observe your horse well from above. A slip-resistant and stable grooming stool box is good for this. Or, an upside-down milk crate will work as well. Just make sure that any larger openings on the side are covered, so that your horse can't get his foot caught in them.

> ### My Tip
>
> **If you trigger a pain reaction, try stroking this area with much less pressure. Breathe in deep as you do so and stay relaxed. This behavior will transfer to your horse.**

Pain or Discomfort

For many horses, stiffness, muscle pain, and sore muscles are a part of their long-term daily life. As a rider, you'll most often first notice how painful and hard the muscles are by palpating and massaging the horse. It may be, however, that your horse has been trying to communicate his pain or discomfort to you for a long time with his body language. Watch for signals during grooming, tacking, untacking, palpation, and massage. With their body language, horses will directly convey where it's painful for them. Try to adjust for this and to accept what they can tolerate.

Are Side Effects Possible?

As with any healing treatment, there can be "side effects." These won't be of a pathological nature, but rather will present as physiological processes that can differ from animal to animal. You should tend to interpret them as positive reactions.

✋ **During massage, a painful reaction may be triggered. As a result, your horse is likely to be more sensitive to touch and move worse for a few days.**

✋ **For a day or two, the horse is tired and lackluster at work.**

These "side effects" are physiological in nature and should only occur after the first few treatments, if at all. After the third massage, the "side effects" should be noticeably lessened.

When Shouldn't You Give a Massage?

You should only give a massage when there are no major physical symptoms or injury. Regard this form of treatment as preventive. When your horse is injured, it's important that you consult his veterinarian, or your horse is first treated by a physical therapist. The physical therapist can show you how to best support the horse's rehabilitation.

When the following symptoms are present, don't massage your horse:

✋ **He has an acute injury, swelling, or localized hot spot. You should leave out these parts. Wait at least five to seven days to allow the tissue to heal. With such symptoms, please first consult the vet or physical therapist for advice!**

✋ **The presence of fever (a normal temperature is 99–101 F/37.2–38.3 C). A fever should always be taken seriously as fever accompanies illness.**

✋ **He has a skin infection.**

✋ **A tumor is present.**

✋ **He has neuritis.**

✋ **When thrombosis is suspected.**

You'll notice that your horse will show you where he likes to be massaged and where he doesn't. If there's a place the horse doesn't like to be touched, you should check your grip and reduce the pressure significantly. Please monitor the temperature in this spot. You can best feel this with the back of your hand. Slowly glide your hand over a large area and feel for any difference in temperature. It can be a sign of local inflammation or a hematoma. You know from your own experience that you don't want to be massaged on a bruise. You can avoid this spot for now and try again in two to three days. If this spot always remains sensitive and feels warmer, I advise you to consult a professional.

Hint: If you're not sure whether it's appropriate to massage your horse, always consult your veterinarian or physical therapist first.

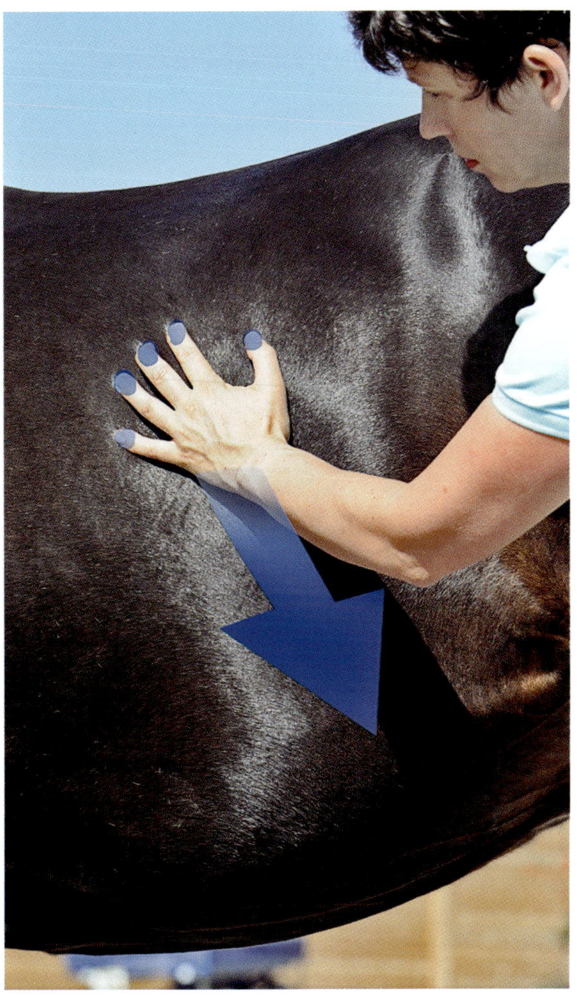

Massaging the intercostal muscles.

Massage in Practice

Hint: At the beginning of a treatment, you should first touch the horse with a light pressure. If the horse tolerates the pressure, you can slowly increase it.

There are many massage techniques that will relieve blockages and tension in the soft tissue, but touch can also increase muscular tension. I'll introduce you to the main techniques that I use, which belong to my standard practices. These techniques are:

1 **Long strokes**
2 **Long strokes with the fingers**
3 **Compression**
4 **Kneading**
5 **Twisting**
6 **Direct pressure**
7 **Circling**
8 **Shaking/vibration**
9 **Knocking/chopping**

Choosing Your Technique

What technique you select will depend on the "therapeutic" goals you have set. For example, when a horse is experiencing a lot of muscular pain, those techniques that lower tension would be most relevant. For these reasons, you'd choose from the first seven of those techniques listed above.

In contrast, the last two techniques can be applied before work in order to warm up the muscles and encourage quicker muscular contraction. These techniques can also be suitable for relieving tension, if they are applied carefully.

Always work with both hands. If you only need one hand to give the massage, it's advantageous to always keep your other hand in contact with the horse as well. This has a calming effect on the horse. With this hand, you can also feel how the horse is doing. Is he relaxed or tense?

> **My Tip**
>
> In the beginning, allow yourself time for each treatment. The horse will relax more quickly, when you are calm around him. When giving a whole-body massage, it's advisable to begin at the head/neck. Doing so fosters the horse's trust.

Always begin with long strokes over the entire body. Next, treat individual body parts; for example, first the

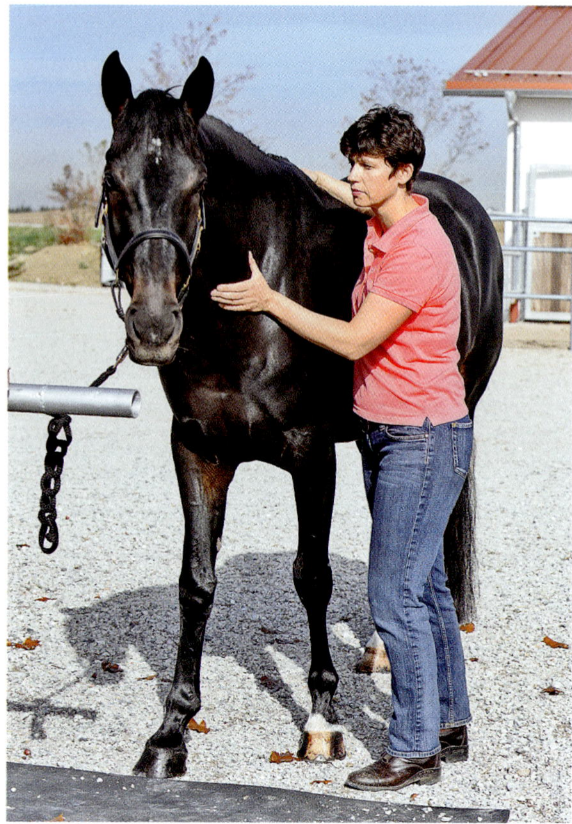

It's more comfortable for your horse if you always have contact with both hands.

neck and shoulder region on both sides, then both sides of the back and continue along until you reach the hindquarters. The order in which you apply specific techniques doesn't matter, except that long strokes should always be used to begin the treatment.

Massaging your horse can be exhausting for you, the therapist. Try to work ergonomically; this means with good posture, so that you don't need a massage yourself the next day! Use your whole body, which will require less arm strength and allow you to massage longer.

To protect your back, it's good to stand with a slight bend in your knees. In addition, when you massage the legs, you should bend at your knees (not from your back), so that your trunk remains straight and stable.

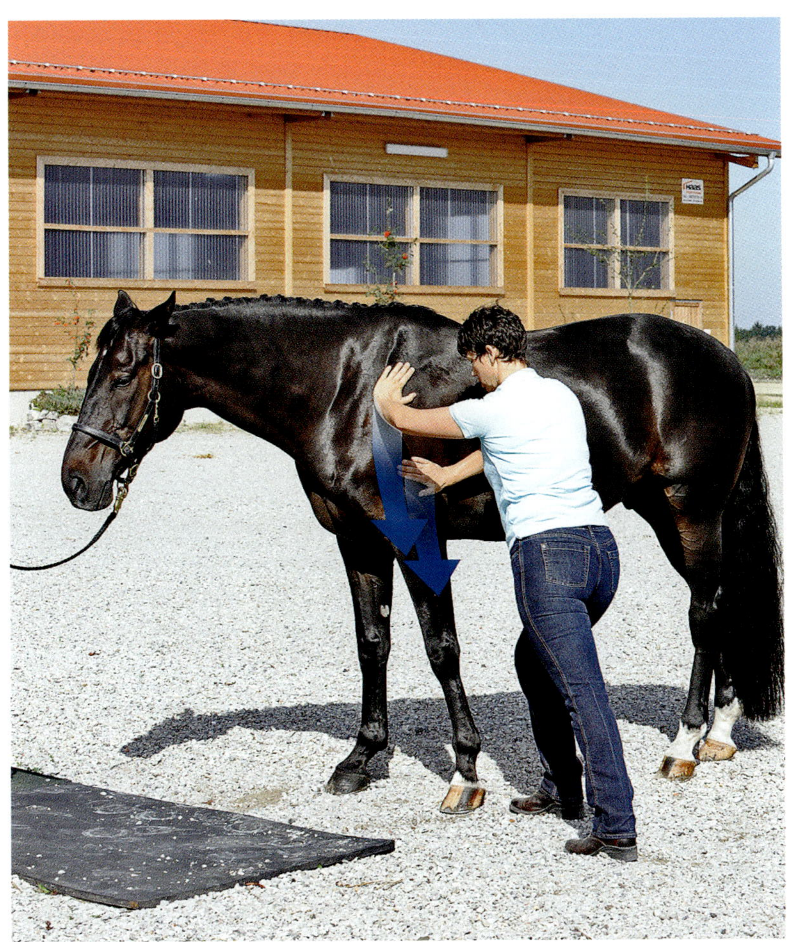

Use your whole body when you give a massage, as shown here with a long-stroke technique. This will save you lots of strength.

1 Long Strokes

How-To

Always begin with long strokes. Stroke with long, quiet movements that last two to three seconds. If your horse is nervous, you can also go even more slowly with this technique. Always switch back and forth between both hands. When one-hand strokes, put the other hand on the horse, so that one hand is always "busy" with stroking. Use the whole flat of your hand. As you do so, your hand will adopt the shape of your horse's body. Follow the direction the hair grows. This technique is the perfect preparation for a massage, during which your horse can get used to this new touch.

Effects

When applying long strokes, you are manually influencing the body fluids, such as blood and lymph, to drain. Thereby, these fluids are activated, and their backflow is increased and supported. As a result, the tissues are supplied with increased blood flow. In turn, this means

HInt: Keep your trunk straight and stable (like you do when you ride).

My Tip

Don't forget: your horse is an individual. Horses respond differently to various massage techniques and not every horse will tolerate every technique. Please pay close attention to your animal!

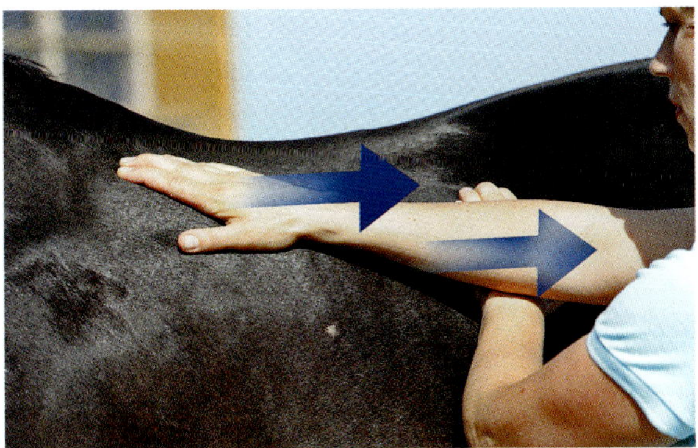

Always stroke with the whole flat of your hand and in the direction the hair grows.

increased delivery of oxygen and nutrients while more "waste" is transported out.

Long strokes influence the nervous system and relax body tissue. They improve tissue mobility (think about muscular connective tissue) and lightly stretch the muscle fascia.

When applying this technique, make sure you're not overstretching with the middle and end joints on your fingers. The whole hand should glide flat over the horse.

If your horse is oversensitive or uneasy, stay with light, rhythmic strokes until he relaxes.

Hint: Long strokes should be the technique you use most often. Always go back to this technique during your treatment and in between other techniques.

2 Long Strokes with the Fingers
How-To

Long strokes with the fingers are like the last technique, except that here the grip of the fingers comes into play more. You'll keep your fingers spread and bent slightly, and the whole palm of the hand should still have contact with the coat. Your fingertips apply

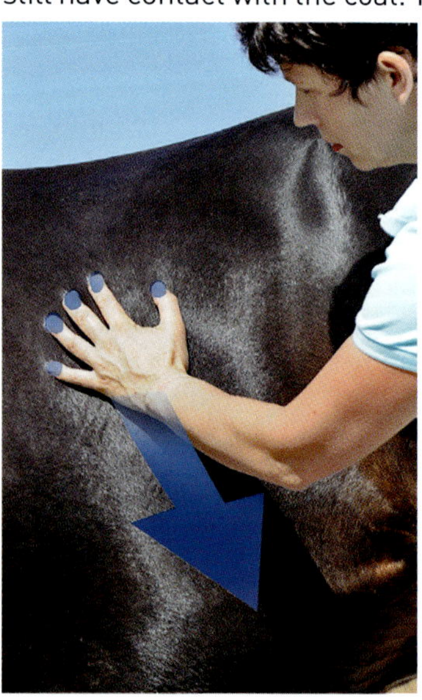

more pressure now. With this technique, I like to alternate which arm is leading as this rhythmic change in touch relaxes and calms the horse. Many therapists work with their hands parallel when executing long strokes, and long strokes with fingers. I personally don't find this to be advantageous, but you'll simply need to try it for yourself. With this technique, each stroke should again last two to three seconds.

Effects

Long strokes with the fingers soothe and calm the muscles you're working on. In addition, there will be a light, localized stretch of the muscle fibers.

3 Compression
How-To

Compressions are rhythmic, pumping movements directly on the belly of the muscle. Use the heel

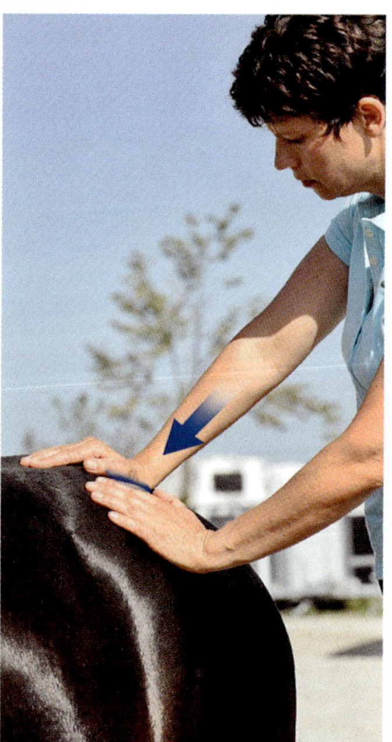

of your hand or your fist. The pressure will also move the skin, a little like you're kneading dough. (The movements are not gliding or stroking.) This massage technique should compress the muscle. In order to be able to apply more strength, you can use both hands.

At the beginning of the treatment, work with less pressure, which can gradually increase. Your horse will show you whether he's comfortable with the amount of pressure in that he'll push into the pressure or move away instead. This technique is suitable for the large muscles of the neck and shoulder. I especially use compression on the muscles of hindquarters. Always execute this technique in a rhythmic manner, about one second per compression and not longer than two to three minutes in one spot. In between compressions, use long strokes.

Physical Therapy for Horses

Effects

With this technique, you're also stimulating the deep musculature. It's intended to loosen tension there and especially to "pump" toxins (lactate) out of the muscles. As a result of compression, the muscles' metabolism is again activated.

> *Hint: You'll quickly notice that this work on the muscles will make them looser and softer. Despite the "strong" handling, horses enjoy this form of touch. It's a good idea to use this technique before applying "direct pressure."*

4 Kneading
How-To

Put both hands on the area you intend to treat and use your thumbs to make a rhythmic, circular movement toward your pointer finger.

I recommend using this technique in a one to two second rhythm to relax your horse. Going more quickly, approximately one touch per second, is more stimulating and often uncomfortable for the horse. Typically, we use both hands for kneading and the thumbs do the work. However, for small places such as on a tendon, we might use one hand and work with just a finger (see p. 138).

For larger surfaces, you can add your body weight in order to apply more pressure. And please don't forget: always return to long strokes.

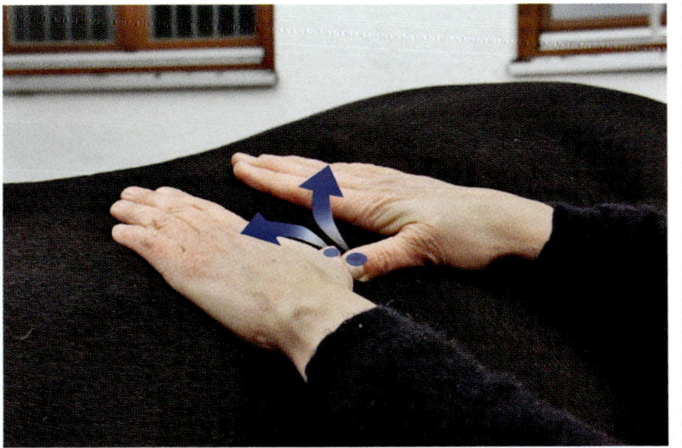

Effects

Kneading is really effective for muscular tension, knots, blockages, scar tissue, and small muscle spasms (trigger points). Kneading is enormously stimulating to circulation and metabolism. You can apply this technique for relaxation, but also to prepare for a performance, such as at a competition.

5 Twisting
How-To

Lay the palms of your hands a bit apart from one another on the muscle you wish to treat. Move both hands away from one another, just a little, and then push the muscles toward one another. You'll use the heel of your hand when you're pushing away, and the pads of your fingertips when pulling toward you. As you do so, try to lift the muscle lightly.

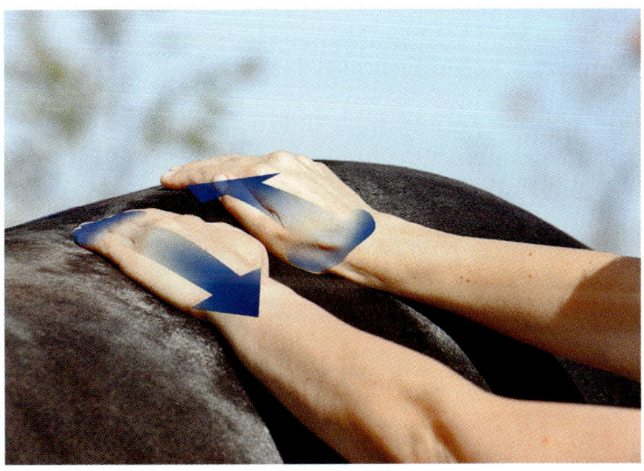

You can also loosen up the crest this way. Hold the crest with both hands. One hand brings the crest toward you, while the other hand pushes it away from you. Hold both sections for two to five seconds and then release them again. Then, switch.

Effects

With this connection, you mobilize the tissue, possibly dissolve adhesions and improve circulation. Use this technique all along the crest and you'll be astounded at how loose the neck and back muscles become!

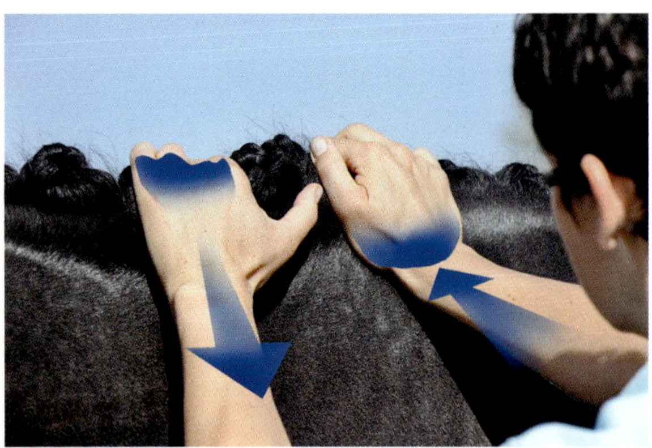

6 Direct Pressure
How-To

Using your finger, your thumb (for small, superficial pain points) or your elbow (for larger, deeper pain points) apply direct pressure to the musculature and adding your body weight.

Direct pressure should be held for between 30 and 60 seconds, so muscle fibers that have become stuck together and accumulated tension can release. It's a good sign when you get the feeling that the tissue is gradually giving way beneath your fingers. Develop the pressure, as you did with the compression technique. Meaning, you begin with less pressure and increase it slowly and steadily. When finished, you want to slowly reduce the pressure again. Finally, take the pressure off and apply long strokes.

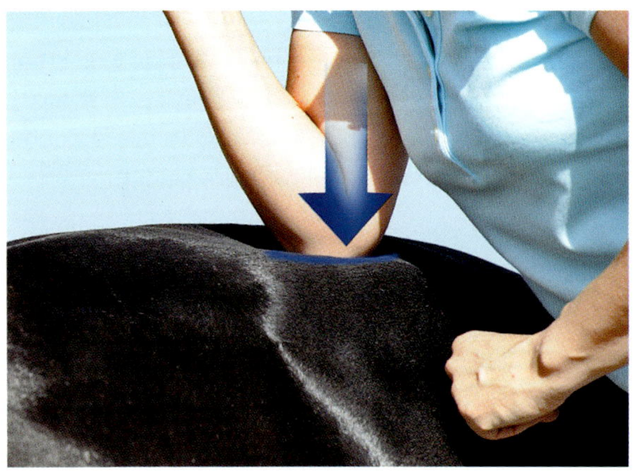

> *Hint: You'll figure out which areas of the body require direct pressure based on your horse's reactions. And you can sense it beneath your fingers. There are small knobs or knots and the tissue will be harder in these places. When the horse moves away from pressure and his skin "shivers" at your pressure, you need to lighten up.*

Effects

With this massage technique, you can relieve deep adhesions and accumulated tension. When the adhesions and tension dissolve, circulation in this area will increase again and the muscle will be restored to full use.

> *Take Note: Always begin carefully. Increase the pressure slowly. As you do so, always observe your horse's reactions.*

7 Circling
How-To

In contrast to direct pressure, where you focus your pressure on just one point and work without movement, circling is a technique that maintains a constant medium pressure and where the fingers move in small circles. Use your thumb or finger. You can stay at a pain point or massage all along a muscle. When you're staying in one spot, then don't massage for longer than three to four minutes.

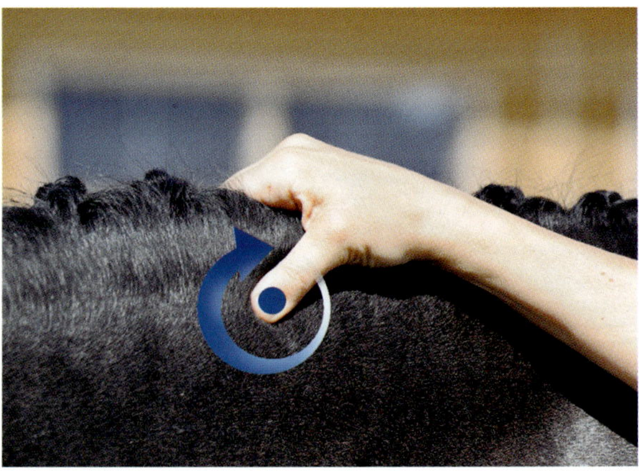

Effects

This technique relieves tension that doesn't lie as deep. It's appropriate for directly relieving pain, reducing tone and rapidly increasing circulation.

Hint: When you work on just one point, this rubbing massage can bring about a little inflammation, which stimulates the body to begin a healing process. Therefore, you may find the horse has a little pain in this area the next day. Until your horse is pain-free, you should administer this treatment only every other day in order to continually reactivate the healing process. Over time the horse should be less sensitive. Please don't strain your fingers.

8 Shaking/Vibration
How-To

You place your whole hand flat against the muscle belly with light pressure and push the muscle (the skin) back and forth quickly (a vibrating movement). Where the skin and muscle are harder, use your fingertips. Where you can grasp the muscle easily, such as with the *brachiocephalicus*, crest or hamstrings, you can hold on with your whole hand and shake. We call this a "C-Hold," because you're forming a half-circle with your hands. You can stay in one place, but please not for longer than three to four minutes, or you can glide your hand over the muscle shaking/vibrating as you do so. Then, you may keep it up even longer. (If you'd like, you can shake until your hands "fall off.")

Effects

Shaking is often used in sports medicine, since it uses mechanical stimulation. This is highly effective as a preparatory massage prior to a competition.

You can also apply vibration to arthritic joints. Thereby, you'll provide this joint with relief, regardless of whether it's an acute or chronic injury. This specific technique can be used, although generally speaking, massage is not recommended for this type of injury. (But, please, as always, consult with your veterinarian before you use it!)

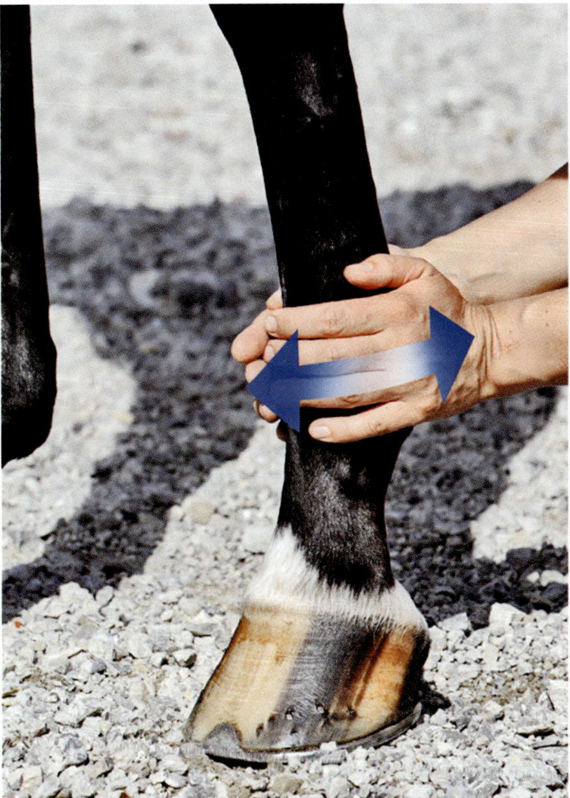

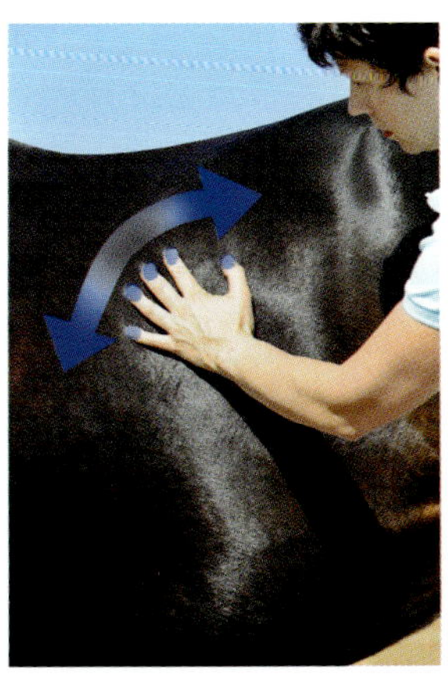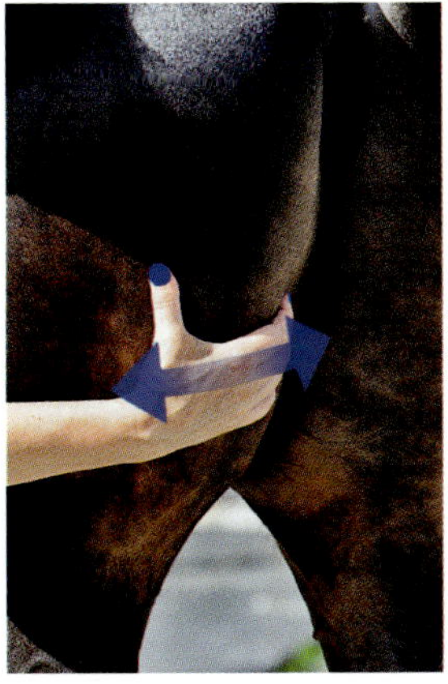

Hint: You've certainly seen this technique on TV, being used on soccer players! The player lies on the ground with his legs out in front of him and the therapist shakes his leg musculature—the metabolism is maintained/increased and the muscle tissue gets loose. This also works really well on horses.

9 Knocking/Chopping

These two techniques are really similar, so I'll describe them together. The one difference is how you hold your hands.

How-To—Knocking

This massage technique is done with the whole hand. You hold your fingers together lightly and slightly cupped. Your thumb is pressed against your pointer finger. The movement comes from your shoulder and your elbows are bent. The hand joints stay loose, and you knock on the horse's muscle, switching from right to left hand. On the larger muscle groups, such as the croup, you can work with more swing, while on smaller, flatter muscles, such as the shoulder blade, you'll use less swing. This movement is done rather quickly, two to four knocks per second.

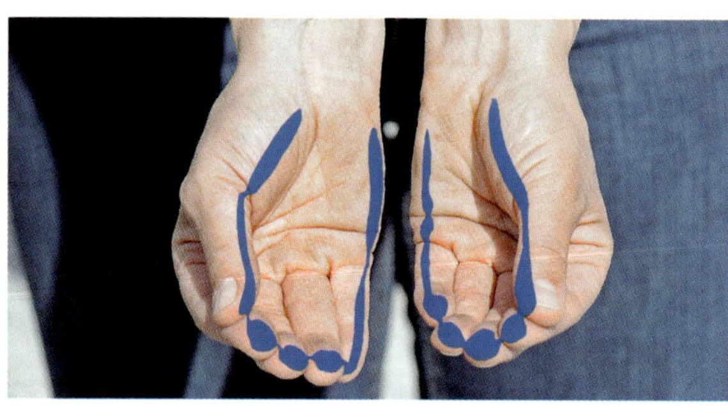

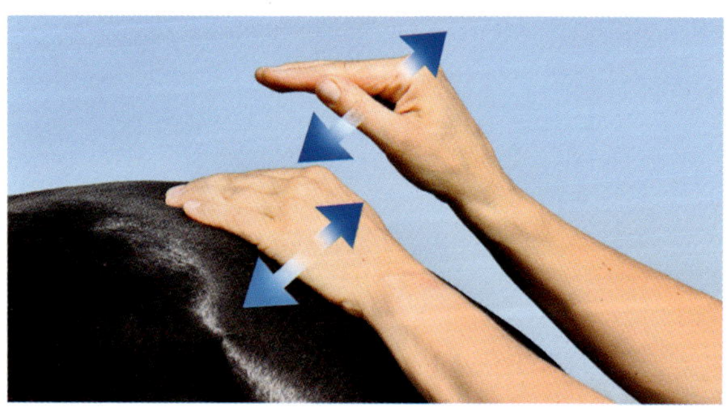

Hint: Knocking should never become painful for you. If your hands begin to "burn," your horse will also experience pain from the treatment. Check how you're holding your hands. You should be able to hear a hollow knocking sound!

How-To—Chopping

This technique is done with the side of the hand or a loose fist. Otherwise, it's just like knocking.

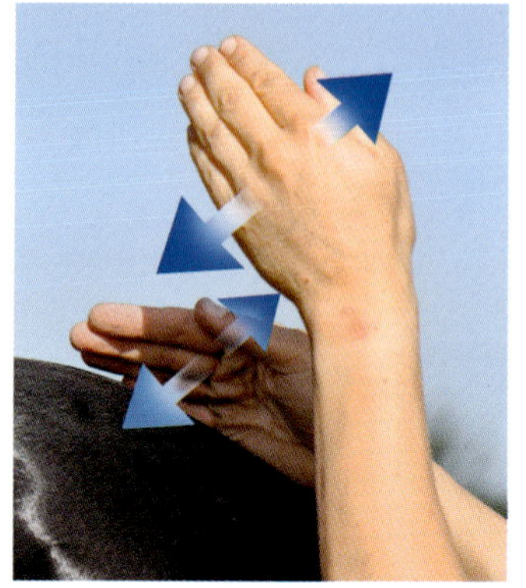

Effects

Knocking and chopping are used to increase muscular engagement/tone. It brings about small contractions in the musculature, which stimulates metabolism. Heat rises in the muscle. Knocking and chopping are good preparatory measures before a training or competition.

Contraindication

Please don't use knocking or chopping techniques in the loin region on pregnant mares and don't do this too strongly above the internal organs.

Special Massages

I've already described the basic techniques that can be applied to the neck, trunk, and hindquarters. Now, I'll provide a couple of additional tips for other areas of the body.

The Head

The head doesn't have many large muscles, but a head massage is still highly relaxing for your horse and this will indirectly affect his entire body. Only apply light pressure in this area, as you're massaging over many bones, nerves, and reflex points, and 15 to 20 minutes is enough time.

Using one or both hands, you can apply massage techniques such as stroking, kneading, and circling to the head. If you are using just one hand, place the other on the bridge of the horse's nose or hold the head from beneath, so that your horse is supported.

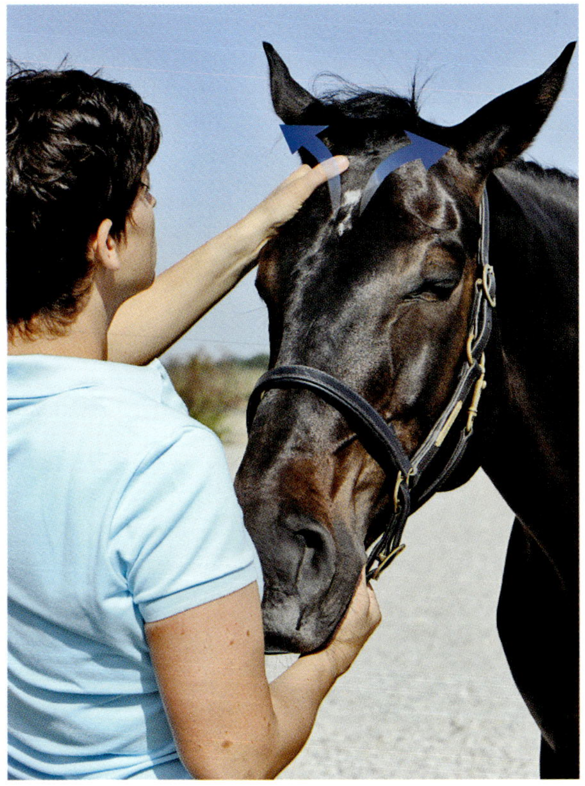

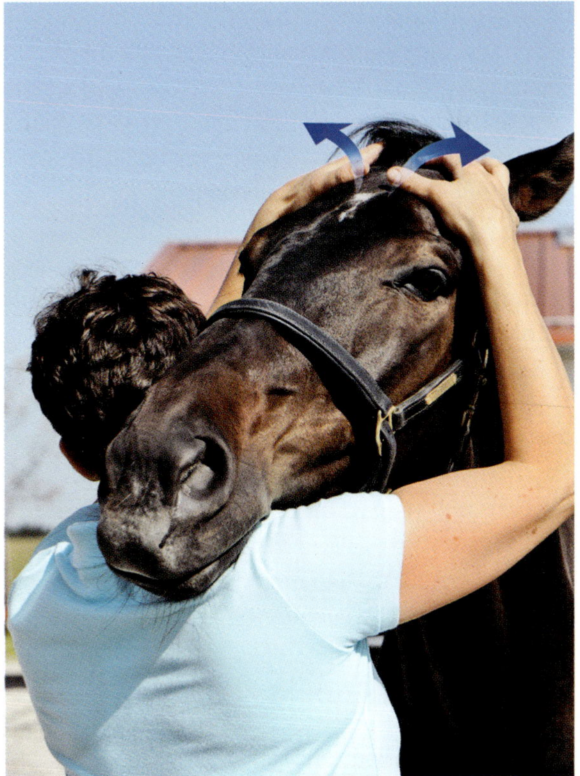

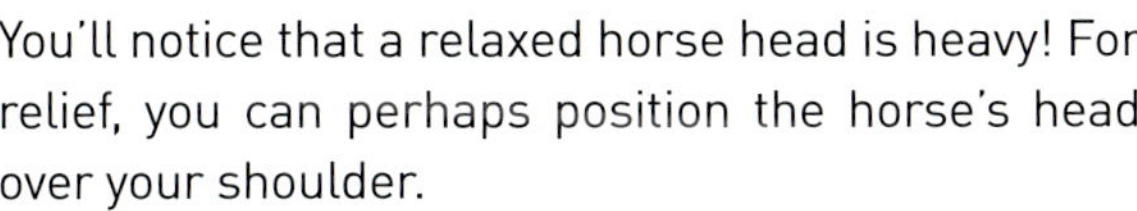

When you support your horse, he can relax even more.

You'll notice that a relaxed horse head is heavy! For relief, you can perhaps position the horse's head over your shoulder.

When you massage the muzzle area and gums, endorphins (hormones) are set free in the body, which relax and calm the horse.

Massaging the ears can work wonders. I've often experienced that nervous horses suddenly become relaxed and calm, thanks only to a light stroking of the ears. However, the ears can also be really sensitive, and a horse may not want the ears or surrounding area massaged at all. The reason may be tension in the poll or a bad experience. You need to respect this defensive behavior; in this case, skip massaging this area. After four or five massage sessions, you can try again, as the pain, discomfort, and fear may now be reduced. Your horse has become accustomed to massage and realized its comfortable and pleasant effects.

The Limbs

A horse's limbs work really hard and "enjoy" a good massage. You'll likely remember the relevant anatomy: the muscles that move the joints lie around the forearm. There's no muscular tissue from below the knee to the hoof. There, you'll find only tendons, joint capsules, blood vessels, and nerves. The blood supply to these soft tissues is poor.

Massage is highly suited for improving circulation in the limbs. Those techniques that are appropriate include long strokes, long strokes with fingers, compression, kneading, circling, shaking, and vibration.

You've certainly already experienced that your horse's legs become stocked up as a result of stall rest or unusually hard work on a warm day. Lymphatic fluid has built up in his legs. When this occurs, massage can really help as it stimulates the lymphatic pathways. When these symptoms occur, it's truly important that you massage *against* the direction the hair grows, meaning upward. You're trying to relieve the swelling and move the lymphatic fluid out. This path only runs upward.

Leg massage also begins with long strokes. Because you're trying to support the lymphatic pathways, you're going to apply a very light pressure, as if you're lovingly stroking someone on their face. You can also apply a compression massage. Place both hands around the leg. Push both hands together lightly, move your hands a half-hand higher, and repeat the pressure. The pressure should be as light as if you were holding an egg that you were not allowed to break between your hands. In this way, you'll travel up the entire leg. In doing so, you're pressing from the outside and supporting the lymphatic pathways as they transport lymph back to the lymph nodes, which can be found between the forelegs and hind legs.

the tug on the tendon, it's indispensable to massage the related muscle. Thereby, you can apply the techniques described above. Circling and shaking are suitable here. It's also helpful to lift the leg and bend it slightly, to relax and relieve the muscle.

Even once a tendon injury is no longer acute, you can massage it directly with circling. Because the tendon is smaller than a muscle, use your thumb and pointer finger. In this way, you'll use a "C-Cup" hand position to massage here. This helps prevent adhesions between the deep and superficial flexor tendons.

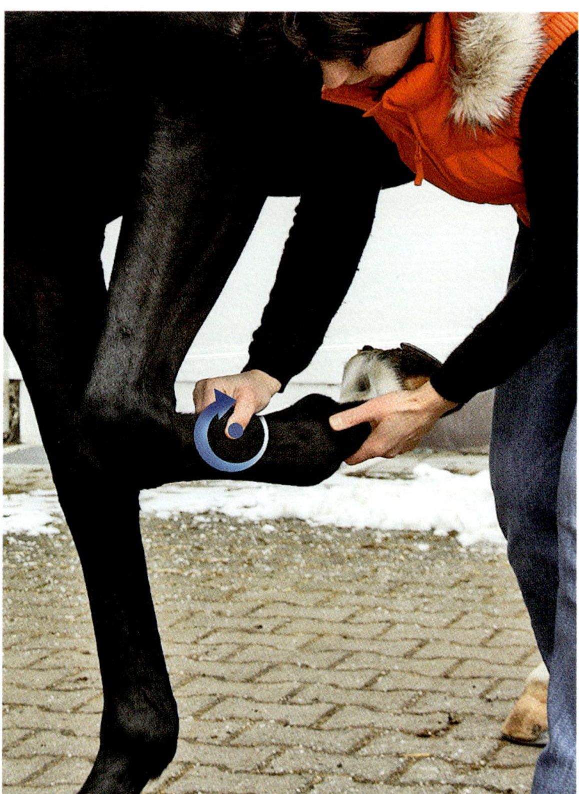

Massage the tendons. Working carefully, you can apply the circling technique using your thumb and pointer finger.

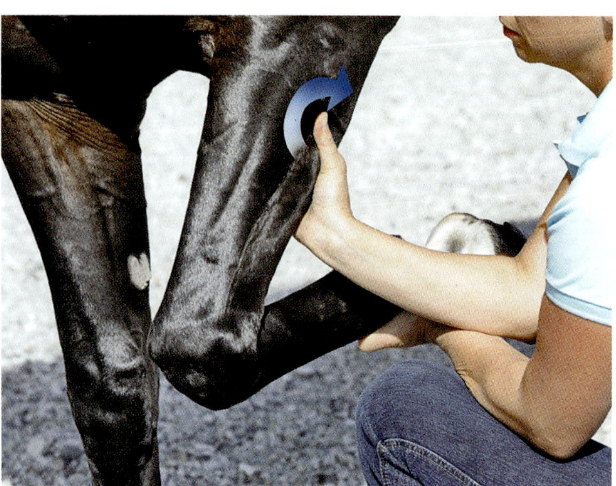

Massaging the forearm muscles. Here you can apply the circling technique using your thumb or your fingertips.

If your horse has a tendon injury, the related muscle, which is found on the forearm, will be tense as a result. There will be a constant, uncomfortable tug on the tendon, which can slow healing. To relieve

In addition, massage can be helpful for other injuries, such as ligament injuries to the lower limbs, in order to increase circulation and prevent the various structures from adhering to one another. For this, circling would be the first technique I'd use, but then shaking, vibration, and the "do-all" long strokes are also good. Vibration is perfect for joint injuries. But, for acute injuries, there's always the same rule: please consult your veterinarian before you begin massaging!

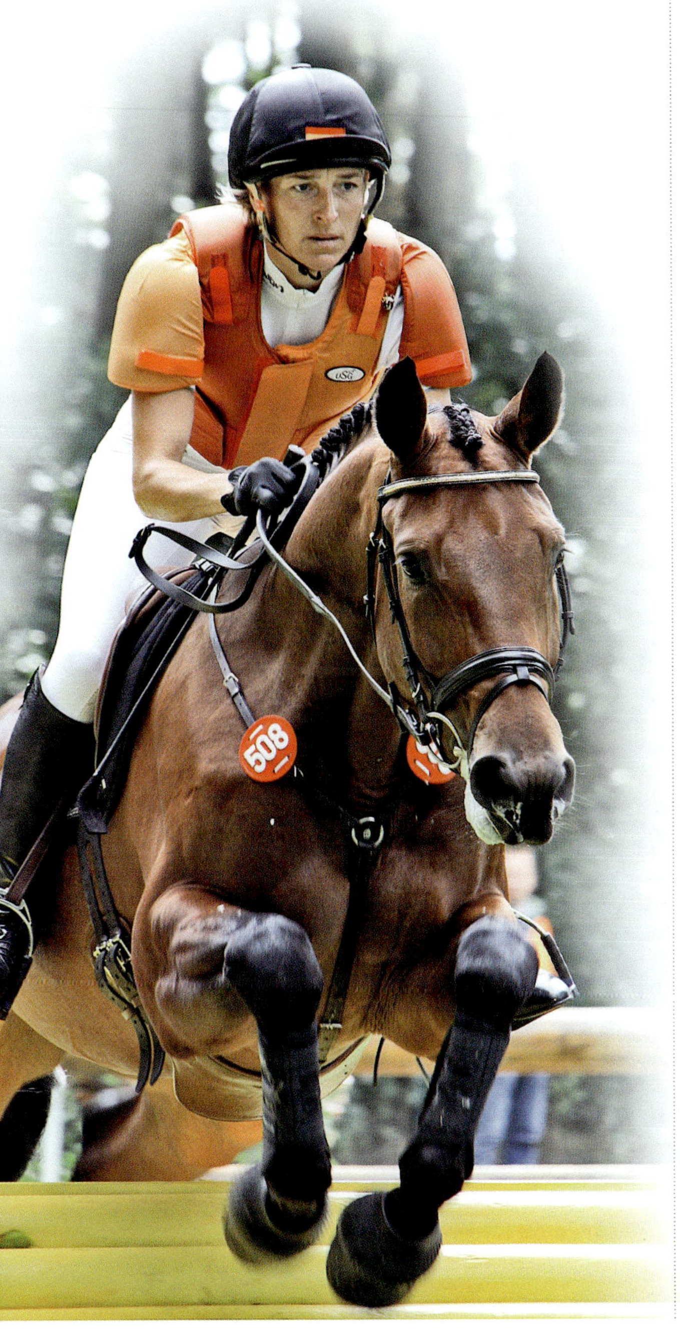

The Longissimus Dorsi and Abdominal Muscles

Over years of practice, I've realized that not all massage techniques should be used when the long muscles of the back are tense. The best techniques are long strokes and twisting. If the pressure in this area is too strong, you'll feel the muscle get tight under your hand. This muscle is tensing up as a reflex and your massage has become useless. This muscle absolutely responds well to a good back stretch, which I'll describe in the next chapter.

For the abdominal muscles, long strokes are also a great technique, though long strokes with fingers work well here, too. There are definitely horses that don't like to be touched in this area and get defensive. If your horse feels uncomfortable, you'd best just skip this area. Just like with the head, you can try again after four or five massage sessions.

To sum it up, all of these massage techniques are basic. You can modify them slightly, without losing the effects of the massage. By massaging your horse regularly, you'll quickly develop the ability to feel problems and also be able to select the right technique for solving the problem. Before each treatment, consider what goal you're hoping to reach with the selected application. To support the treatment, you could—and should—incorporate stretching exercises after the massage.

You are now familiar with many techniques within massage, but you don't need to use every one of them each time you massage your horse. Pick the most suitable technique for your horse. And, one thing is clear: there is nothing more satisfying than being able to relieve a horse (or person) from pain.

Mobilizing and Stretching

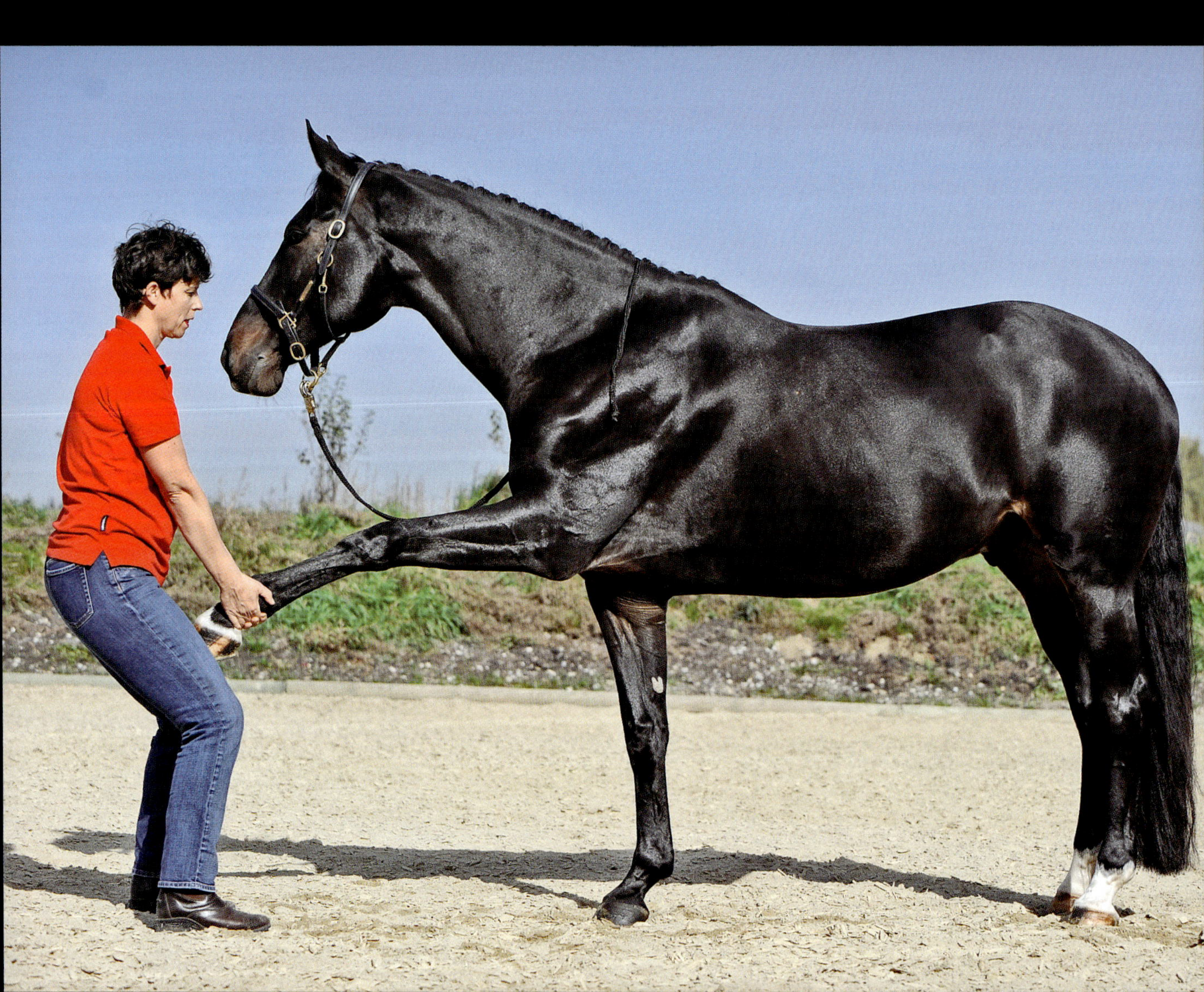

Do you want to be fitter? Slow down the aging process? Become more agile? With mobilization and stretching exercises, you can ensure your musculoskeletal system stays healthy and supple. For athletes, it's unthinkable to train without mobilizing and stretching. It's a routine element for the prevention of injury and a good opportunity for improvement in your sport of choice. With these two components, you're helping your horse's musculoskeletal system become more supple, looser, and more mobile and ensuring that your horse can move with more control, coordination, and speed. In this way, the horse's performance improves while the chances of injury and long-term damage to the musculoskeletal system greatly decline.

> *Fact: Mobilization exercises are intended to improve the mobility of one or more joints. Stretching is a way of improving the elasticity of the muscles.*

With a little smile, I consider that we riders are those athletes who spend the least amount of time mobilizing and stretching our own bodies. Or, do you see lots of riders who do these types of exercises before and after they ride? But we certainly need to be doing them! One example is the muscle group that lies along the inside of our thighs—our *adductors*! Riders always have tight adductors. Over time, without regular stretching, these muscles get short. Try doing a split. How far do you get? Probably not very far as almost all riders have shortened adductor muscles.

Studies have shown that we riders have much more pronounced adductor fascia than non-riders. Without stretching, the mobility of your hips will be reduced, which can lead to back problems/pain. And, both factors can severely limit your riding ability. What do you need to do in order to have a better seat in the saddle? That's right, you must stretch out this shortened muscular group.

It's not any different with animals. When dogs or cats stand up after a long nap, the first thing they do is stretch. The reason is that dogs and cats are hunters. These animals rest a lot, relatively speaking. When they stand up, they stretch in order to prevent shortening of their soft tissues and to prepare their muscles to react quickly. In contrast, horses, as flight and prey animals, need to maintain suppleness in their musculoskeletal system by moving constantly.

Unfortunately, however, many horses suffer from a shortened musculoskeletal system. When you consider that a large percentage of horses stand in a stall for 23 hours a day, it's clear that they're not getting enough movement to maintain their musculoskeletal systems. In addition, the work that horses do today is much different than in earlier times. Today, their main job is being sport horses. To manifest maximum performance, training for strength and endurance should be part of their standard training program, along with mobilizing and stretching exercises. Sure, regular gymnastic work and daily schooling require active mobilization, but often it's not enough. If we expect to have equine athletes, we need to treat them that way.

The point of mobilizing and stretching is to improve or maintain the maximum length of the fascia and muscle fibers. When the muscle fibers get longer, they are also more supple. Because the muscle belly is more pliable, the related tendons experience less pull and strain. Well-stretched muscles have improved blood circulation, so that metabolism can be optimized. In contrast, a shortened muscle will constantly pull on the place where the muscle attaches, where the tendon inserts on the bone. Through this constant pulling, this location will become strained, inflamed, and painful; for example, the tendon insertion of the neck muscle at the poll (for a horse), or tennis elbow (in a person).

The fascia also responds negatively to immobility. If not regularly moved or used, the fascia adheres and/or mats together and the entire musculoskeletal system is affected.

Example: Fasciae of the trunk, which are plaited, tend to be thicker and stronger. Through this tight connection, they reach over the entire back, beneath the sacroiliac area and run down into the hind limbs. Out to the side, they reach the oblique abdominal muscles and are also connected to the forehand.

These fasciae are the first thing you'll feel when you palpate the back. Fascia lies directly beneath the skin. Amazingly and unfortunately enough, many horses are already reactive to a light pressure on fascia due to pain. This is typical among horses who can no longer swing through their back and that are demonstrating an altered way of going due to back pain. They also react defensively to pressure when you touch the back.

When we ride, we're "sitting" on fascia. When the saddle doesn't fit well, riding is incorrect, or there's lameness present, the fascia will be affected sooner or later. Here's the good news: you can wonderfully treat the fascia and shortened musculature through the massage, mobilizing, and stretching exercises

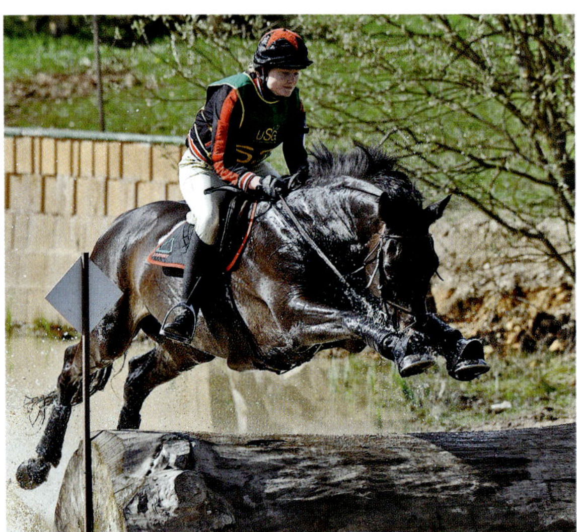

Here, the horse has jumped too early and must stretch really far in order to make it over the jump without hitting it. He'll only be able to do so if his musculoskeletal system is mobile and flexible.

as described in this book, helping them to become loose again or as a preventive measure.

Fact: You can improve your horse's overall performance and reduce the risk of soft tissue and joint injury with regular mobilization and stretching.

What Causes Shortening of Soft Tissue?

Muscles shorten for various reasons. Examples include:

- **Inactivity, Injury, Tension, and Pain**
  Your horse has sustained an injury and is now confined to his stall. Or he's experiencing acute or chronic pain, which has "forced" him to compensate by altering his way of going. As described above, adhesions or matting occurs when fascia or muscle accumulate tension and tighten up; then, muscle fibers stay bound together and are no longer able to free themselves. The individual muscle fibers get stuck in this contracted position, which will significantly reduce the muscle's ability to stretch/extend. The related joints will become less mobile.

- **Hard Training, Overuse, One-Sided Work**
  As I described in the introduction, muscles shorten really quickly during strength training or they can build up knots when overstretched in order to protect themselves. When worked one-sidedly, certain muscles are constantly developed, when those that are not involved, atrophy and shorten. For example, endurance and racehorses, that only train straight ahead over longer distances, lose their ability for longitudinal bend in the spine. Dressage horses that are worked in collection for too long (and often held there with the rider's hand), lose their ability to stretch over the long muscles of their back and/or in their neck muscles. As a result, they can no longer stretch forward and downward (long and low).

Physical Therapy for Horses

- **Poor Coordination, Bad Rider Posture, Unbalanced Rider**

These three conditions lead to a horse moving with shorter strides in order to keep his balance. You try taking long, relaxed steps while carrying a big, awkward backpack, or taking long steps on a slippery surface. It just doesn't work. In order to maintain your balance, you take smaller steps and tense up. Thereby, your active stretch will reduce. Over time, the muscles will become less and less able to stretch, as they are not being stimulated to stretch during movement. In addition, the joints will be affected, and their range of movement reduced.

I will now explain the difference between mobilization and active and passive stretching.

Mobilization

The term mobilization comes from the Latin *mobilis*, which means "moveable." Through mobilization, the range of movement of the joints and/or other body parts will improve. This is achieved through both passive movements (no effort required from the horse) and active movements (the horse himself does the stretch). These exercises can be done preventively but are also recommended when movement has become restricted. Mobilization exercises, such as carrot stretches (see p. 150) and back lifts (see p. 156) are active mobilization and stretching exercises: this means, the horse uses his own energy to execute them. On one hand, they're mobilizing, but on the other, they're also strengthening the muscles that are working. Thereby, the range of motion is large so that the opposite side of the body is being stretched. As a result, you're reaching three treatment goals with just one exercise!

Active Stretching

Active stretching takes place constantly when your horse moves. When moving forward, your horse

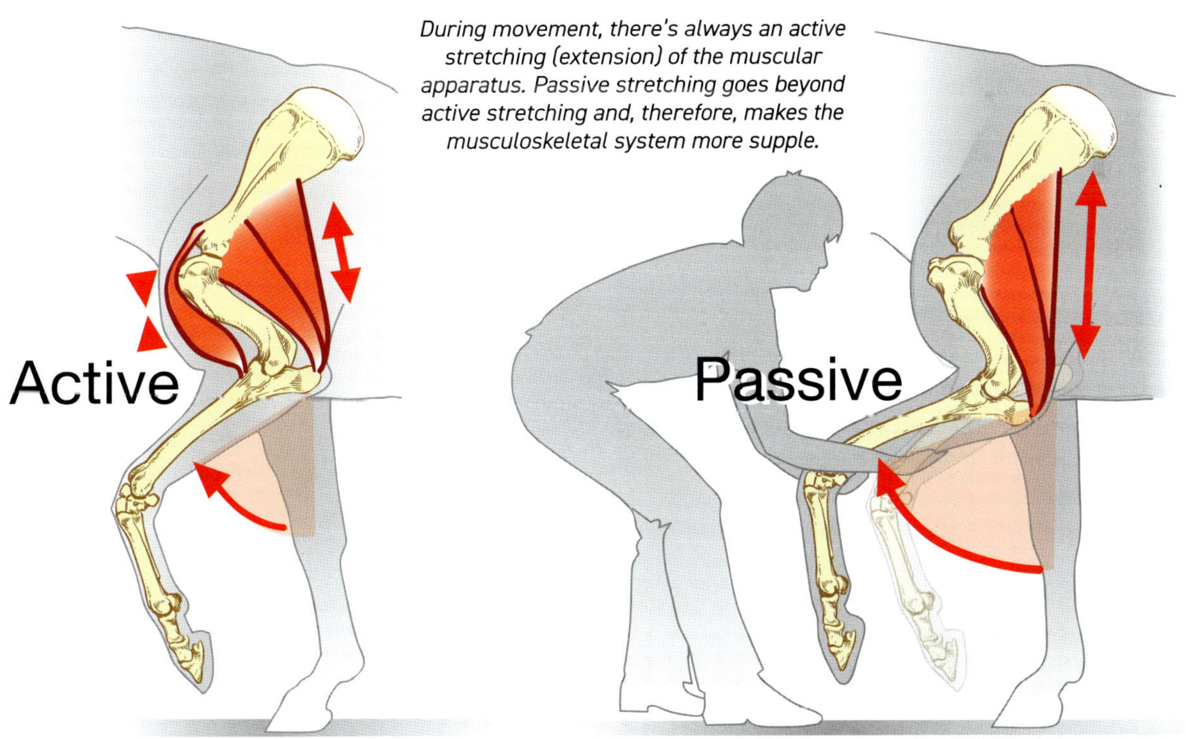

brings the active foreleg forward. One of the muscles responsible for moving the leg forward is the upper arm muscle (*m. biceps brachii*). Here, this is the active muscle—the *agonist*.

Its counterpart, the *antagonist*, is the triceps muscle (*m. triceps brachii*). When the agonist contracts, as the biceps do here, the antagonist automatically gets longer: the antagonist is actively stretched by the agonist. Therefore, active stretching is a kind of stretching that the horse carries out himself when he moves.

How intensely the muscle is stretched depends upon a few factors:

- **The range of movement.**
- **The physiological mobility of the joints.**
- **The agonistic contraction (of the active muscle).**

Unfortunately, a muscle won't achieve its maximal elasticity through the naturally occurring (active) stretch alone. In order to reach this, you must help with supplementary passive stretching exercises, meaning controlled "over-stretching."

Fact: When a muscle is shortened over a long period of time, it can easily lead to injury.

Passive Stretching

Passive goes beyond what active can do. During passive stretching, the origin and insertion points of the muscle must be carefully spread as far from one another as possible. Your horse can't execute this movement on his own: you must support him.

The muscle fibers will lengthen and allow the joint greater mobility. The outcome is a larger stress-bearing area in the joints, which spares the cartilage. The soft tissue also benefits from passive stretches, as their chance of injury is greatly reduced.

The Stretching Reflex

Every muscle has receptors, the so-called muscle spindles that measure the length of the muscle. If the muscle is overstretched too quickly, for example when a horse slips, these receptors are responsible for the reflexive contraction of the muscle. This reflex should prevent overstretching and also an injury to the soft tissue and joints.

During passive stretching, the protective mechanisms aren't usually active. The muscle is slowly stretched until you encounter light resistance and then held there. You must ease into the stretching position very lightly; otherwise, the muscle spindles will activate to protect the muscles and the muscle will contract. Very gently and slowly, you can make an almost invisible seesaw movement, which will improve mobility.

Fact: During movement, the stretching reflex protects the muscles and ligamentous apparatus from overstretching. During passive stretching exercises, these reflexes are "shut down."

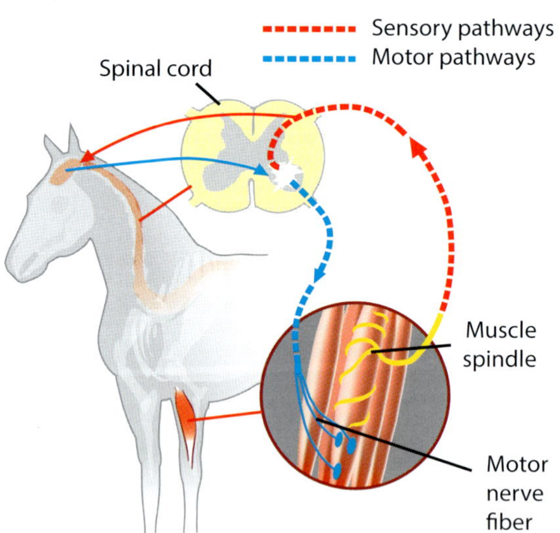

The muscle is overstretched. This sensory nerve channel carries the signal to the central nervous system, to the spinal cord. Here, the information is evaluated. A message (signal) is then carried back to the affected muscle, via the motor nerves, which tells the muscle to contract quickly to avoid injury.

When Should I Mobilize/Stretch?

There's a lot of discussion about whether it's best to mobilize and stretch before or after a training session. Studies have shown, generally speaking, you can do these exercises anytime, meaning before, during, and after a training session. And all three options have their advantages. In the following section, I've identified the right time for stretching exercises in reference to application and effects.

● To Prepare for a Training Session

The advantage to mobilizing and stretching *before* a training session is that the joints and musculature are prepared for the stress to come. The mobility and flexibility of the musculoskeletal system are significantly improved. This makes it easier for the horse to get loose and the training session will be more effective.

However, with cold muscles, you're going to think about mobilizing more than stretching. Just as with joints, the fluid that lies between the muscles (and muscle bindings) is still in a cold state and hasn't yet warmed up to "working temperature." This fluid is still viscous, so please proceed carefully; otherwise stretching can lead to muscles rubbing up against one another. In addition, the muscle fibers are not yet optimally prepared for stretching. You'll also notice that the horse's mobility is not as good as it will be when his musculoskeletal system has warmed up.

> **My Tip**
>
> **It's advisable to massage first, which prepares cold muscles for mobilization, stretching, and work.**

● After the Warm-Up

Once the musculoskeletal system has warmed up, you can mobilize and stretch more intensely, reaching a higher level of mobility and capacity for work as described above. This is preferred over the "cold start,"

but it's often difficult to embrace in practice as it means the rider needs to dismount after the warm-up.

● After the Training Session

Through movement, muscular engagement/tone is temporarily heightened. Stretching exercises after exercise lend themselves to bringing the muscles back to their normal level of engagement, while maintaining and improving flexibility. You should do mobilization and stretching exercises a maximum of 30 minutes after exercise; any later and the muscles will have already cooled down. At that point, you would need to treat the muscles as you would to "prepare for a training session."

● After an Injury

There's the danger that injured or damaged muscle fibers (for example, after a muscle tear), caused by the pain-induced non-use of the muscle, don't build up in the correct fiber direction. (This is because the muscle has taken a resting position due to pain.) To correct orientation, the fibers need to be stimulated. You can get this stimulation through purposeful movement (active stretching) and, very important here, by supplementing with mobilization and passive stretching. The affected, newly built structures will be more resilient as a result.

> *Fact:* If there's an acute injury, these exercises should only be done under the guidance of a qualified physical therapist or veterinarian, as they can easily cause the muscle to overstretch.

In the case of soft tissue injury, horse owners themselves should employ rehabilitation measures at the earliest two weeks after the injury, in order to avoid restricting the building up of new blood vessels. At three weeks out from injury, you should certainly execute a purposeful mobilization and stretching program, in order to influence the newly formed tissue.

> *Fact:* To handle work/stress, it's not only important for a muscle to be strong, but also flexible.

How Often Should I Mobilize/Stretch?

If your horse is naturally elastic and supple, it's enough to mobilize and stretch after hard work. With lower intensity work, it still makes sense to mobilize/stretch about two to three times a week as a prevention against joint immobility/muscular tightness.

When you feel less mobility in one direction, you should purposefully stretch this side, twice a day if possible (for example, before and after riding), until mobility is reestablished.

When your horse is on stall rest due to illness, you should mobilize and stretch the parts of the body that are not painful/sick once a day if possible, in order to counteract contraction of the musculature. Massage, mobilization, stretching, and stabilizing (see chapter 9, p. 166) of the injured area can be done under the advice of your veterinarian, depending on the reason for the stall rest or extent of the injury.

How Long Should I Mobilize/Stretch?

• As a Preventive Measure

Stretches of the extremities are held for at least 10 to 20 seconds, but not longer than 45 seconds, for three to four repetitions, two to three times per week.

• For Tight/Contracted Musculature

Stretches are held at least 10 to 20 seconds, but 45 seconds at the most. This should be repeated five or six times a day. The exercises can also be repeated more frequently throughout the day.

• As Rehabilitation

Stretches in the affected, painful area should not be held for long, but for at least 10 to 20 seconds. Repeat five to six times. If possible, spread the repetitions out over the course of the day.

When Not to Mobilize/Stretch?

You'll notice if stretching causes your horse to become sensitive or have pain. He'll behave similarly as he would during an uncomfortable massage.

Never stretch your horse if:
- **He has an acute injury.**
- **He has a fever.**
- **He has nerve inflammation (neuritis).**
- **There is a suspected thrombosis.**
- **He exhibits ataxic or uncoordinated movement.**
- **There is hyper-flexibility in his entire body or just in one joint.**
- **There is a lameness with an unclear source.**

An important hint!
With a horse that is too flexible, you should avoid stretching, as this can result in major difficulties when riding and the horse becomes even more elastic. With these horses, you can do the exercises in chapter 9 for strengthening and stabilization (see p. 166).

But how do I recognize that a horse has too much elasticity and movement?

This horse will often have a very soft, more hypotonic (low tone) musculature. A further clue is very weak pasterns. Without much effort, the forelegs can extend to be almost horizontal. When stretching his spine, the horse can arch his back very strongly (like a cat).

When ridden, there may be challenges with keeping straight, as the horse weaves side to side. These horses tend to be good at lateral movements.

Hint: Are you unsure whether you should stretch your horse? Consult first with your veterinarian or physical therapist.

What Should Be Avoided When Mobilizing/Stretching?

Please never:
- **Provoke pain.**
- **Make big or fast "springing" movements during a treatment.**
- **Stretch muscles that are already acutely over-stretched or injured.**
- **Provoke compression in the joints.**
- **Make movements that are too quick.**
- **Apply too much strength during a stretch (it's correct to stretch just to the point of light resistance).**

If you don't follow these guidelines, you can actually trigger microtrauma in the soft tissue. Therefore, it's always better to think "less is more" when it comes to stretching. Above all, you want to avoid overstretching.

When you work closely with a horse, always observe him closely and execute the exercises as described. Then all will be well. At the first sign of the horse feeling uncomfortable or unwilling, you must immediately reduce the pull into the stretch. If you stretch too much, your horse will show you, for example, by pulling his limb out of the stretch. You can then repeat the exercise, but with less pull.

Fact: To put your mind at ease a little, I've never received feedback from a customer or reader that she has injured a horse with stretching exercises!

Are There Side Effects?

You won't encounter true side effects here, though horses may become sensitive from stretching as they can from massage. When this is the case, you've mobilized/stretched too much!

The best "side effect" is for your horse to feel really good after mobilization/stretching and for his movement and impulsion to be much improved. I've also got feedback from many horse owners that their horses feel so good because of their "new" mobility that they buck for joy in the first days after treatment. So, hold on please! Should your horse have a shortened muscle, you'll see him become clearly more mobile after a short amount of time (at the most 14 days).

Implementation

Just like with massage, choose a quiet, familiar place with secure footing and a wall for this treatment. In addition, the horse should not be tied the first time you stretch him.

Mobilizing the extremities is good preparation for stretching. The advantage lies in the excellent loosening action. You can do this every day for every horse, from pleasure horse to sport horse.

If you notice that your horse is not ready to cooperate during the actual stretching, or that the muscles you want to stretch are simply too short, you should continue mobilizing the affected limbs until the resistance goes away. You'll notice that mobilization is extremely effective. In addition, you'll get a feel for which limbs have more limited mobility and flexibility.

Learning a new skill is often challenging so be careful with mobilization/stretching in the beginning. You and your horse both need to get used to this new form of treatment. Begin with one or two exercises and don't try to practice every exercise from this book at one time. Gradually increase the number of stretches. Try to feel when the passive stretch reaches its limit. It's really important to recognize the limit of the stretch and not to stretch beyond this point. You'll notice that the resistance of the tissue definitely increases.

In practice, you'll stretch until you can feel a light resistance, then slightly move the limb back toward its original position. Hold this position for 10 to 20 seconds. This time is sufficient to achieve an effect. It won't hurt, however, for you to hold the stretch a little longer, but not longer than 45 seconds. If you notice the resistance lessens during the stretch, you can also take the stretching position a bit farther. As you do so, pay attention to your horse's breathing. Only go deeper into the stretch as your horse exhales. During an exhale, the muscle relaxes more. After about 45 seconds, relax the engagement and slowly guide the limb back into its original position. You should never just "let go" of the limb from the stretching position.

> ### My Tip
> **The effects of stretching will improve with frequent repetition.**

When the horse is restless and doesn't allow the stretch, it might be that the stretch is unexpected, uncomfortable, or even painful. You should then work with even less resistance, so that your horse will tolerate the exercises.

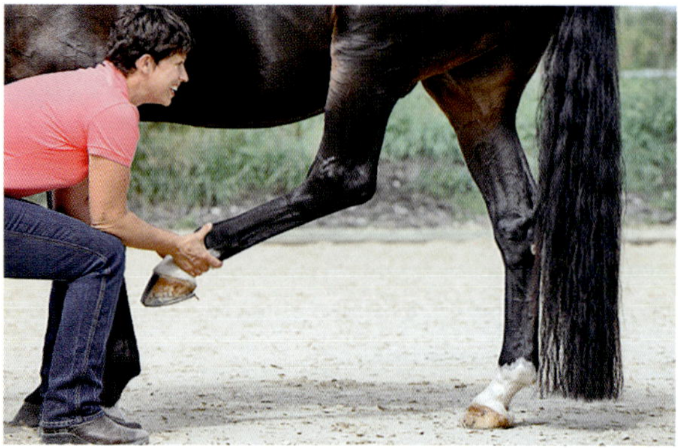

When you support your elbows with your thighs, you can effectively relieve your back.

A Hint for You!

When executing stretching exercises, attend to your own well-being by using your body correctly and effectively.

A few important tips:

- Always position yourself toward the horse in such a way that you can't get injured if, for example, he kicks. If your horse tends to kick or is really nervous and restless, forego the stretches of the hindquarters that go toward the back and, likewise, the tail stretch.
- Many stretching exercises require you to assume a bent position. Always try to keep your back

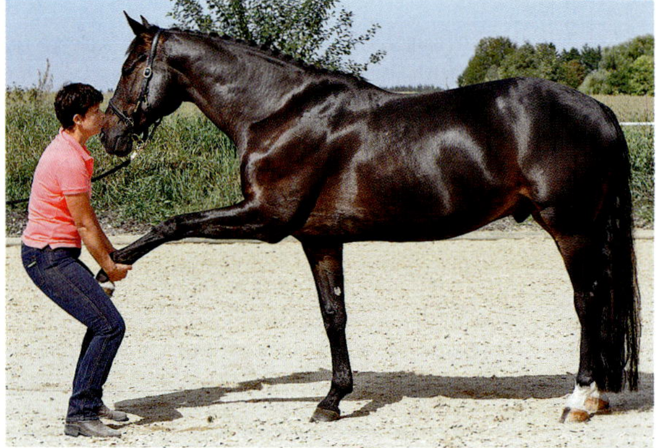

Correct body position

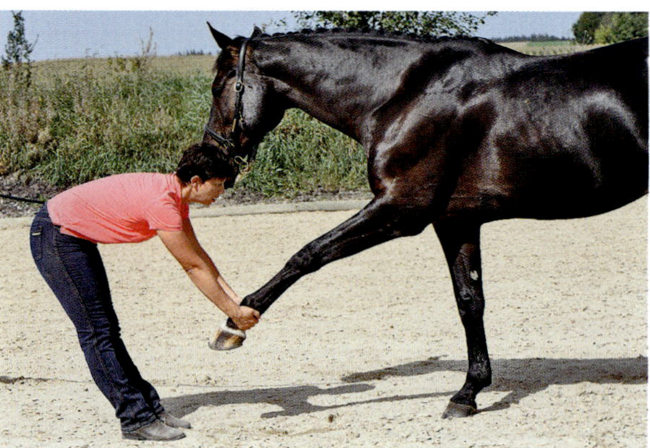

Incorrect body position

straight (and without a stretch of your spinal column) and use just your knees and hip joints to bend. Execute the stretch by using just the stretch of your upper legs, in that you move up and down by bending and stretching your knees. If you find this position too difficult, you can also support your elbows above your knees (see photo left).

- Don't interlace your fingers. Instead, put one hand over the other so that you can quickly let go if needed. It can happen that your horse shifts his weight on you during a stretch. If you notice that it's too much for you, immediately end this stretch—before you hurt yourself.

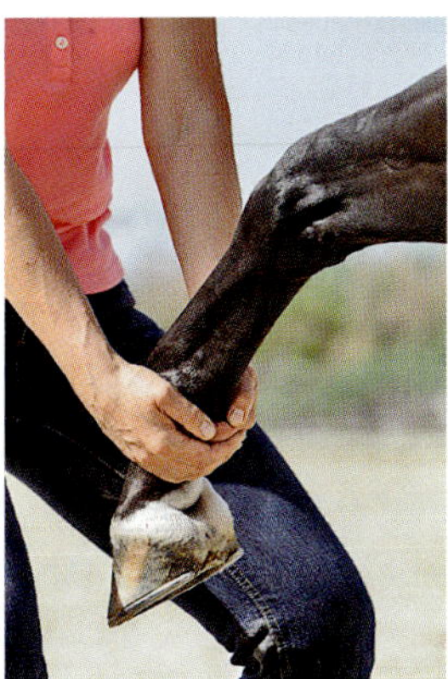

The hands are correctly positioned here.

The Effects of Mobilizing and Stretching

The stretches:
- **Improve mobility.**
- **Improve elasticity of the soft tissue.**
- **Improve body awareness.**
- **Improve coordination and reflexes.**
- **Improve circulation in the musculature.**
- **Loosen adhesions and accumulated tension in the soft tissue.**
- **Are relaxing.**
- **Are a preventive measure.**
- **Lessen the risk of injury.**
- **Relieve muscle pain.**

Exercises for Mobilization and Stretching

Ideally, you'll first do the exercises for about a month. Afterward, you can do the easier stabilization exercises for another month (see chapter 9,

p. 166), before you begin the advanced exercises. With young horses, I recommend staying at each stage for a longer period of time.

I've divided the exercises into two parts for practical application:

1 Mobilization
The forehand
The hindquarters
The jaw
The spine
The tail

2 Stretching the Extremities
The forehand
The hindquarters
The tail

Before you begin to practice, I want to share the following guidelines:

- With some stretching exercises, there are two or more variations.
- Additionally, I've assigned each exercise a degree of difficulty.
- It's best for you to begin with the "Basic Exercises." Once you and your horse have become used to the stretching exercises, you can move on to the level of medium difficulty.
- I also show which superficial muscles are being stretched with each exercise. Of course, more deeply lying muscular structures are also being stretched, which I'm not going to go into here.

Mobilizing Exercises

Mobilizing the Forelimbs

Lift up the front leg as if you were going to pick out the hoof. Holding the leg on the fetlock joint and stretch it by moving yourself backward, toward the horse's head. The leg will be stretched forward, as this movement is more natural for the horse. At the end of the movement, change your hold. You want to hold the limb above the knee joint and lift it up until the forearm is almost parallel to the ground. Simply allow the cannon bone to hang down.

Variation 1

This exercise mobilizes the shoulder and the elbow. Hold the leg by the forearm and guide it in circling movements. Begin with a small diameter and slowly allow it to get bigger. A good rule of thumb is three to five rounds to the right, then go the other way. Change direction several times. To conclude the exercise, lower the leg back to its starting position and set it down. You can certainly do all three variations as a sequence.

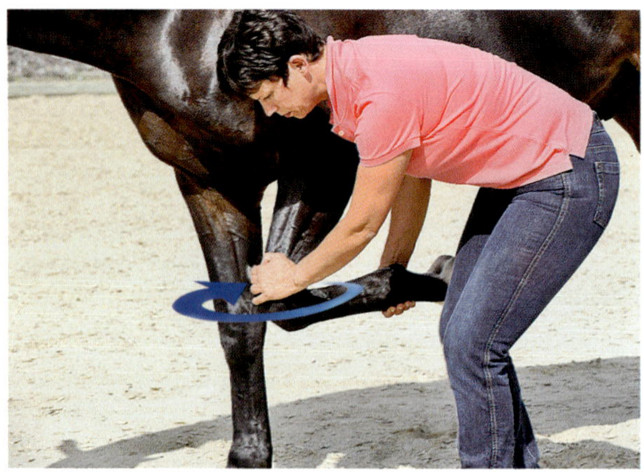

Mobilizing the shoulder and elbow joint.

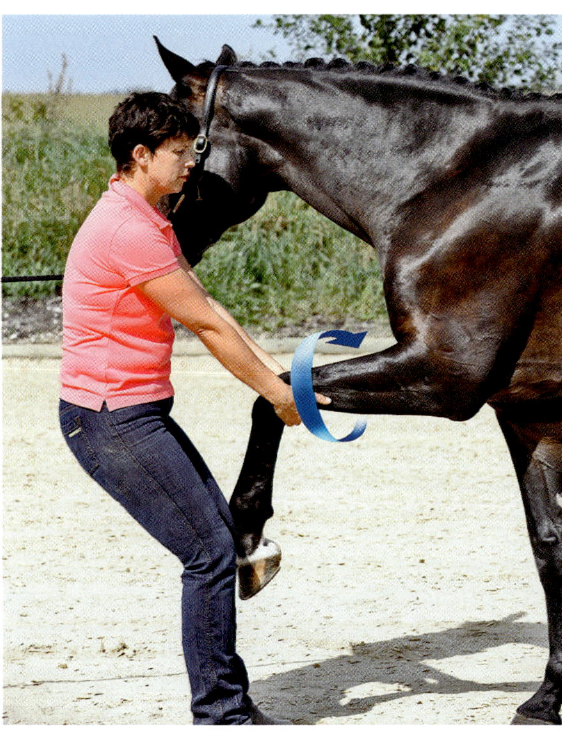

Mobilizing the shoulder and elbow joint. The hold is correct. However, you don't need to bring the leg as far forward as it is here in the photo.

Variation 2

This is likewise an exercise for shoulder and elbow. This time, you stand beside the horse, looking toward his head. You hold the leg by the cannon and forearm. You move the leg in a horizontal circular movement.

Variation 3

Here, you're mobilizing the knee joint. The starting position is the same as above, but now one hand holds the forearm and the other, the cannon bone. You circle the leg, as if you wanted to draw a circle on the ground with your horse's hoof. Here, too, circle three to five times to the right, then circle the other way. Continue to allow the circle to get bigger.

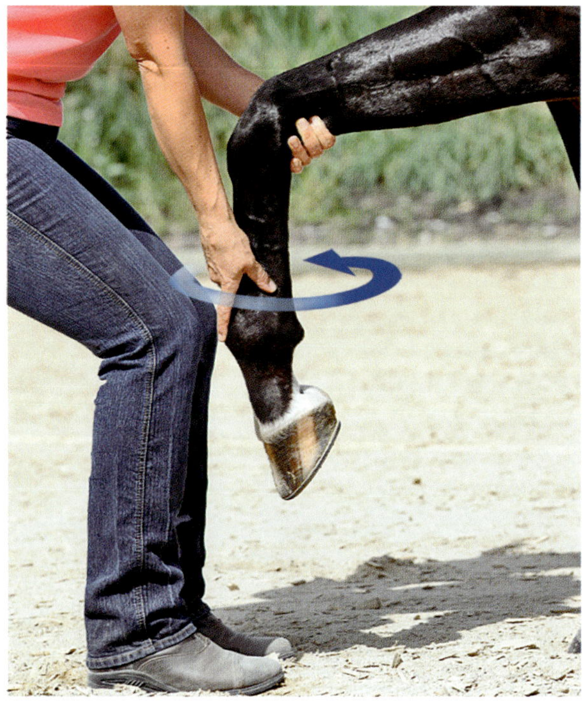

Mobilizing the knee joint.

Mobilizing the Hind Limbs

The muscles of the hindquarters are your horse's motor. They are responsible for most of the forward thrust; horses depend on having highly mobilized joints as well as well-stretched, flexible muscles in this area.

Basic Exercise

Stand beside your horse and to the side. Lift the hind leg and hold on with one hand around the fetlock joint and the other around the hoof (see photo below).

As you did with the forelegs, guide the hind leg in a circular movement as if you were drawing a circle on the ground. Begin with small circles and gradually allow them to get bigger. Three to five rounds to the right, then change direction. Do this a couple of times. To end the exercise, bring the leg back to the starting position and set it down.

Mobilizing the Jaw

Surely, you're familiar with this: you're stressed or tense and so you clench your teeth together, which causes your jaw to tighten. Horses do the same exact thing. When they're physically tense, they lock their jaw together. As I described in the section on biomechanics, this has significant consequences in terms of your horse's *losgelassenheit* (p. 12).

You can relieve tension in your horse's jaw by sticking your fingers in his mouth. Carefully put the fingers under the tongue, between the incisors and back teeth. In doing so, you'll trigger a reflex and the horse will begin to make large chewing movements. Through the large chewing movements, tension in the temporo-mandibular joint (TMJ) will be relieved.

You can switch sides, right to left, and see on which side it's easiest to open the joint. You'll recognize this by the sideways shift of the lower jaw.

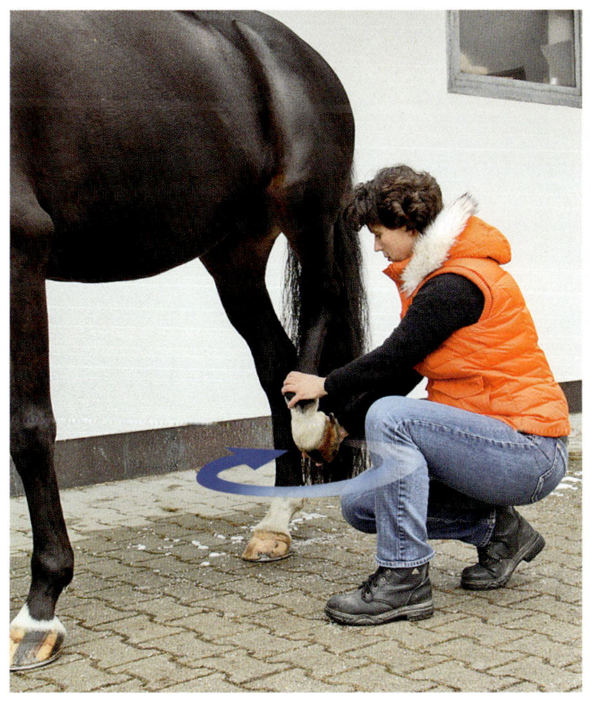

A loosening exercise for the coffin joint and hindquarters musculature.

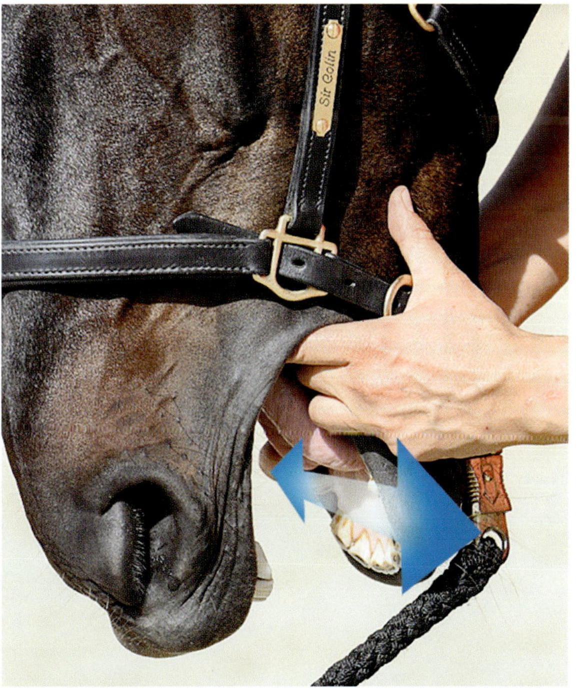

Please be careful that you don't hurt your horse's gums with long fingernails or rings.

Mobilizing the Spine

Exercises that gently mobilize the spine can work wonders against accumulated tension and immobility. Thereby, you're mobilizing and stretching all the joints of the spinal column as well as the muscles of the head, poll, neck, and back. When tension is present, you'll notice this reduces the pain sensitivity in the back muscles and significantly improves mobility in the spine, often within a short time—even just a few days. You'll also observe that your horse walks with much more supple movement, his longitudinal bend improves, and even the mobility and impulsion of the limbs will benefit.

Fact: *Scientific studies have shown that these mobilizing and stretching exercises help with chronic back pain. The horses that were studied became significantly more mobile and were less sensitive to pressure.*

■ Mobilizing the Head, Poll, and Neck in Flexion

Variation 1 (Basic Exercise)

This stretching exercise influences the head, poll, and neck extensors. For this exercise, bring a treat, play with it near your horse's mouth, and at the same time, bring your hand...

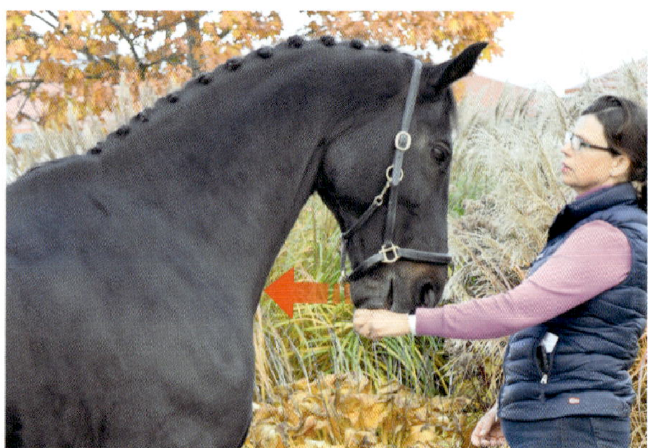

...straight back toward the center of his neck (for mobility of the upper neck).

Variation 2 (Basic Exercise)

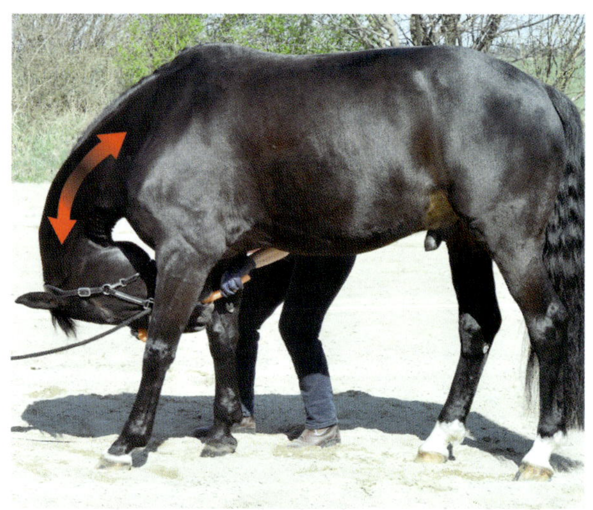

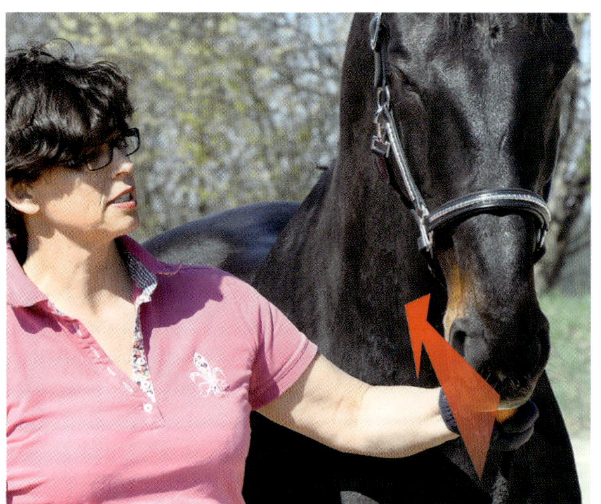

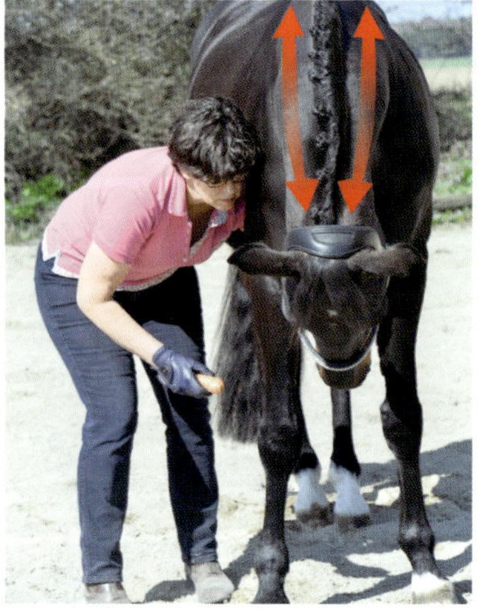

...directly toward the lower part of the breastbone (for mobility of the middle neck).

Physical Therapy for Horses

Variation 3 (Basic Exercise)

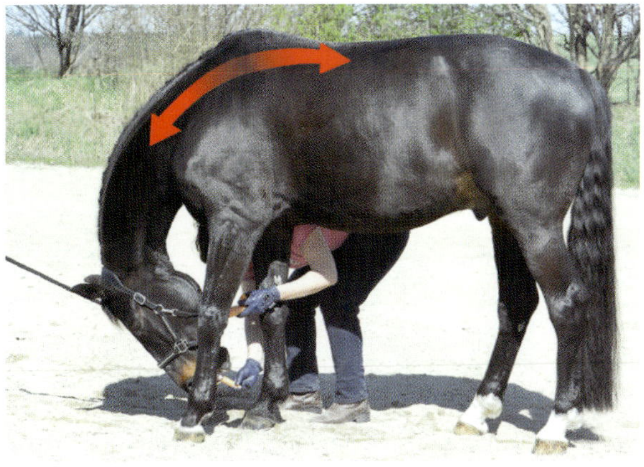

...to the ground between the forelegs (for mobility of the lower neck all the way to the hindquarters). As you do so, please make sure your horse doesn't bend his knees too much.

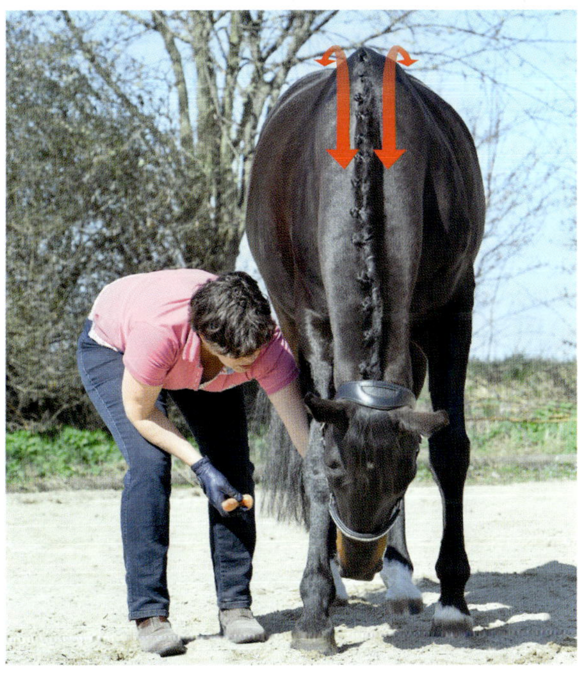

Hint: With this exercise, it's important that your hand always stays close to the horse's mouth, since your horse can't see the treat that remains right under his nose. You're motivating him to keep his head and neck straight. Try to maintain this position for a few seconds by not giving him the treat immediately.

My Tip

In this exercise, try to keep the head and neck straight. If it's not working, you can support your horse by "guiding" his head.

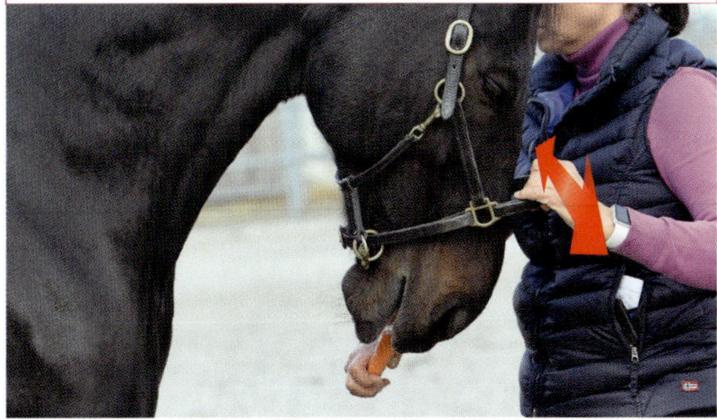

My Tip

In the beginning, carry a treat in each hand, so that you can use both hands. Hold one hand in front of the forelegs and one behind, encouraging the horse to stretch far down.

■ **Mobilizing the Head, Poll, and Neck in Longitudinal Bend (Basic Exercise):**

Variation 1 (Basic Exercise)

In order to get your horse to bring his head to the side in the direction of his hindquarters, you can encourage him with a carrot or treat. To prevent the horse from turning around, position him against a wall.

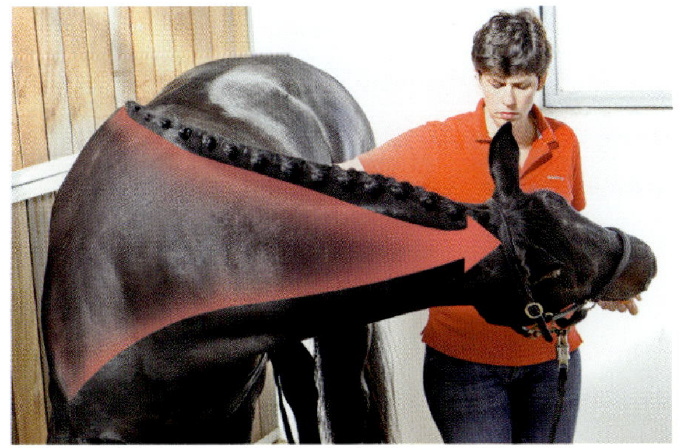

Position yourself at the trunk, an arm's length from your horse, and stretch your arm toward his mouth, encouraging him to turn his head and neck toward you because you're always keeping his "treat" near his mouth. Continually play with the treat on his lips, so that he doesn't lose his desire to follow the movement. Draw a large arch with the treat to prevent the lower cervical spine from compressing too severely.

When he's gone as far as possible in terms of backward and sideways bend, continue to play with the treat on your horse's mouth for another two to five seconds or so, in order to prolong the stretch.

My Tip

Make sure that your horse doesn't bite your fingers. Hold the treat between your thumb and forefingers and make a fist. This way you can always keep your hand near the mouth, without getting bitten. At the end of the exercise, your horse gets the treat as a reward.

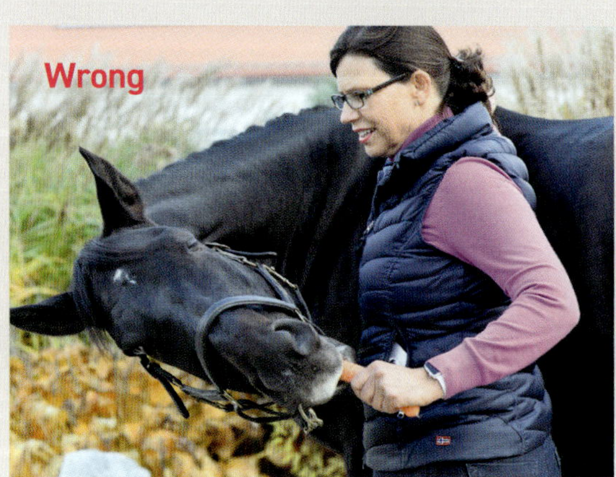

This exercise can be practiced at different heights, but never higher than the point of hip.

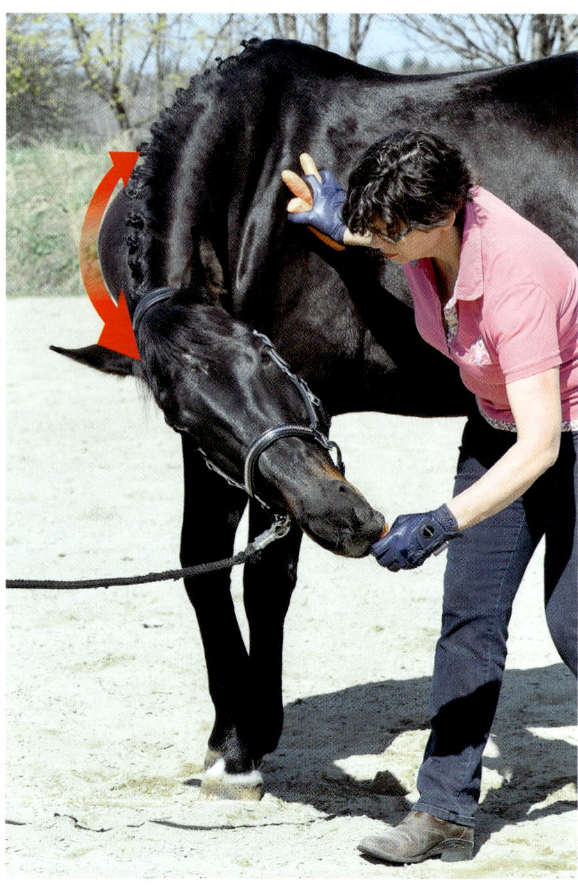

Hint: During this exercise, the horse may not tilt his poll (downward). If this happens, stop the exercise and try again, but with less longitudinal bend this time.

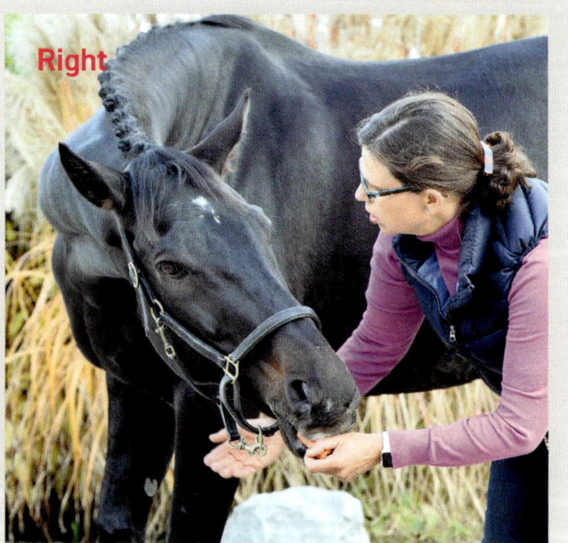

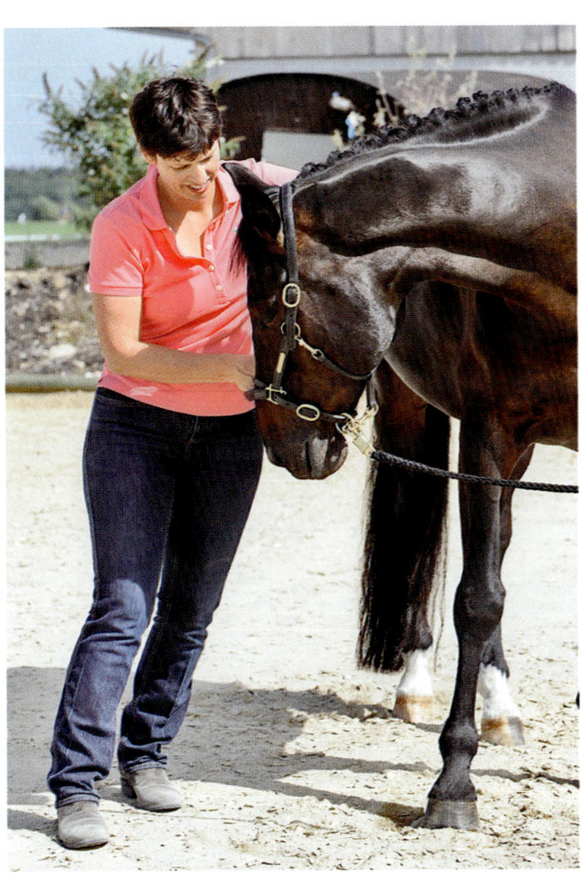

Position the neck in longitudinal bend.

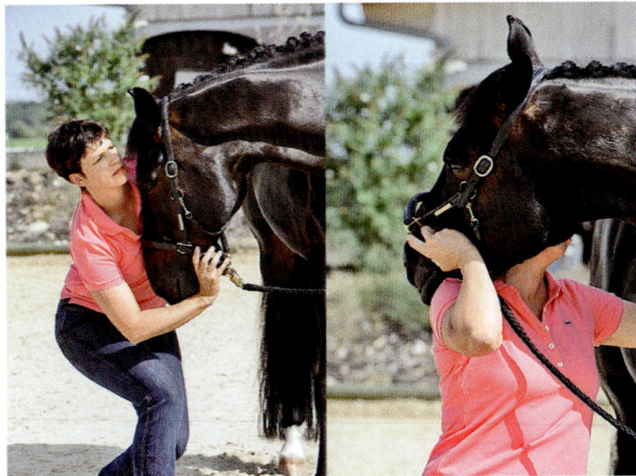

Bend your knees.   *Place the horse's head on your shoulder.*

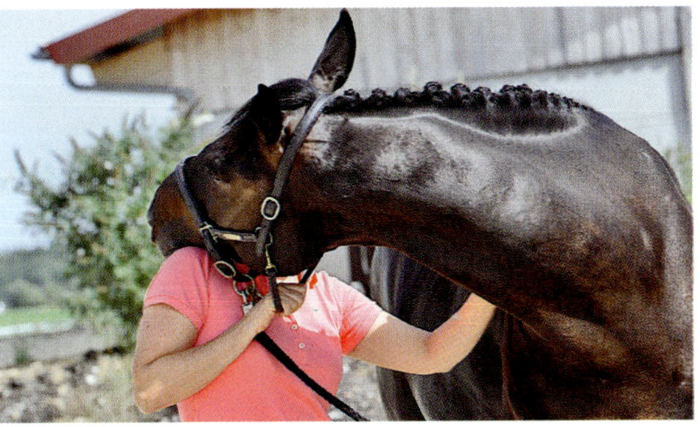

Slowly stretch and straighten your knees.

Variation 2 (Medium Degree of Difficulty)

This exercise should achieve longitudinal bend from the neck, poll, and head. Horses love this stretch as they can relieve the weight of their head, but you as their "helper" need a little patience and dexterity in the beginning.

Stand near the shoulder and use the halter to guide the head into longitudinal bend. Bring the horse's head to the height of your chest. Now, bend your knees a bit and place the horse's head on your shoulder. Slowly straighten your knees until you can feel a light resistance on your shoulder. Hold the halter with one hand or place your hand behind the ear on the C1 vertebra (atlas) and apply a slight pressure. With your other hand, apply light pressure to the *brachiocephalicus* muscle, just above the shoulder joint. This is a point that helps the horse relax.

With this exercise you accomplish a stretching of those muscles responsible for extension, turning, and longitudinal bend of the neck musculature on the opposite side. Often the horse will "fall asleep" during this exercise—he will close his eyes and relax. You are just the helper, the horse executes the stretch by himself. He will show you through shifting back and forth in which position he likes to be stretched. You can hold this exercise until your horse wants to end it by himself.

Some horses will not allow this exercise. In these cases, it is possible there is a blockage in one of the upper cervical vertebrae or the muscles are too short. In this case you should repeat the exercise with the carrot (see Variation 1, p. 153) a few times to improve mobility of the poll.

■ Mobilizing the Head, Poll, and Neck in Extension

Variation 1 (Basic Exercise)

Position your horse so that he can't avoid the exercise by moving forward; for example, behind a stall door (obviously one that's open on top and not too high). Hold the treat (i.e. a carrot) in front of his mouth and slowly draw it away from him. As you do so, it's important that the treat remain close to his mouth so it motivates the horse to stretch his head and neck. When he reaches his maximum stretch, play with the treat near his nose for 10 to 20 seconds before you give it to him.

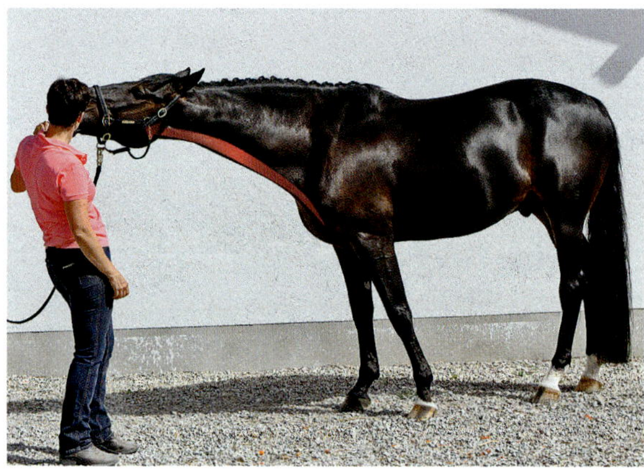

My Tip

When you're working with treats, protect yourself by wearing gloves and use a specific food container. This prevents the horse from constantly looking toward your pockets. Your horse will know immediately when it's time to practice.

Fact: This exercise is perfect for horses that crib.

■ Mobilizing the Thoracic and Lumbar Spine While Lifting

• Lifting the Back

There are two variations to this exercise, as you'll see on the page that follows. One is for the area at the front of the withers and the other is for the lower thoracic and lumbar spine.

• Lifting the Withers

Stand at a foreleg and face the hindquarters. You'll achieve this stretch by applying your fingertips along the midline of the abdominals. You're triggering a reflex that lifts the back. The back/withers lift slightly, causing the spinous processes of the withers to move forward. This relaxes the nuchal ligament and the head lowers.

You'll keep your fingers bent. You can either travel along the abdominal midline until about the middle of the horse's belly, tickle your horse's breast bone or try, through a gentle lift, to raise the withers from below. You should try out the different techniques, as horses respond to them very differently.

My practice has shown me that many horses are highly sensitive to this, and most of them are blocked and "locked" at the withers. In this case, they can no longer lift through the withers (so how should they be able to move forward and downward?) and find it uncomfortable when I trigger this belly reflex. As a response to this uncomfortable stimulus and the "offending" hand, they step their hind legs forward under the abdomen, therefore, it's important that you keep an eye on the hind legs and stand near the shoulders, so you don't encounter a hind hoof.

Fact: Horses can also be sensitive when they have stomach problems. When the breastbone lifts, it creates pressure on their stomach, which is uncomfortable and/or painful.

Generally, Thoroughbreds will need less pressure on their breastbone than Warmbloods in order to lift their withers. With cold-blooded horses, you'll often get no reaction at all. This doesn't necessarily mean that there are no blockages present. More likely, the horse has fewer reflex points and is not reacting.

When you have a more sensitive horse, begin with little pressure and movement. If the horse reacts, which you'll see by the movement of his muscles, continue with the exercise; it will be worth it.

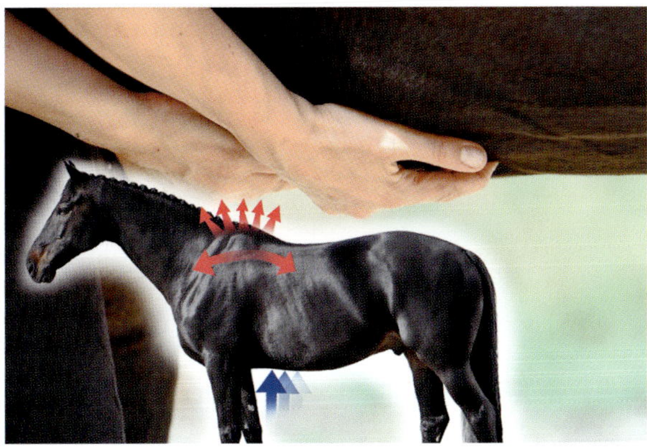

• Mobilizing the Thoracic and Lumbar Spine While Lifting

Variation 1 (Basic Exercise)
Stand to the side near the hind leg. Using the pointer finger on both hands or two rounded wooden dowels (as in the photo), about one hand-width apart from one another, push against the loin musculature to the right and left of the spine. Next, with light pressure, pull along the croup toward the tail. In the

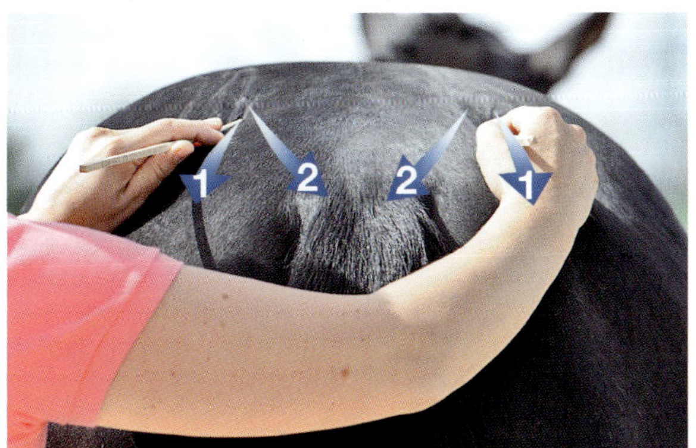

lumbar area, you'll first see the horse push away with his back, so use less pressure. When you stroke over the croup musculature, the back lifts up. From here, you can apply more pressure. The most sensitive reflex point lies to the right and left of the tail dock. This is also the end of the exercise; please don't stroke further.

If this reflex isn't triggered, try it again using more strength. Horses that are tight in their back or have fewer reflex points in their hindquarters will need you to apply more pressure. But, the first time, you should begin with little pressure and then gradually increase it.

Variation 2 (Medium Degree of Difficulty)
This is a good exercise for longitudinal bend and stretching the long muscles of your horse's back.

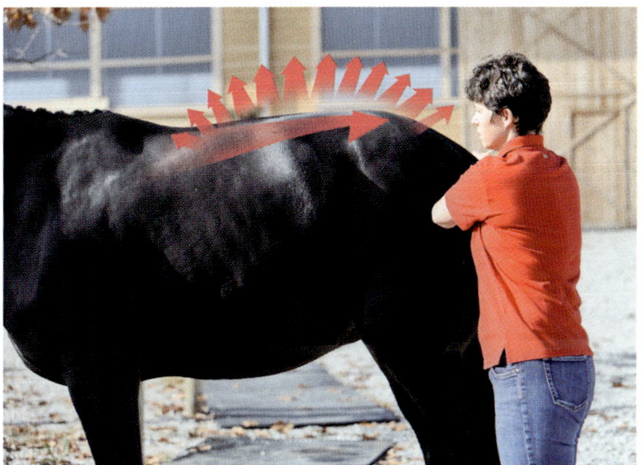

Your position is again to the side of the hindquarters. Using your bent finger, pull from the opposite point of hip in an arch toward the tail. The spine responds by lifting and moving sideways toward you. Be aware that your horse might take a balancing step in your direction: pay attention to your feet.

My Tip

Firm brushing at this reflex point can also trigger a lifting and sideways movement here. If your horse doesn't respond by lifting when you use your finger, try with a brush.

Should the horse show no reaction during the back exercises, find a dull instrument, such as a pen cap or wooden chopstick. Use this tool to apply a stronger pressure than your fingers. Draw the tool slowly over the reflex points. But, again, begin with a low level of pressure.

■ Mobilizing the Thoracic and Lumbar Spine in Extension

Although you don't want your horse to travel with a hollow spine, there are actually many horses that cannot hollow their back at all. This affects their biomechanics, as in various phases of movement, the spine must go into extension: for example, when the hind limbs are stretched backward at a gallop or when the horse lands after a jump.

To activate the extension, you don't want to stretch the spine so much as you want to mobilize it.

Again, hold your wooden chopstick or pen cap and make light, small, quick strokes perpendicular to the spine: Tick, tick, tick. Complete 5 to 10 strokes on each side with three to four repetitions.

Fact: This has a mobilizing effect, but at the same time also activates and strengthens the musculature of the spine.

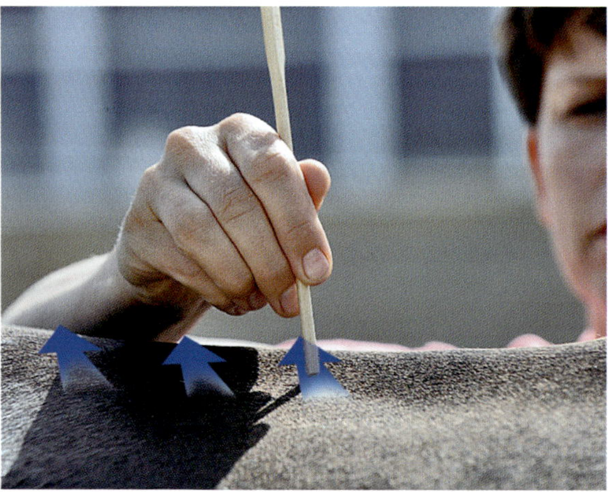

The horse briefly twitches and tenses the *longissimus dorsi*, which seesaws the spine. This is a sign that all is well with the extension. If this doesn't happen, the muscle and the mobility are restricted. Please don't start pressing harder: every light twitch of the muscle leads to release. You'll see that your horse reacts a bit more each day.

My Tip

Change it up when treating the back: first mobilize with extension and then return to lifting the back (see photo on p. 157). This up and down is great for the mobility of the back.

■ Mobilizing the Tail

The tail is an extension of the spine. As with a head massage, a tail massage can have indirect effects on the entire body, all the way to the muzzle.

Basic Exercise

This is an easy exercise. You take the dock of the tail and move it in a circle. Begin with small circles and allow them to get bigger. Three to five circles to the right, then change the rotation to the left. Here, you can also apply massage techniques: stroking the entire dock of the tail or circling where the tail attaches to the body both work wonders. You'll notice that your horse gets very relaxed.

Mobilizing the tail in this way has a loosening effect on the whole spine and horses enjoy this treatment.

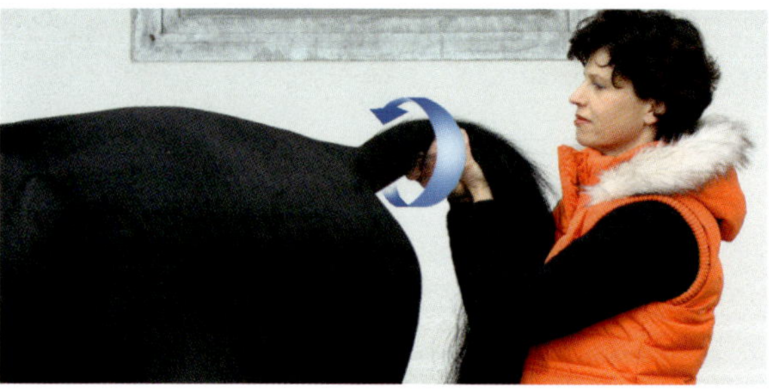

Physical Therapy for Horses

Stretching Exercises

Stretching the Forelegs

■ Stretching the Forelegs to the Front

In these exercises, you're stretching those muscles that move the forelimbs toward the back. There are three variations to this exercise.

Basic Exercise

Pick up the front leg as high as you do to pick out the hoof. Move slowly backward toward the horse's head, carefully bringing the foreleg forward as you do so. Position yourself in front of the horse. The leg is pulled in the direction of movement toward the front and the knee joint should be at almost full extension.

You're now standing with a straight back and bent knees in front of your horse, your hands around his fetlock joint. By straightening your bent knees, you'll lightly bring the foreleg up and farther into the stretch. The stretch will continue until you feel a slight resistance. Now hold for at least 10 to 20 seconds. If you notice that the resistance gets less, you can bring your horse farther into the stretch as he exhales or back out of the stretching position for a brief moment (relax) and repeat as above. When finished, put the leg back down.

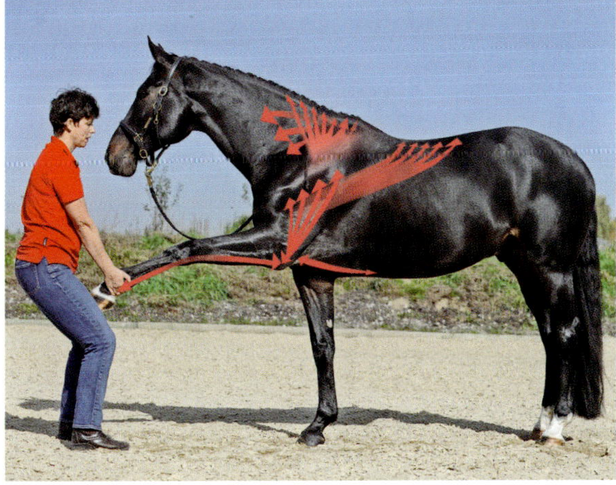

At the maximum of mobility that you might reach, the foreleg will be almost parallel to the ground. If your horse has this level of mobility, you don't need to stretch this muscle group every day. I'd suggest only doing so after hard work.

If the foreleg comes even higher, your horse is hypermobile and should never be stretched in this direction.

Variation 2 (Basic Exercise)

When your horse has an injury to the lower limbs, such as joint inflammation or a tendon injury, you can benefit these joints by only stretching the muscles of the upper forelegs. Pick up the leg as described above, hold on to the knee joint, and allow the joints of the lower leg to hang down. Move toward the horse's head, and in doing so, stretch his shoulder.

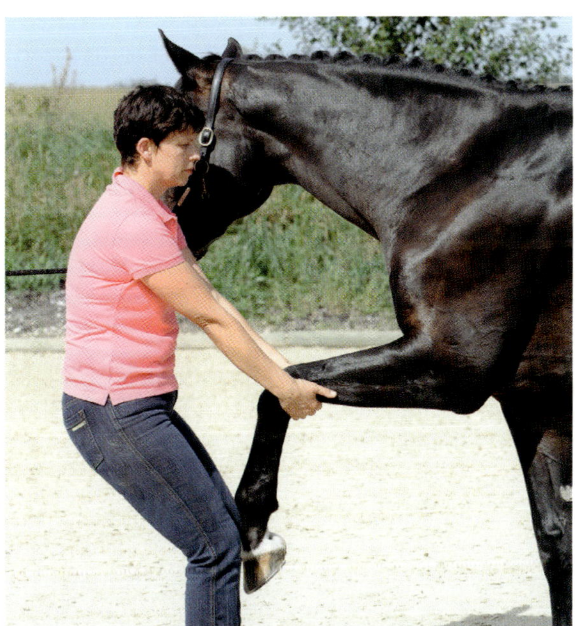

Hint: The chest muscles stabilize the shoulder joint against the ribs when the foreleg is suspended. While the foreleg is extended, you shouldn't make any movements that also bring the leg outward, as this can cause the shoulder joint to become unstable.

■ Stretching the Forelegs to the Back

These exercises stretch the muscles of the forehand that are responsible for bringing the limbs forward.

Variation 1 (Basic Exercise)

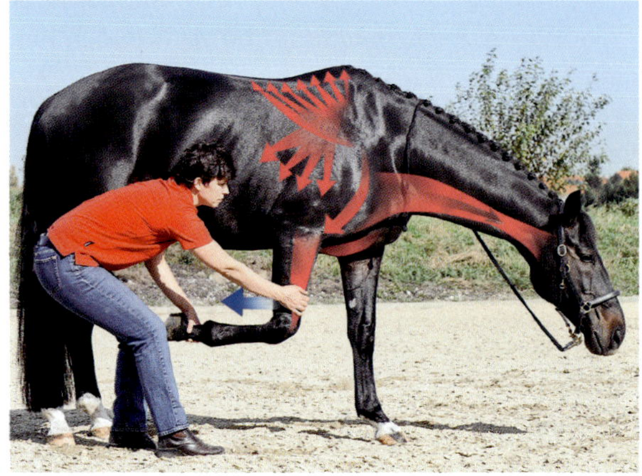

Pick up the leg (as if to clean the hoof) and turn yourself around. Now, you're looking in the same direction as your horse, and standing parallel to him.

One hand should loosely support the weight of the leg at the fetlock joint. Don't pull. The other hand wraps around the leg above the knee joint and pulls it just so far back as to feel resistance. Hold for at least 10 to 20 seconds, then go more deeply into the stretch or gently come out of the stretch and repeat. Often, horses like to put their legs back down in this position, where their legs are stretched far back underneath them. Allow the horse to do so, as he's now taking over the stretch for himself.

Variation 2 (Basic Exercise)

This exercise is a targeted stretch for the extensors of the lower limbs. Take the foot and look in the direction of the hindquarters. As you do so, you're standing perpendicularly to his longitudinal axis. One hand wraps around the cannon bone; the other around the hoof. The knee joint/forearm is fixed in place by the outside of your thigh. The hoof is lifted gently in the direction of the elbow. As this takes place, the fetlock, pastern, and coffin joints are stretched to a max.

My Tip

This exercise is really good for horses that tend to "give way" in the front.

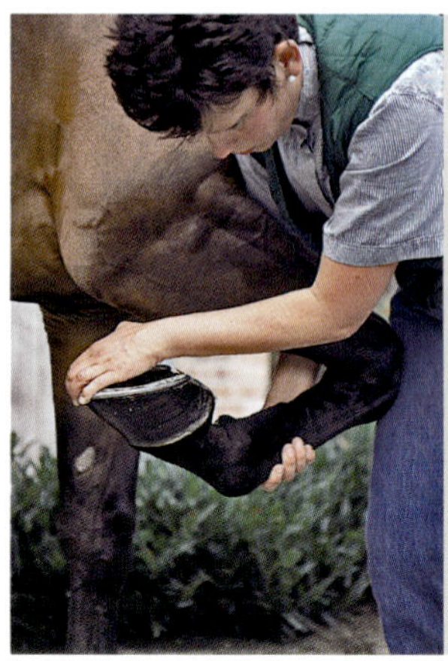

Hint: This position can be held for 10 to 20 seconds at most; otherwise, it can put too much compression on the joints.

■ Stretching the Forelegs to the Outside

This exercise stretches those muscles responsible for moving the forelegs to the inside (the *pectorals*).

Basic Exercise

The mechanics of the limbs do not allow for large sideways movements (to the outside or inside). With lateral movements, the movement comes primarily

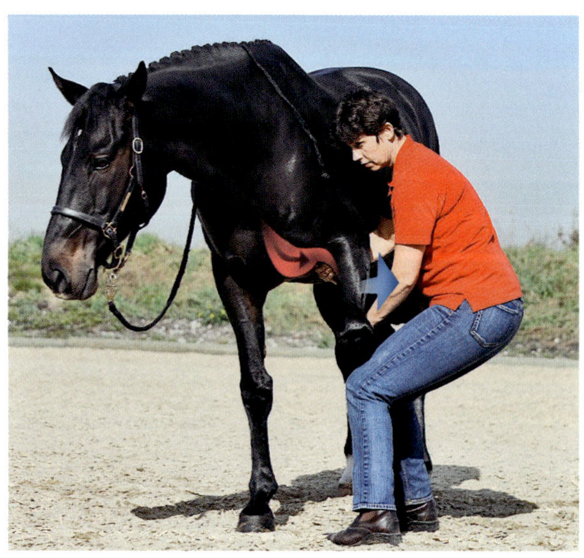

Physical Therapy for Horses

from the shoulder/elbow joints. To allow this movement, the *pectorals* must be extremely elastic.

Pick the leg up with one hand and bend the knee joint. Turn toward your horse and bend your knees. Place the cannon bone on your upper thigh and hold it firmly with one hand. With the other hand, grasp the forearm at about elbow height. By leaning back slightly, use your body weight to pull the leg outward. When you feel resistance, maintain the position.

■ Stretching the Forelegs Forward and Across

This exercise stretches those muscles responsible for backward and outward movement of the limb (needed for lateral movements).

Basic Exercise

Standing at your horse's shoulder, take the opposite foreleg and pull it toward you about 30 centimeters (about a foot) in front of the standing leg.

> **My Tip**
>
> For all exercises that require crossing of the legs, it's helpful to have an assistant available who can pick up the leg in the beginning.

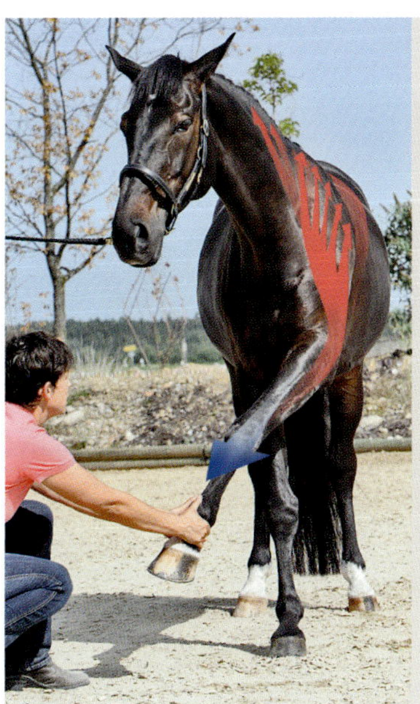

Hint: Be careful with this stretch in the beginning, as your horse could have balance problems.

■ Stretching the Forelegs Back and Across

This exercise stretches those muscles responsible for forward and outward movement of the limb (also needed for lateral movements).

Basic Exercise

You stand near your horse, take the opposite foreleg below the fetlock joint and pull it about 30 centimeters (about a foot) behind the standing leg, toward the hind leg.

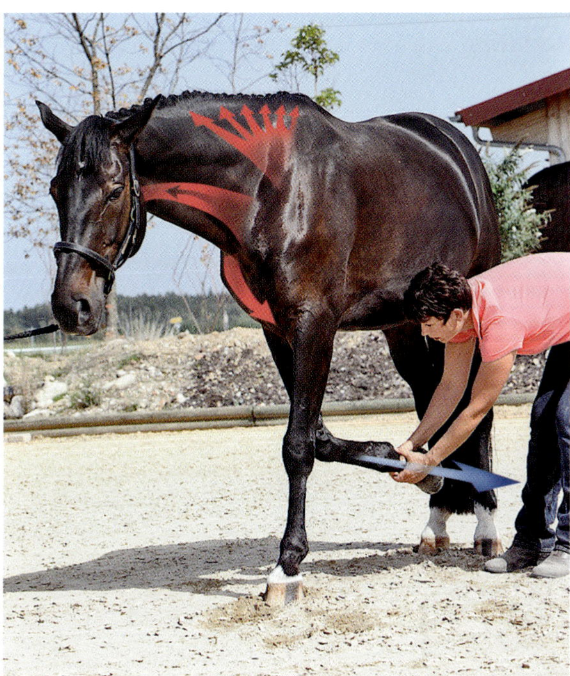

Stretching the Hind Limbs

■ Stretching the Hind Limbs Forward

Here, the muscles that bring the hind limbs back are stretched.

Variation 1 (Basic Exercise)

Stretching the Hamstrings

Pick up the hind leg and place your hands below the fetlock joint. Bend your knees and, keeping the leg above the ground, bring it briefly forward toward the foreleg. At the same time, move it a hoof-width to the outside, so the horse doesn't hurt himself.

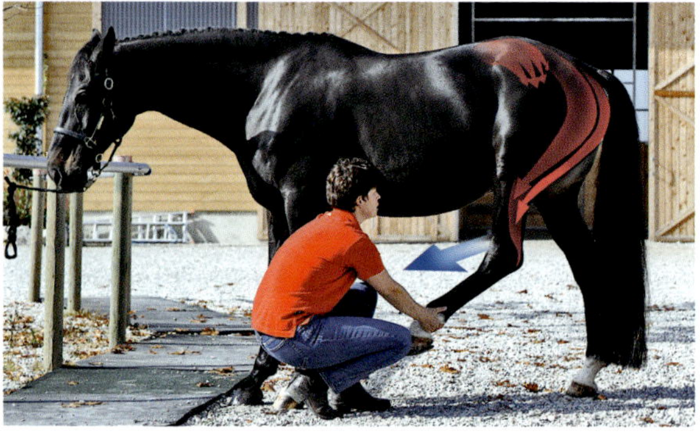

Variation 2 (Basic Exercise)

Stretching the Croup Muscles and the Biceps Femoris

Begin in the same position as with Variation 1. Then, slowly unbend your knees and draw the leg toward the horse's belly. Hold the stretched leg there for 10 to 20 seconds, as usual. Your goal is for your horse's hoof to almost reach his belly.

Hint: If your horse pulls his leg back with either of these exercises, you know the stretch is too intense. Lessen your pull toward the front. For all exercises, pay attention to your posture (see "A Hint for You!" on p. 148). If holding the leg in position is too difficult for you, protect yourself during the exercise by resting your elbows on your upper thighs. This will protect your back.

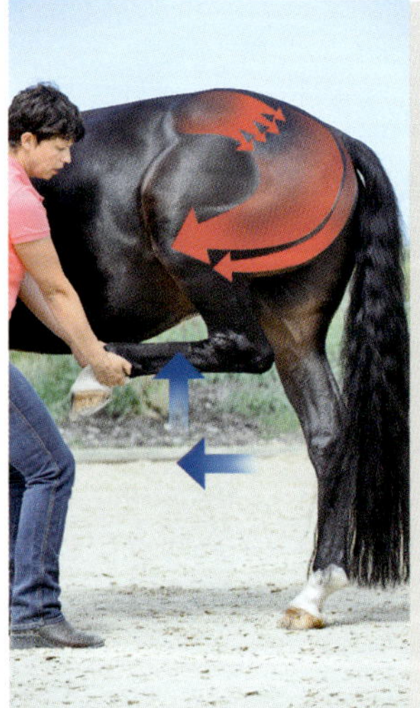

Hint: You're now stretching muscles that are closely connected to the back musculature. My experience has shown that when the back muscles are tight, it affects all the muscles that are behind them. If I can loosen shortened muscles of the hindquarters, then I'll also notice the back muscles get looser right away.

■ Stretching the Hind Limbs to the Back

Here, you're stretching the muscles of the hind limbs responsible for moving the limbs forward.

Variation 1 (Medium Level of Difficulty)

Quadriceps

Lift the leg as if you were going to pick the hoof, then turn so that you're facing forward and remain parallel to the hoof as you move toward the back. With the stretched hind leg, you'll stand directly behind the horse, holding the limb in this stretched position. Your hands hold the hock or cannon bone. Always keep an eye on the horse's reaction. If you hold the hoof low to the ground, you're stretching the thigh and gaskin muscles.

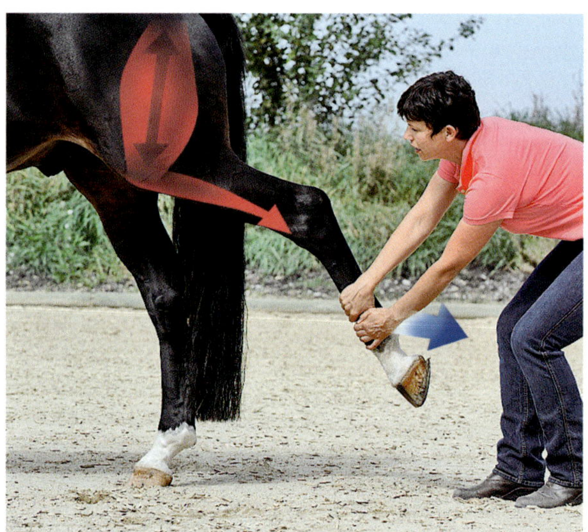

Variation 2 (Medium Level of Difficulty)

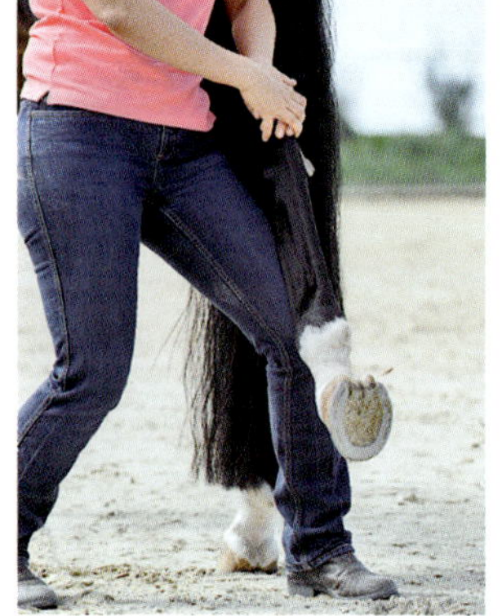

Pick up the leg and pull it backward and away from the horse. Keeping your leg slightly bent, place the horse's leg lightly on your thigh, like a farrier would. Keep your back straight as you do so. Place your hands on the point of hock

Physical Therapy for Horses

and press downward lightly. If there's give in the stretch, move a couple of centimeters (half an inch) farther back. At the end of this exercise, move the leg forward again and place the leg down. The disadvantage of this stretch is that you won't be able to see how the horse is reacting.

My Tip

My experience has shown that pelvic misalignment is often caused by shortened muscles in the hindquarters, in particular the loin musculature. This muscle group is so strong that it can actually pull the pelvis out of alignment. By regularly stretching this muscle group, as described above, you can remedy this condition.

Variation 3 (Advanced Level of Difficulty)

Loin Muscles

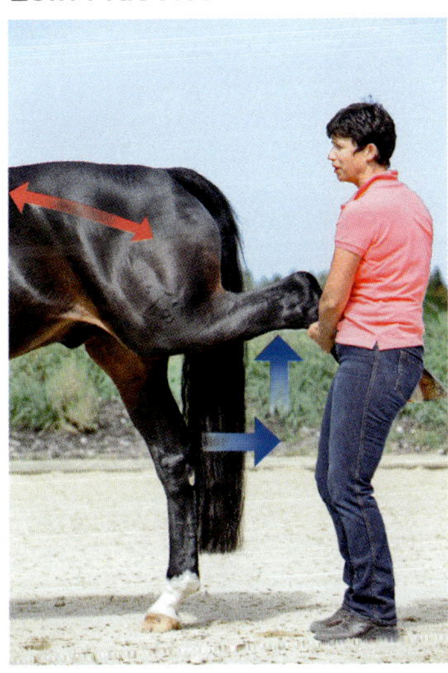

Your starting position is as described above. Here, the leg will definitely be guided upward; this means, the lower thigh (gaskin) will be parallel to the ground, which gives you a heightened stretch of the inner loin muscle. Please proceed very carefully with this stretch and only go backward really slowly. Many horses have tight muscles here and don't like having them stretched.

With a horse you don't know or if your horse tends to kick, this exercise should not be used for your own safety.

■ Crossing the Hind Limbs Under the Belly

Here, the muscles that move the leg backward and outward are stretched.

Variation 1 (Medium Level of Difficulty)

Pick up the leg from the opposite side and pull it toward you, under the belly, and diagonally to the horse's longitudinal axis. Pull the leg directly in front of the other leg. When the resistance lessens, you can stretch it farther toward the middle of the belly.

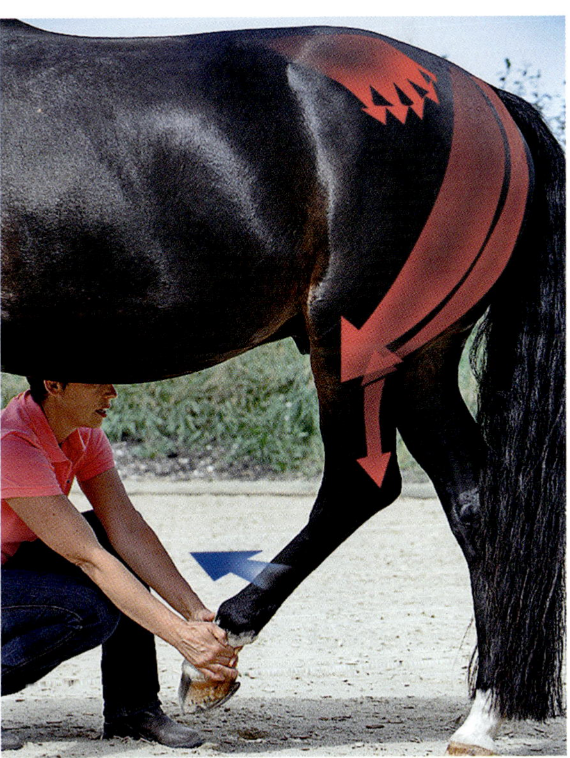

If the horse has a problem with picking up his leg, find an assistant who can hand the leg over to you. However, as soon as she's done so, the assistant should move back toward the horse's head, so that she's not standing in a place where she might get kicked.

Fact: Please keep in mind that most muscles involved with sideways movement work together with muscles that move the limbs forward or backward. This means that a single muscle can have two jobs. For example, the loin muscle (hip flexor) flexes the hip in the lifted phase and simultaneously brings the leg to the inside, and the croup muscle extends the hip joint and at the same time brings the leg to the outside. This means that when you stretch the muscles responsible for sideways movement, you're also providing a stretch for the muscles that move the limb forward and/or backward.

■ Stretching the Hind Limbs to the Outside

These exercises stretch the muscles that move the leg to the inside.

Variation 1 (Basic Exercise)

Pick up the limb at the fetlock joint. The limb should stay slightly flexed and you'll bring the whole leg to the outside and forward.

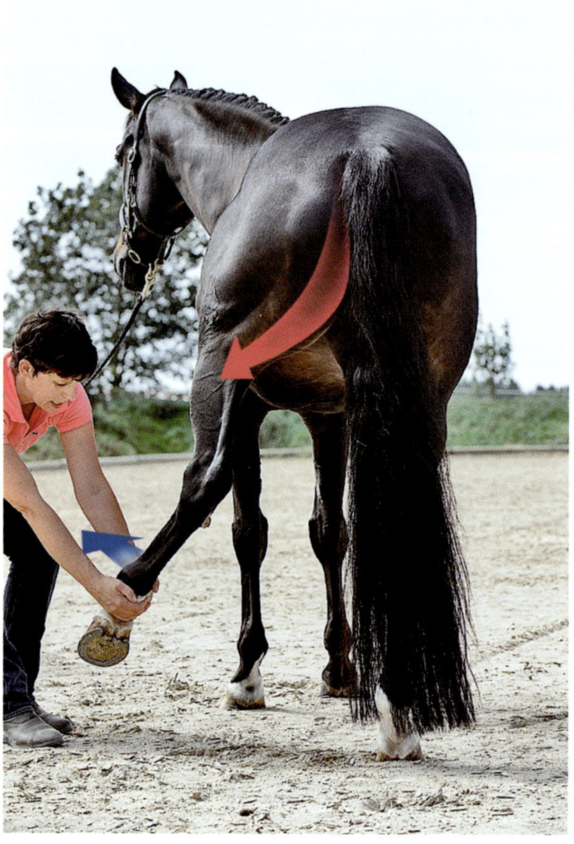

Stretching the Tail Back

This exercise directly stretches the small, stabilizing muscles directly along the spine.

Stand behind your horse and place your hands on the dock of his tail. Slowly and carefully, pull the tail toward you until you encounter a light resistance. The tail affects a lengthening of the sacrum.

Pulling on the tail dock is great for relieving tension in the spine. You can hold this pull for up to a minute. Please begin slowly and also go slow when you let go. Often, horses will begin to pull against you from their own accord because they find this pull so wonderful, relaxing, and full of release. Allow this to happen. You can hold against them, but please don't forget to go slowly when you let go so that the horse has the chance to shift his weight back into balance again.

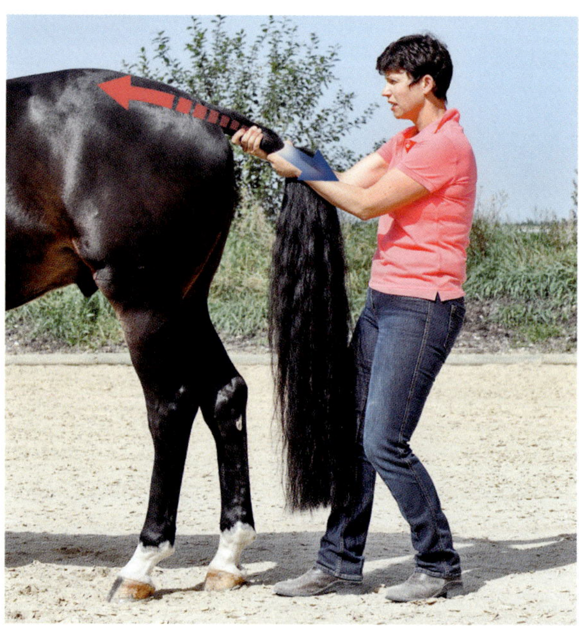

If your horse becomes restless or threatening, stop the exercise, and skip the tail pull.

Hint: Should your horse move worse in the one to three days following these stretching exercises, it may be a sign of an underlying problem. You should definitely have this horse examined.

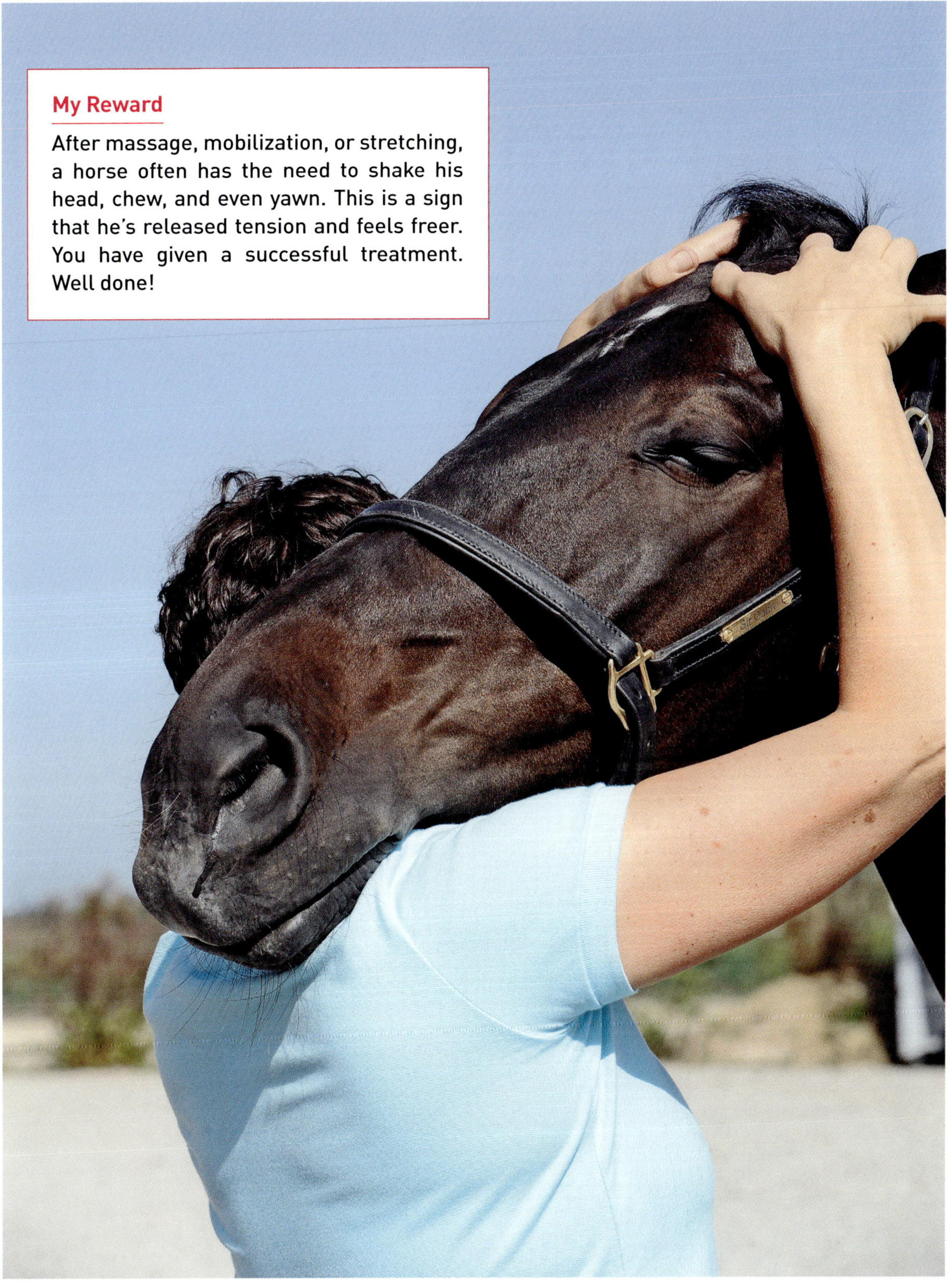

My Reward

After massage, mobilization, or stretching, a horse often has the need to shake his head, chew, and even yawn. This is a sign that he's released tension and feels freer. You have given a successful treatment. Well done!

Stabilization and Strengthening

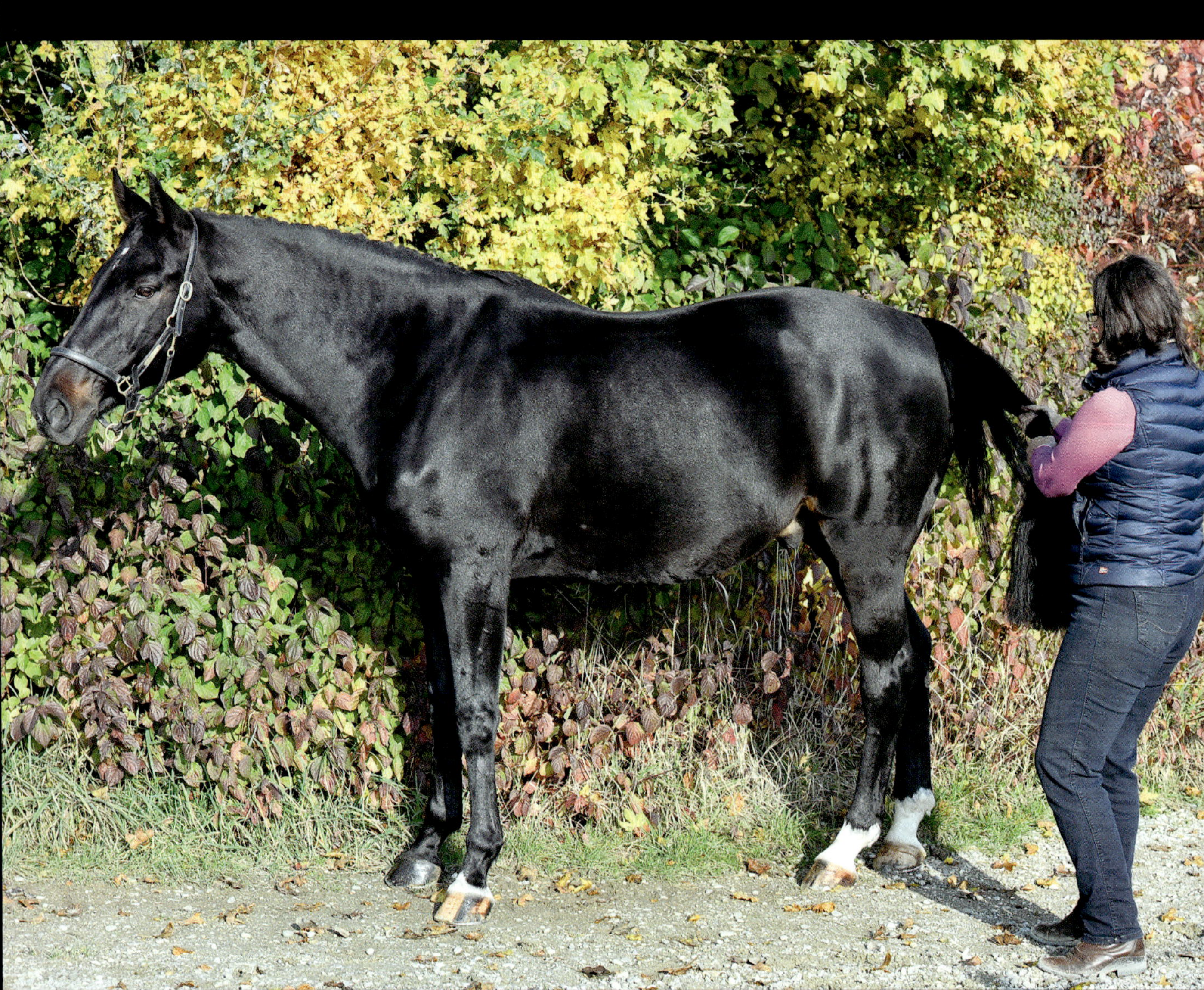

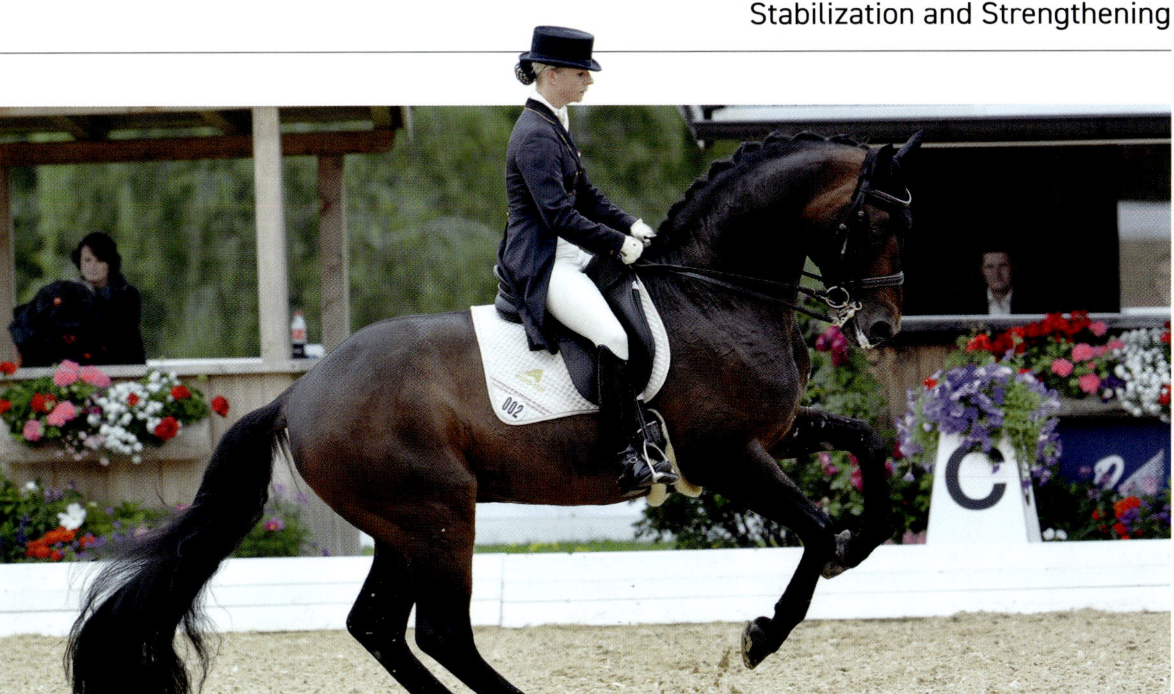

Riding promotes physical stability.

Have you ever tried Pilates or yoga? If so, can you remember how your back and/or abdominal muscles felt after your first practice? Yes, exactly. They hurt—your muscles were sore! I'm sure you thought, "These are muscles I didn't even know existed!"

Pilates and yoga encompass many fantastic exercises, specifically strengthening the stabilizing trunk muscles. It doesn't matter what sport you engage in: 100-meter sprint, golf, gymnastics, riding.... The same principle holds true for all sports: athletes need excellent body stability. This is as true for the hobby sportsman as it is for the Olympic athlete. An unstable body will lead to a loss of performance and, even worse, to a heightened risk of injury.

This is not only true for humans. For your horse to carry weight correctly and perform consistently, he has to be physically balanced and stable. Unfortunately, this is not always the case. The reasons for this vary but might include illness, conformation, or even riding discipline. In addition, breeding practices have changed horses' physical balance. Most riders are looking for rideable horses with a lot of movement potential. However, the spectacular movement demonstrated by many dressage horses of today can compromise stability: their back has become more mobile so they need more strength in order to balance and stabilize themselves. Often, they are unsuccessful at doing so. I would like to remind you at this point that, in nature, the horse's back is less mobile, which is what makes it more stable.

What Is Physical Stability?

Way back when, it was believed that muscles stabilize the body. Today, we know that muscles and fasciae form a unit and both are important for posture and balance.

The fasciae hold the human body upright and support it. Many medical doctors use the image of the mast on a sailing ship to explain the way in which the back is simultaneously mobile and stable/upright. Following this image, the mast consists of the spine and the deep stabilizing musculature. The rigging that supports the mast runs diagonally—like

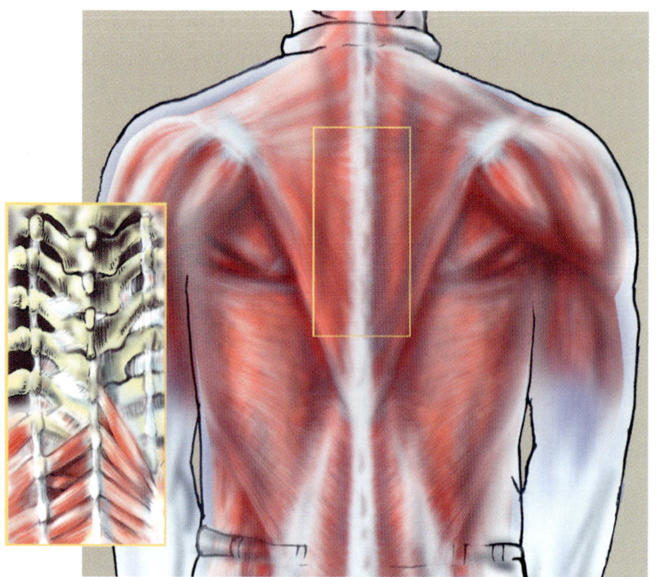

The spine forms the mast while the muscles and fasciae form the rigging that supports the mast.

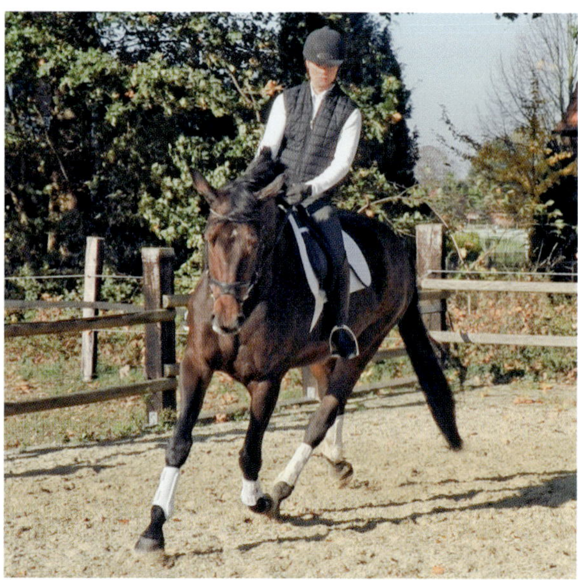

A young horse needs time and variety in his work in order to build stabilizing muscles.

the muscles along the trunk/barrel. The tension in the rigging/muscles provides stability for the mast/spine. This way the spine stays supple and can withstand pressure and pull when under the strain of movement.

The stabilizing muscles and the fasciae can be imagined as a corset that keeps your body upright. Important muscle groups include the deep muscles close to the joints of the spine, the abdominal muscles, the hip flexors and the shoulder and pelvic girdle muscles, among others.

When you consider the horse's body, all these muscle groups and fasciae support the trunk/barrel when the large, strong muscles of the hindquarters develop their forward thrust, or when the horse shifts his weight. On the one hand, they stabilize and, on the other, these muscle groups carry out movement in a controlled manner.

Fact: The body needs stability in order to perform at a high level, absorb stress caused by movement, and buffer concussive impulses.

When young horses are first ridden, they are not well balanced and have little physical stability. They

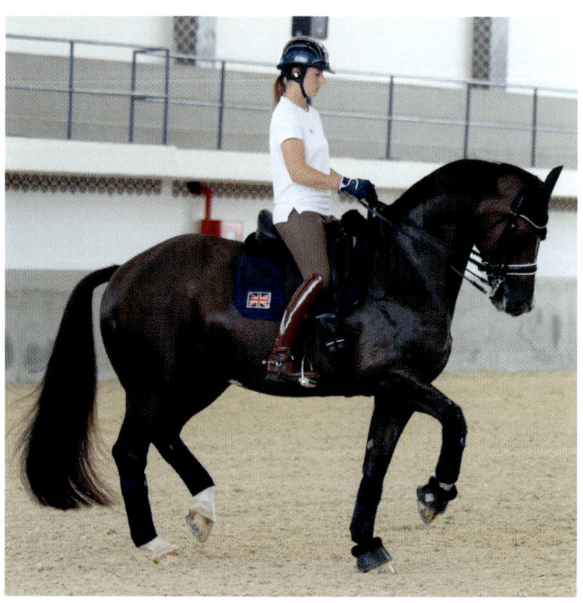

Gold-medal winner Valegro, during training in Rio. Here, you can very clearly see how he is able to stabilize his spine and carry weight with his hind end—a great example of physical stability. (Valegro is slightly behind the vertical in this very moment. Therefore, the poll is not the highest point.)

Physical Therapy for Horses

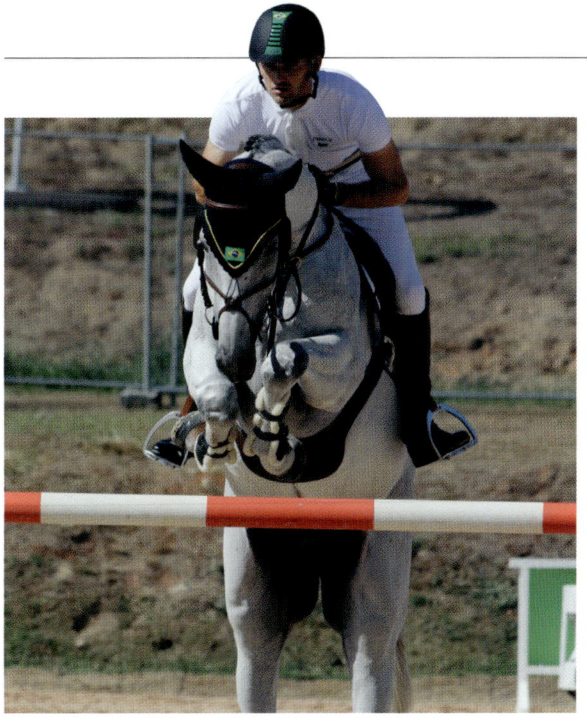

During takeoff, the horse also needs to stabilize himself in order to use strength from his hindquarters correctly.

will gain these skills throughout their training. If the rider doesn't allow for enough time, the horse is not given the chance to develop stabilizing musculature. This missing link in the education of the horse can cause weakness further down the road. You often see the result in dressage tests. Let's take the piaffe as an example: the horse performs a beautiful trot, but the moment he starts to piaffe, he loses rhythm and cannot lift his hind legs. This can be a sign of lack of stability in the trunk and pelvic girdle muscles, which will not allow the horse to carry weight on the supporting pair of legs and hold them until the other pair touches the ground again. So, too, in the pirouette, when jumping or executing a spin, the horse needs the strength of the stabilizing musculature.

One of your responsibilities during the education of the young horse is to mobilize his body through work but also to strengthen and stabilize him. The more advanced the training becomes, the more the body needs to be stabilized. This is the requirement for controlled movement patterns and it reduces the risk of injury and improves performance.

What Causes Instability?

From medical research, we know that for people who suffer from back pain, the deep stabilizing muscles are no longer functioning. As a result of the back pain, the muscles become inactive! They lose mass and strength, changes that are already visible in ultrasound images after just three days.

When the patient is pain-free, these muscle groups do not just automatically start working again. The probability that the back pain will return is around 80 percent. When the patient receives physical therapy and learns to reactivate the deep muscles, the percentage of recurrence is as low as 30 percent. It is assumed that the same is true for horses. In the same context, it was found that the fasciae in the back also change: they adhere and become matted, lose their mobility, and become painful.

In the United States, a study was conducted that followed horses over several months that participated in mobilization, stretching, and stabilizing exercises. The results were astonishing: after just a few weeks the horses exhibited better posture, the withers lifted, and performance was much improved, especially in the collected exercises. In addition, ultrasound images showed that the deep stabilizing musculature gained mass and strength. It is scientifically proven: working your horse from the ground pays off!

Since horses have the same muscle groups as humans and those muscles can quickly be reduced (atrophied), you need to act fast when pain or injury occurs. You need to provide those muscles with new stimuli to strengthen them again.

Back pain is not always the cause for instability. Other causes can include illnesses related to changes in the horse's training schedule, such as tendon or ligament injuries, or colic surgery. Instability can also be genetic.

When to Stabilize

The following stabilizing exercises constitute a continuation and progression of the mobilizing and stretching exercises described in chapter 8 (see p. 140). You should practice mobilizing exercises for about four weeks before beginning the stabilizing exercises. The following specifically strengthen the muscle groups responsible for posture and weight-bearing (trunk, shoulder, and pelvic-girdle musculature). They are uniquely suited for horses in rehabilitation as well as horses with weak abdominal muscles and horses with swayed backs.

I am convinced that most of us have seen a horse lose muscle mass very quickly due to an injury. We also know how long it takes to rebuild muscle strength. In cooperation with the treating veterinarian, the stabilizing/strengthening exercises (following the mobilizing phase) can be practiced during rehabilitation: they are in fact indispensable as they maintain mobility, strength, and stability. Studies have shown that horses were able to gain muscle mass through these exercises, even when they were not being ridden. With regular practice, horses will emerge in a better condition from a break in training and the rehabilitation phase will be shorter.

In addition, these exercises are very helpful for young horses. We know through experience that focused administration of exercises helps young horses to balance the rider's weight. They don't just help the horse carry the rider, they also benefit the horse's coordination and balance. These stabilizing exercises are also very well-suited for horses being schooled at a very high level. These horses have to perform but should not be overwhelmed. Especially when the collected exercises are not yet confirmed, stabilizing exercises can lead to improvement. You will see the difference even after a short time!

How Often and for How Long?

If you have the opportunity, you should do these exercises regularly and, if your horse is particularly weak, even several times a day. I know that most of us don't have the time to get out to the barn more than once a day. My advice: always do the exercises after riding the horse. This will guarantee that the horse is warmed up and well-prepared.

With a very unstable horse, it is worthwhile doing the exercises before riding.

My Tip

Daily training is recommended, which is not always possible, but the more, the better. Even if you only get to the exercises three times a week, it is still so much better than nothing!

When *Shouldn't* Strengthening Exercises Be Applied?

- When ataxia or other neurological disorders are present (poor coordination).
- In the case of severe trouble with balance—for example, when the horse needs to lean against a wall to pick up one foot.
- In the case of fresh injury or after surgery. When your horse has an injury affecting his musculoskeletal system, please clarify with your veterinarian and physical therapist as to whether or not you should do the exercises.
- Should you observe that your horse gets worse from the exercises, rather than improving, please contact your veterinarian. A secondary problem may be present that has not yet been diagnosed.

Safety

- As with all exercises in this book, it is important to practice on non-slip footing.
- Until you and your horse are familiar with the exercises, you should ask an assistant to hold him.

Implementation

You already stabilized your horse by practicing the mobilizing and stretching exercises, since it is not possible to mobilize or to stretch without stimulating other areas.

You can easily test how effective the next exercises are: ask another rider to "push" you in different directions, while you stay upright and still like a tree. Do you feel how much muscle strength you must activate? And you probably also feel how many different muscle groups are working all over your body to maintain your balance. This is the positive aspect of these stabilizing exercises: they are effective.

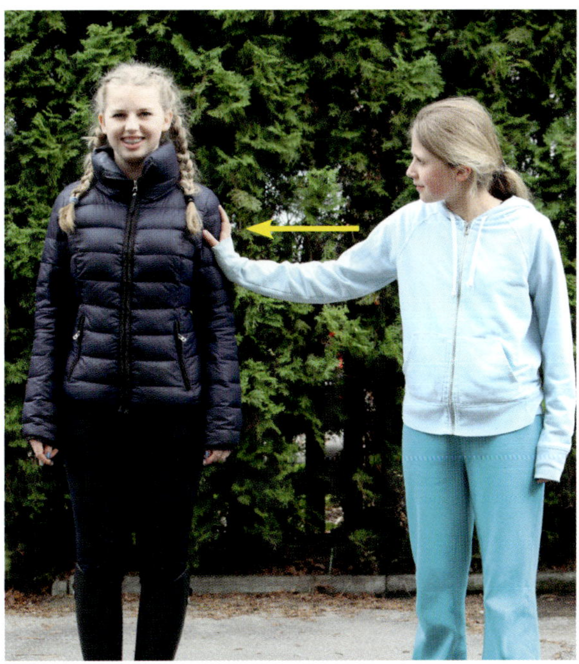

Through this simple exercise, you can experience how many muscles have to be activated to stay stable and avoid losing your balance.

Every position within the individual exercise can be held for up to 20 seconds. Here too, a variety of signals should be administered. Sometimes the signals can be given in shorter intervals to activate the horse's reaction.

Exercises for Stabilization and Strengthening

Stabilizing the Forehand

These exercises serve to strengthen the shoulder girdle and abdominal musculature. There are two variations.

■ Lifting the Withers

Stand next to the front leg, looking at the hind leg. You achieve the lifting of the withers by activating the reflex at the abdominal midline with your fingertips. This causes the front part of the back to slightly rise and the rib cage to move upward between the shoulder blades (compare to the exercise on p. 156).

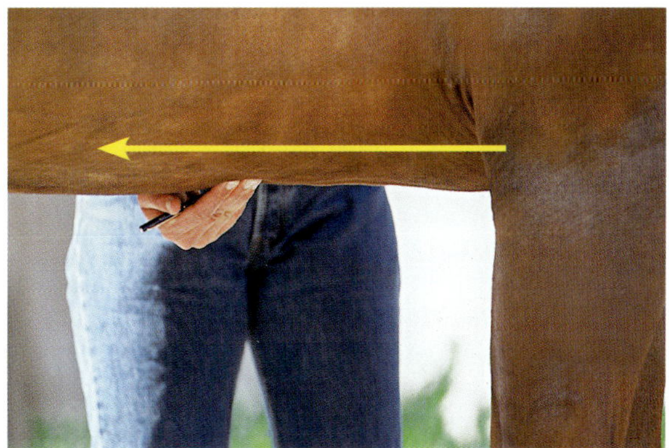

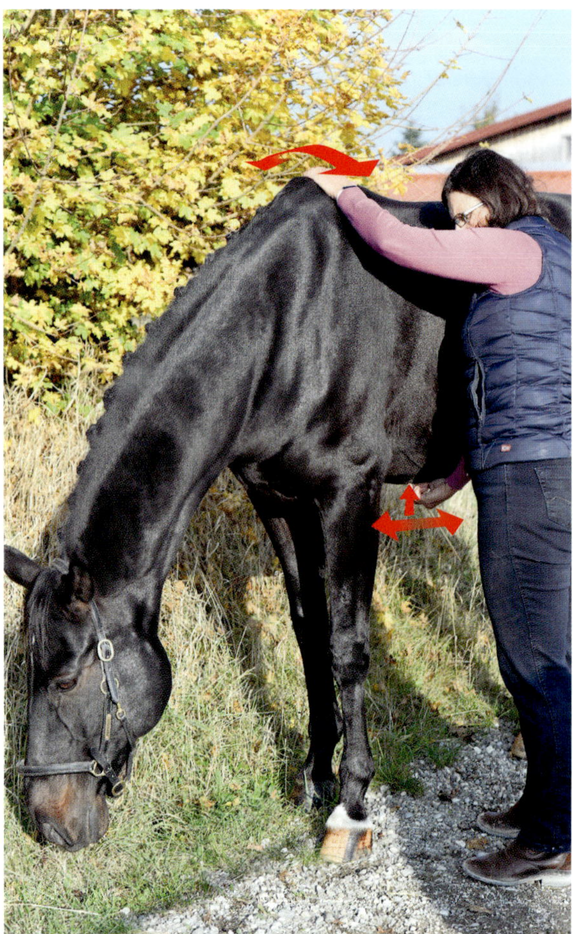

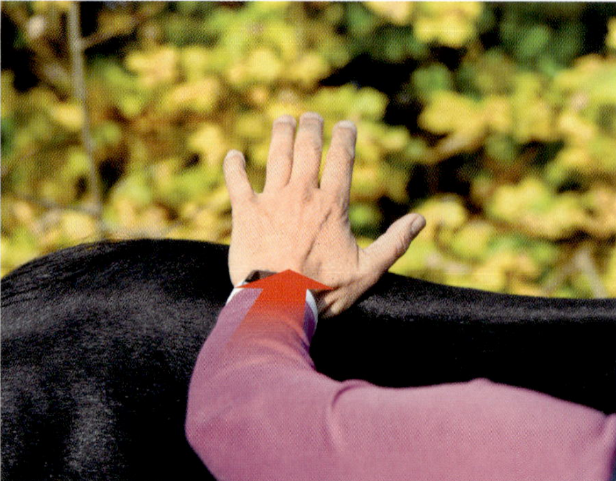

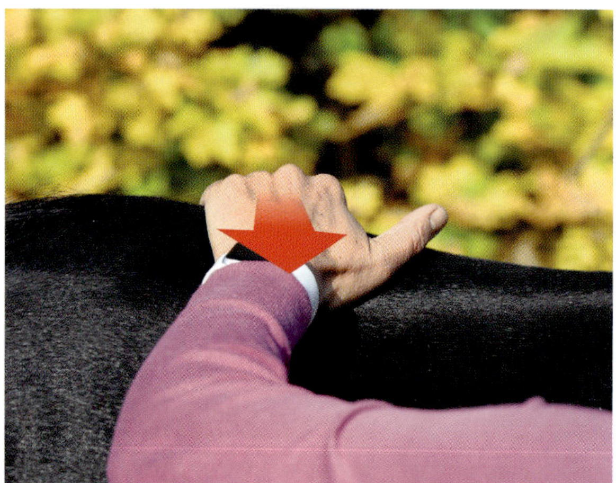

Variation 1

With continuous light pressure at the sternum and lifted rib cage, the horse is being positioned back and forth with short signals with the other hand at the withers (as shown in the pictures above). The intensity and scope of the movement should be varied. This exercise stabilizes the shoulder-girdle musculature. Make sure that the withers stay lifted between the shoulder blades during this exercise. That means that you must repeatedly give a signal at the sternum.

When the horse does not cooperate during these exercises, only perform the easier ones, the mobilization exercises that are described on page 149 and the following pages.

Variation 2 (Medium Degree of Difficulty)

The basic position is the same as in Variation 1, but you lift one front leg with your hand closest to the horse's head and hold it in a relaxed manner. Your other hand activates the reflex at the sternum. The horse has to shift the rib cage to the other side using his shoulder-girdle musculature. This is a great strengthening exercise for the forehand!

Variation 3 (Medium Degree of Difficulty)

An even more difficult exercise is the lifting of one front leg (as shown in photo p. 173, top left). At the same time, you can activate the reflex at the sternum. The standing on one leg and the activation of the reflex at the same time causes the horse to lift his trunk, and stabilizes the shoulder musculature on the side of the supporting leg.

Physical Therapy for Horses

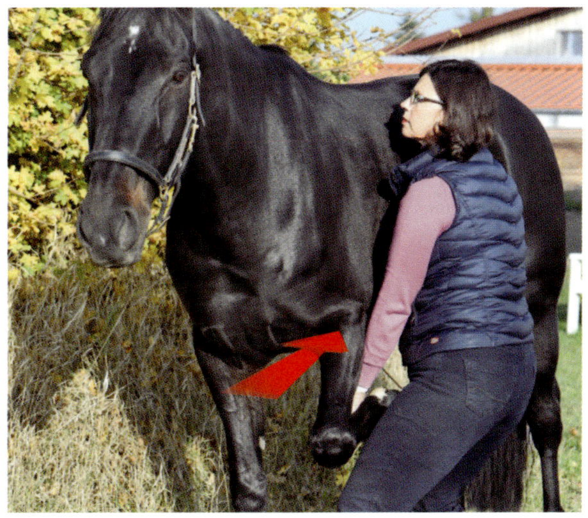

■ Shifting Weight to the Forehand

Starting Point
Stand to the side of the hindquarters.

Implementation
Push the horse forward using light pressure. When shifting his weight to the forehand, he has to activate his shoulder-girdle musculature.

This exercise can also be modified: an assistant can activate the reflex at the sternum and the horse will lift his rib cage at the same time.

Fact: Many horses that appear to be built "downhill," are actually weak in the forehand. As a result, their trunk is lowered between their shoulder blades.

■ Strengthening the Abdominal and Upper Thigh Muscles

Starting Point
Stand to the side at the hindquarters and stimulate the reflex found to the right and left of the hindquarters (see photo p. 157, bottom left) so that the horse lifts his back. This will stimulate a reflex of the hindquarters, which activates the abdominal muscles and stretches the upper thigh. The upper-thigh muscles as well as the abdominal muscles are being strengthened and the topline is being stretched. In addition, this activates the shoulder-girdle musculature as the horse shifts his weight forward.

Variation (Medium Degree of Difficulty)
This is a great exercise for improving your horse's bending. Again, position yourself to the side of your horse's hindquarters. With a bent pointer finger, draw a line from the direction of the opposite hip point over the croup in the direction of the tail. The spine will react with a lift and sideways bend in your direction. Caution, the horse could take a step in your direction to regain balance—watch your feet.

Among others, this exercise strengthens the *longissimus dorsi*, the *intercostals*, and the *abdominal* muscles on the side the horse is bending toward.

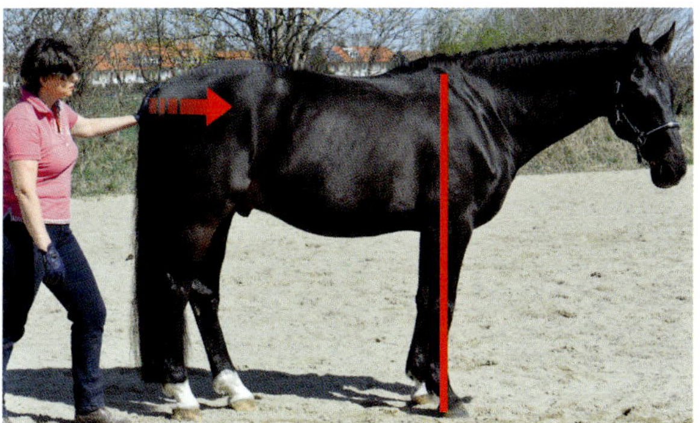

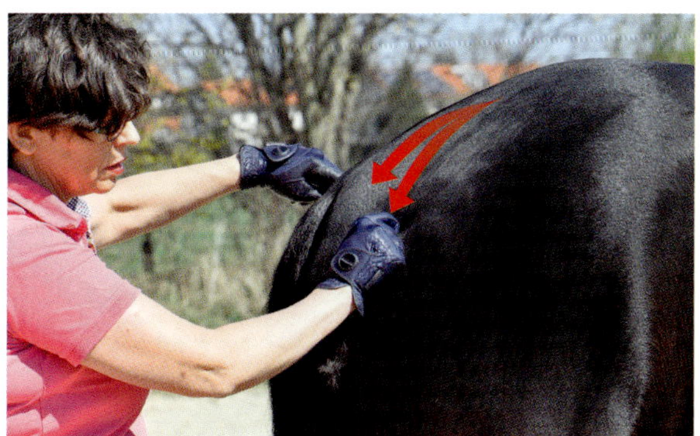

> **My Tip**
>
> **If your horse does not enjoy the lift stimulated by your finger, try using a brush.**

■ Pulling the Tail

This exercise can improve stability and strength of the hindquarters.

Starting Point

Stand to the side at the hindquarters.

Variation 1

Your horse is standing square. Now, pull the tail in a 90-degree angle slowly toward you, until tension in the upper thigh becomes visible. Hold the position for up to 20 seconds. You can give different signals: sometimes hold the tail longer, sometimes for a shorter time.

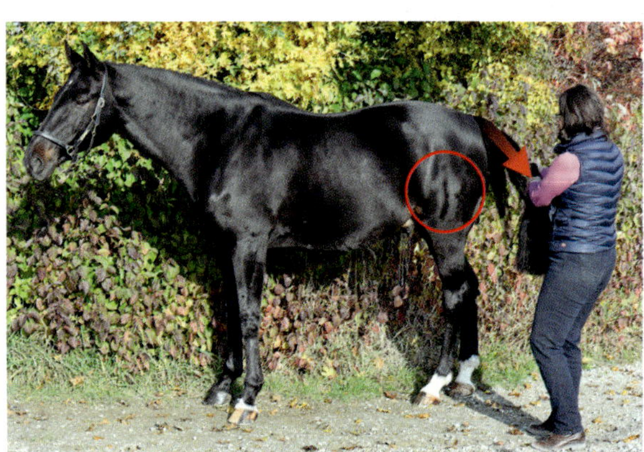

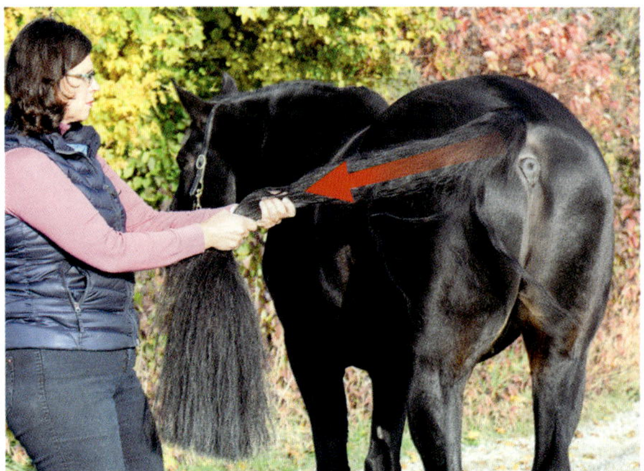

Variation 2

In this exercise, you can increase the difficulty by using one hand to create pulses (small pushes) away from you as you release the pull on the tail. In this way, both hind limbs are stabilized and you avoid the horse simply leaning into the pull on his tail. Important: The pulling motion should never be

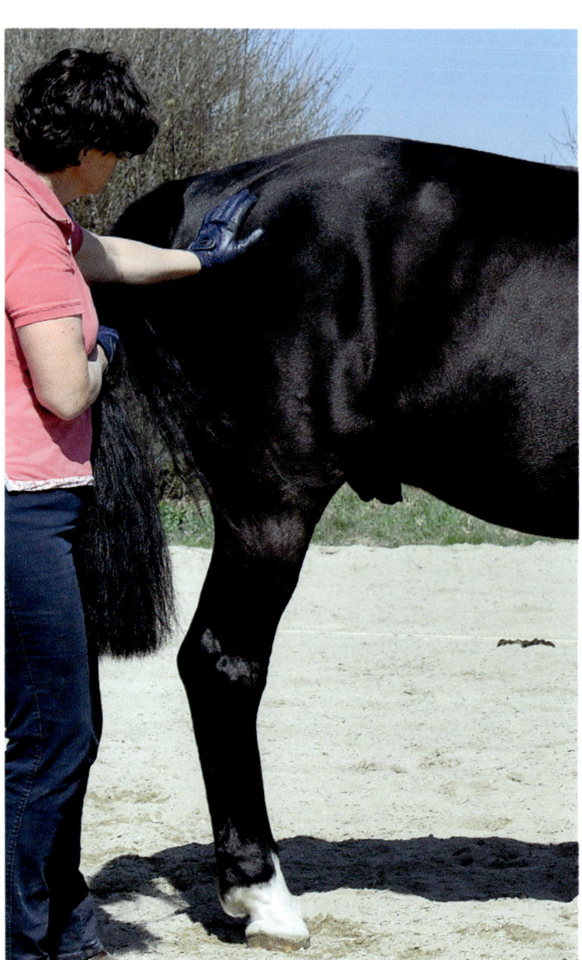

choppy, but rather always applied with caution and by slowly increasing and decreasing pressure.

> *Hint: Please make sure that the horse is not twisting his fetlock joint. If this is the case, you are pulling too hard and the horse cannot withstand the pressure.*

■ Shifting Weight to the Hindquarters

Starting Point
Stand to the side of your horse.

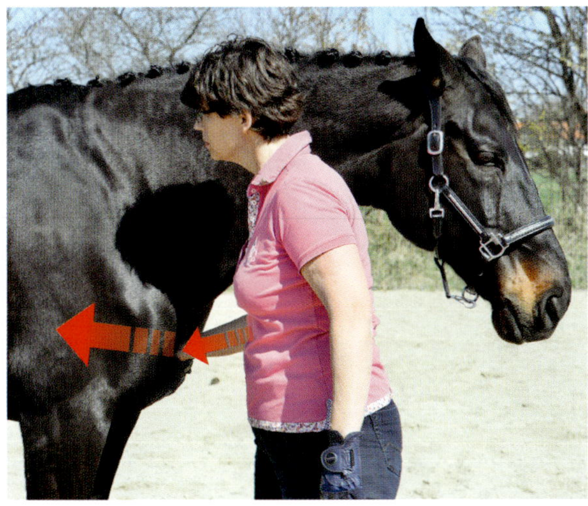

Implementation
Give the horse a push backward at the sternum. The horse will shift weight to his hindquarters and has to activate the pelvic-girdle musculature.

Many horses will step backward during this exercise, as the input you're giving is one he recognizes as a signal to back up. Should that be the case, you can position the horse so that his hindquarters are in a corner. This way, he will quickly learn to stand when you apply pressure to the sternum in this context.

This exercise can also be made more difficult: a second person can pull on the tail at the same time (see photo p. 174, bottom left), causing the horse to stabilize himself even more.

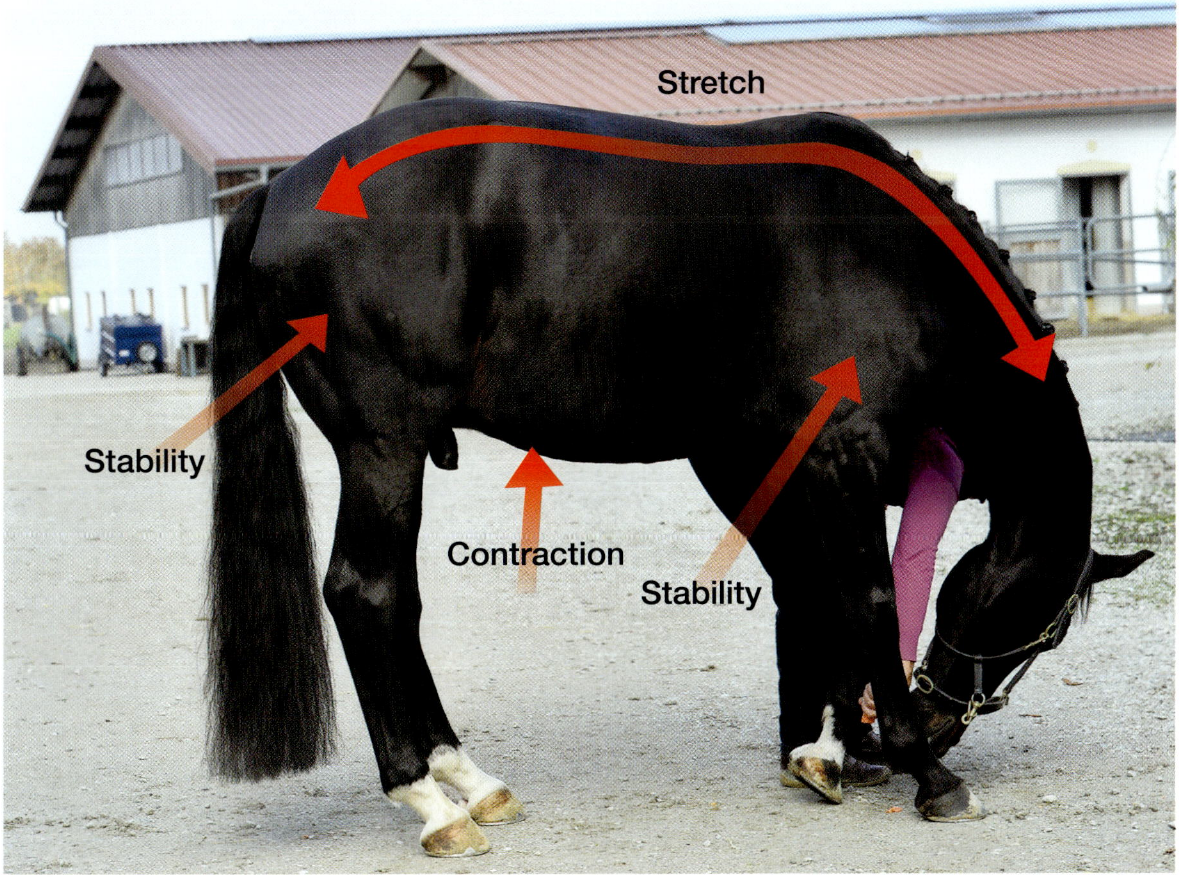

Physical Therapy

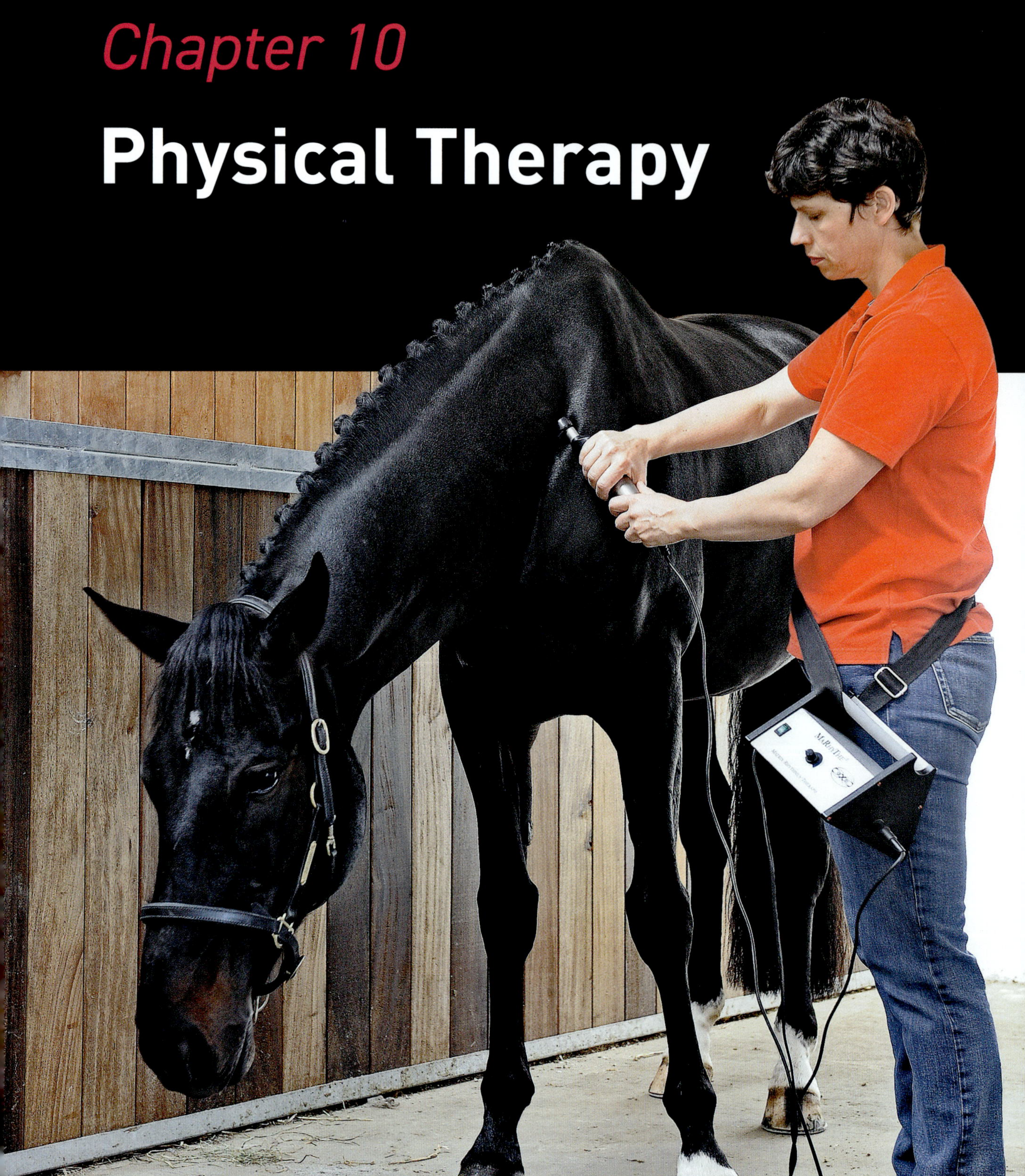

Your horse is injured and possibly needs to be treated by a veterinarian. As horse owners, we often stand by and all we want to do is help our partner get free from pain and healthy as quickly as possible. Physical therapy can be a primary measure for limiting injury as much as possible, supporting the affected structures and assisting in a quick and successful recovery. These measures can be applied during rehabilitation or preventively.

In this chapter, I will introduce and explain the most common tools and equipment used in equine physical therapy:

- Ice
- Water
- Heat therapy
- Matrix-rhythm therapy
- Magnetic field therapy
- Laser therapy
- Ultrasound therapy
- Muscle stimulator
- TENS (Transcutaneous Electrical Nerve Stimulation)
- Kinesiology tape

Important Hint!
This book does not explain the length or dosage of treatments, since they vary greatly between devices. For each device, the manufacturer provides detailed instructions. Here, I must reiterate that competent, professional instruction by a veterinarian, physical therapist, therapist, or the maker of a specific device is very important. Treatment can only be effective and successful when these instructions are being followed correctly. Therefore, always get competent advice for diagnoses and treatment; otherwise, you could cause irreparable damage.

Ice Therapy

Ice therapy is applied for all acute injuries—for example, bone, tendon, ligament, and muscle injuries (bruising, sprains, strains, fractures). In addition, in the case of an acute injury, ice is the most helpful and least expensive application there is.

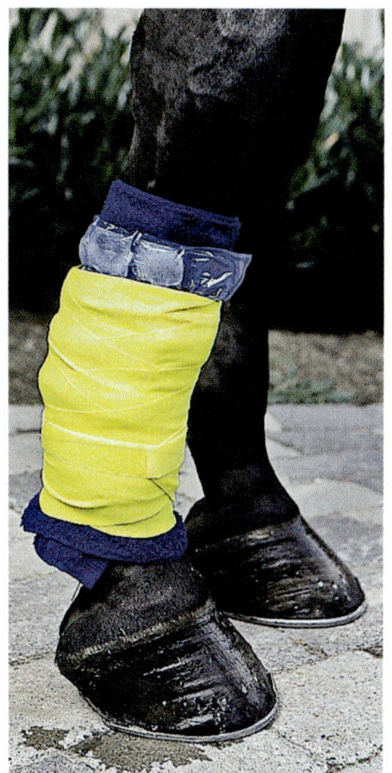

An application of ice done early and correctly can minimize the extent of an acute injury.

Effects
The result of an injury is destruction of tissue and blood vessels. With an open wound, blood exits the wound. With an internal injury, blood enters surrounding tissue. Internal injuries result in swelling and hemorrhaging, leading to pain and a slowing of the healing process. This type of injury can be treated with ice effectively.

How Ice Affects Injured Tissue
The immediate application of ice to an acute injury triggers a response in the blood vessels surrounding the wound. The vessels contract, which leads to less bleeding in the area. And, in order to keep bruising (hemorrhaging) at a minimum, your goal is to stop additional bleeding into the injured tissue.

A few days after an injury, you enter the subacute phase of healing. During this phase, you need to increase circulation again. Ice can be useful here, too, but it needs to be applied with great caution.

Application

> *Important Hint!*
> *Don't use ice directly on the skin. Always position a damp, thin cloth between the ice and the body part to avoid injury to the tissue.*

• Acute Injury

In the case of an acute injury, it is your goal to stop the bleeding into the injured tissue. This means that the quicker you start treating an injury with ice, the better.

First, use a bandage or your hands to apply light pressure to the "internal wound" from the outside. Immediately afterward, apply the ice. In this way, you can compress the blood vessels, which suppresses swelling and bleeding. A superficial injury to muscle, tendon, or ligaments requires an application of ice for about 10 minutes, followed by a 20-minute break. Apply light pressure during the break. Repeat the application until bleeding in the tissue has stopped (two to four times).

Important

It is important to adhere to the times during the application. If ice is applied to the acute injury for too long, the body will register the cooling and will reopen the blood vessels in order to help the cold tissue. The result is that even more blood reaches the injured tissue and even more hemorrhaging occurs.

• Subacute Phase

After a few days, should swelling and inflammation occur, you can continue treating with ice, but with different treatment times. Otherwise, you should stop treating with ice. During the subacute phase, you should use a "short ice" application, meaning, ice is now applied for short intervals only, since your objective is now to *increase* blood flow. The ice is applied for 1 to 3 minutes, followed by a 5-minute break. This pattern is repeated four to six times. The short cooling of the tissue increases cell activity and blood flow, but it also decreases the production of substances responsible for inflammation.

Again, it's important to adhere to the times described here because applying ice for too long can actually injure the tissue: nerves can be irreparably damaged, lymphatic vessels can be destroyed, and cell activity can be decreased.

> *Ice Timing:*
> *Acute muscle injury:*
> *10-minute icing, 20-minute break.*
>
> *Acute tendon and ligament injury:*
> *10-minute icing, 20-minute break, as often as possible during the 48 hours directly following the injury.*
>
> *Subacute injury:*
> *1- to 3-minute icing, 5-minute break, four to six repetitions.*

A Few Tips

Pure ice cubes made of water are well-suited for injuries. I always use the disposable ice cube bags. These can be directly applied by wrapping them around the leg and holding them in place with polo wraps. But remember: please use a damp towel/cloth between ice and leg.

Be careful with gel ice packs. They quickly lose their cooling ability and then actually start accumulating heat from the body. Heat is the last thing you want on an acute injury since it increases circulation!

You can also put **wet towels or bandage liners** in the freezer and then wrap them directly around the injury. They don't hold cold very long and start storing heat after a while.

To create an **"ice lollipop,"** fill a paper cup with water and put it in the freezer. When the water is frozen, cut away half of the paper cup. Now you can massage the affected area of your horse for some time, without your fingers getting too cold. When you move the ice lollipop in small circles, you massage and cool the affected area at the same time.

When You *Shouldn't* Use Ice

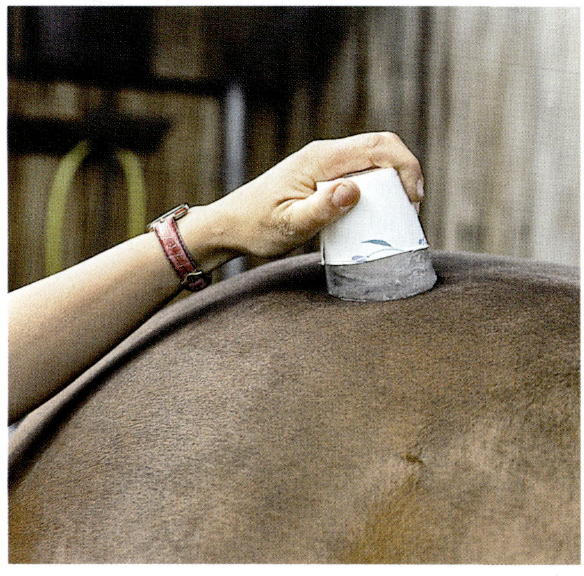

The ice lollipop is a great alternative to other ice applications. Make small circles with the ice lollipop. Since the ice is in constant movement, you can apply it directly to the skin.

The following injuries and changes in tissue are a contraindication to any treatment with ice:

- Open wounds
- Chronic damage to blood vessels and lymph vessels
- Injury to nerves

Hydrotherapy

Hydrotherapy uses the power of water. The effect is aimed at the body's self-healing abilities. The combination of water and pressure on the skin results in activation of the cardiovascular and lymphatic systems. For example, if your horse has swollen limbs as a result of an injury or too much stress, treatment with running water can be excellent lymph drainage. Using the gentle pressure of the water, the lymph vessels get support from the outside and with the deliberate aiming of the water stream you can move the excess lymph upward.

Application

The water is supposed to flow with little pressure against the horse's limbs and the stream is always pointed upward. Splashing should be avoided; the water is supposed to flow softly over the horse's skin. Start at the hoof, then move along the inside of the leg and guide the water stream upward to the knee/hock. Make small circles at the joint and move back down on the outside of the leg back toward the hoof. Start at the hoof again, and guide the water stream upward to the chest/upper thigh area and back down on the outside of the leg toward the hoof.

The principle of guiding the water stream up and down on the limbs is as follows: from bottom to top on the inside of the limb, and from top to bottom on the outside. The water stream should be moved up and down the leg twice on each side, for a total treatment time of 15 to 20 minutes each time (up and down).

Hint: Start treatment with water on the limb farthest from the heart: back right, back left, front right, front left.

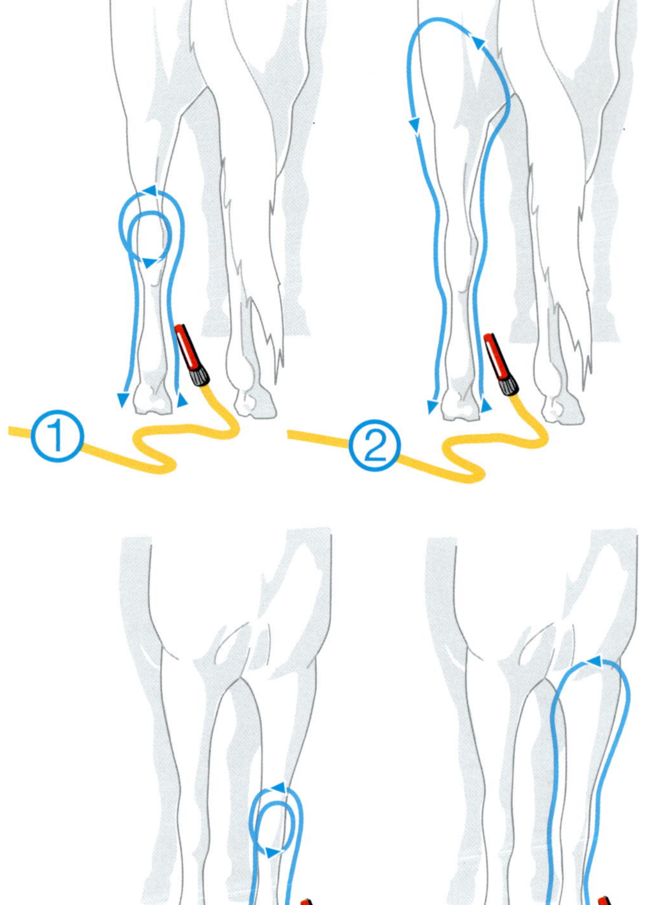

Hydrotherapy has a great effect on the lymphatic system. Swollen and tired limbs can be treated with water with good results.

When You *Shouldn't* Use Hydrotherapy

Under no circumstances should you use water as a treatment for the following problems:

- Open wounds
- Heart problems
- Nerve injuries

Heat Therapy

We all know the feeling: we feel a pinching in our shoulder muscles or back and intuitively we want to apply heat to these tight muscles. This is not a new idea: the use of heat for healing purposes is a practice that has been around for a very long time. Still today, heat plays a large role in human and veterinary medicine. For chronic illness involving the horse's musculoskeletal system, treating with heat promises to be a successful therapy. The muscle tone decreases and tightness, which is often the source for pain, loosens up. The tissue becomes more elastic and vessels open up, which leads to improved circulation.

I will introduce three applications for heat therapy for horses.

Fango

Fango is an Italian word, which directly translates as "healing mud." Originally, it consisted of volcanic mud that is rich in minerals.

Effect

Horses love *fango* treatments and if you've enjoyed one before, you understand why. *Fango* consists either of mud from a bog or a mix of volcanic minerals. The specific benefits are generated by the long-term heat storage and the quality of the minerals in the substance, which strengthen circulation and penetrate deeply. The heat leads to increased circulation, which in turn, leads to general relaxation and decrease of muscle pain and tightness. For example, when the *fango* treatment is applied to the horse's back in the thoracic area, there will be a reflective effect on the inner organs. This deep heat also helps very well with chronic joint changes (arthroses). The heat causes your horse to become more supple and flexible.

You can also use other materials that store heat. For example, cherrystone pillows, warm bran, or mashed potatoes. Put mash in a wet towel, since moist heat penetrates deeper into the tissue. These treatments only provide heat and lack the additional healing benefit of the minerals found in *fango*.

Application

Different versions of *fango* packs are available. You can find mud that can be directly applied to the horse's coat or *fango* that is packaged in a permeable foil. In addition, there are reusable bog and paraffin packs available on the market.

Always follow the instructions included in the package, but make sure that the pack is not too hot for your horse. To check, first put the back of your hand on the *fango* and only move it to your horse when the temperature feels acceptable to you. Keep in mind that the *fango* pack will stay in touch with your horse's skin for a long time, 20 to 40 minutes. You don't need to treat with heat any longer than 40 minutes, since the maximum circulation is achieved after 40 minutes.

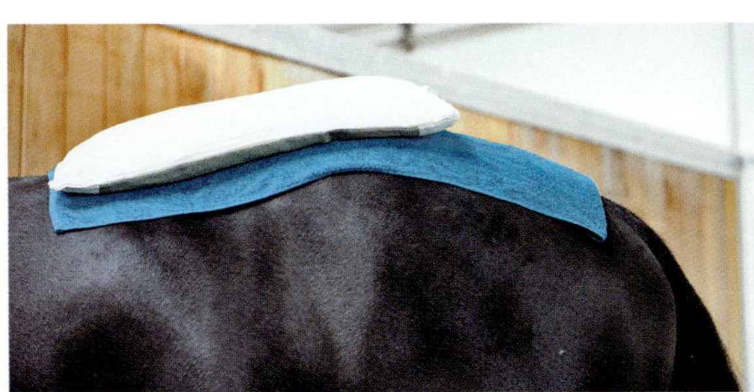

Here chickpeas are used for heat treatment. Using a wet towel helps the heat to penetrate deeper into the tissue.

When You *Shouldn't* Use Fango
- Any type of heart problem
- Acute injury and infection
- Fever
- Pregnant mares (when area of concern is in the loin area)

Hot Rolls

You can treat the same symptoms with a hot roll as you can with *fango*; for example, tightness and muscle pain. The effect is the same, although the heat will not penetrate as deeply with a hot roll, due to shorter application intervals. The advantage of the hot roll: you can apply it to those parts of the body where application of *fango* packs or heat pillows is impossible—for example, the shoulder, neck, and/or the upper extremities.

Application

Fold three towels lengthwise and tightly roll them into one another, forming a chute. Slowly pour hot water into the chute.

This hot roll is applied to the tissue briefly, several times (one to two seconds). Now the towels can be unfolded slowly, so that a part of the warm towel can be applied to the tissue in intervals. The towel touches the skin only briefly to avoid burning. The therapy consists of short heat impulses, helped by the moisture in the towel. The application should last 10 to 15 minutes.

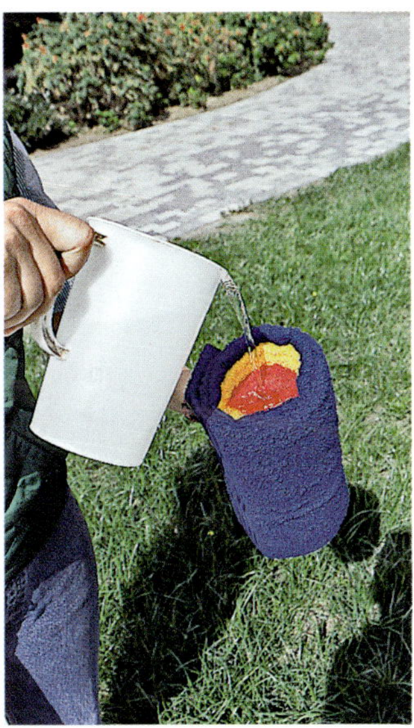

When You *Shouldn't* Use a Hot Roll
- All heart problems
- Acute injury and infection (hematoma, wounds)
- Fever
- Pregnant mares (when area of concern is in the loin area)

Solarium Therapy

The solarium is a very popular device in many barns. It provides infrared and ultraviolet (artificial) daylight, which have a positive effect on your horse's well-being. The infrared sends energy into the deeper skin layers of your horse, which is a pleasant experience. The artificial daylight, the ultraviolet light, supports the production of Vitamin D. Since many horses unfortunately still lack enough exposure to sunlight, the solarium can support their health a little bit, though it cannot replace genuine daylight. First, the solarium helps with horses' recovery after work. They perceive the warmth as pleasant and it helps them to relax after physical work. As a result, the muscle tone is lowered and blood flow in the tissue is normalized.

Application

Horses really enjoy solarium therapy after being worked. It can provide some pain relief in the neck and back areas, but unfortunately, the heat doesn't penetrate deeply enough to loosen chronic tenseness. It is understood that the solarium is also useful in the winter to dry the coat. The optimal application time is around 20 to 30 minutes.

Hint: If your horse ends up under the solarium for more than 45 minutes, be aware that his blood pressure can momentarily drop. After an application of this length, your horse needs at least one hour of rest to allow for him to recover and for optimal therapeutic results.

Often the assumption is that the solarium helps with warming up the musculature before riding and shortens the warm-up time under saddle. This is not correct, since the heat only works on the surface.

When You *Shouldn't* Use the Solarium

There are no contraindications to the use of the solarium. But, obviously, no one should put a feverish or hot horse under the solarium.

Matrix-Rhythm Therapy

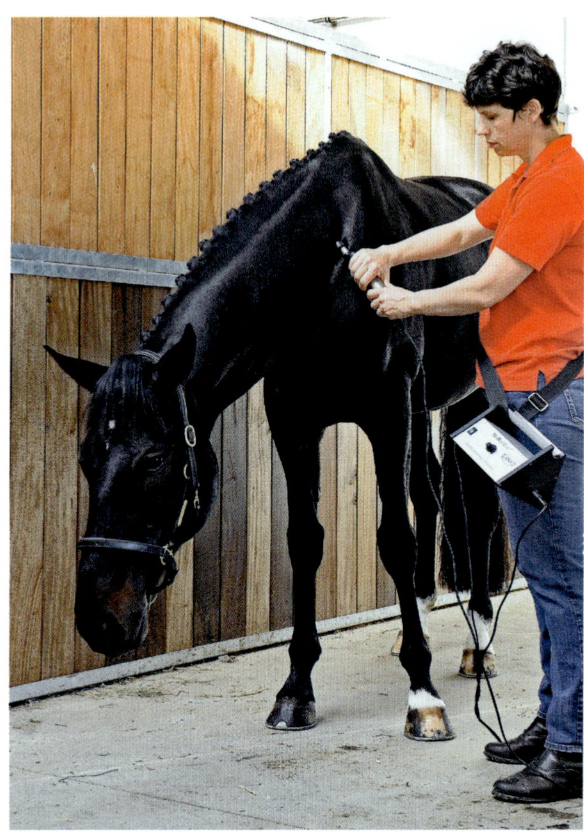

Matrix-rhythm therapy very effectively loosens muscle tenseness and helps the horse to relax.

The matrix is the basic substance of our body. It exists in the extracellular spaces, which means that it is present between each cell in the body. The matrix is interwoven with small, fine, blood vessels, which remove oxygen and nutrients to the matrix and receive metabolic waste. The transport between blood vessels and cells happens through the matrix.

Each cell, even in rest, executes a small rhythmical movement (micro-vibration). When this micro-vibration is disturbed, as in the case of pain and accumulated tension, the matrix quantity and quality quickly deteriorate. The cell supply is reduced and the emission of cell breakdown products is slowed. As a result, metabolism is no longer optimal.

Physical Therapy for Horses

Effects

The matrix-rhythm device creates vibrations. These specific vibrations have a positive effect on the micro-vitality. As a result, blood flow is greatly improved in the treatment area. This "flushing" cleans the organism (matrix) of metabolic wastes and over acidification. In this way, for example, muscle tone can be regulated. The activation of muscle cells leads to a much improved coordination between the individual muscle cells. Many structures in the body can be treated this way; for example, chronic pain, wounds, and scars.

Application

The device consists of a motor and a treatment stick with a specifically formed head, which creates vibrations. This head is applied to the affected tissue, transversely to the orientation of the muscle fibers. Turning the head of the stick creates a slight stretching of the tissue. Superficially and more deeply, tightness and adhesions are gently loosened through this micro-stretching technique. Two minutes per treatment area is enough time.

I personally work a lot with a matrix-rhythm device and have had astonishing results. As a medical layperson, you can also us this device, but you need a very good introduction to be able to use it correctly. The device is "harmless": you cannot do any damage, as long as you pay attention to the contraindications.

When You *Shouldn't* Use Matrix-Rhythm Therapy

Contraindications to the treatment with a matrix-rhythm device are acute injuries (wounds, hematomas, soft tissue injuries), fever, and direct application to skin conditions like fungal infections.

My Tip

When you treat muscle tightness with this device, you'll find that, for example, the *longissimus dorsi* responds excellently to the matrix treatment. You should limit the treatment to two minutes per area, or three to four minutes for larger areas. I've experienced getting the musculature so loose, that horses temporarily became "unstable" in their haunches. I was able to loosen the tenseness, which acts like a "muscular corset," and the horses lost their stance. In my experience, you can achieve better results with short treatment repetitions.

Magnetic Therapy

Magnetic therapy is a very popular treatment option. This is not a new, modern treatment. It is believed magnetic stones were already being used 2000 years ago to support the healing process as part of Chinese medicine. During the same time period, Romans and Egyptians wore magnetic stones as jewelry to improve their health. Even Hippocrates[7] wrote a few words about the use and effect of those stones.

Today, we don't need to put stones on our horses anymore. Depending on the manufacturer, static or pulsing magnets are created with coil mats, small pillows, sticks, and tubes (with different frequencies, intensities, and programs). The magnets are inserted in blankets, splint boots, or into small pillows that you can put on your horse.

There are different types of magnetic therapy. There is the static type, which does not use electricity, and there is a variation with pulsing magnets, which are powered by electricity. The latter allows the user to work with different frequencies.

---

7 Hippocrates (460 to 370 BC) is the most famous medical doctor of ancient times.

Effects

Within and around a cell, there is electrical voltage. The cell needs positive and negative voltage to allow for optimal metabolism. If this voltage gets out of balance (caused by injury, illness, or overexertion) the metabolism of the affected cell is lowered. Through the influence of magnetic fields, this voltage can be brought back into balance, the metabolism and cell activity will be activated and can therefore better support the recovery and healing process.

In trials, it has been observed that cells are able to reestablish their own rhythm (movement), via the application of magnetic therapy.

Application

Magnetic therapy is easy to apply. With static magnetic fields, you can put the magnets on the treatment area. With electromagnetic treatment, you adjust the control unit according to the manufacturer's instructions. You can adjust to different frequencies to produce alternating magnetic fields. This opens the possibility of using magnets selected for different types of tissue, such as bone, cartilage, or muscle tissues, since the tissue types respond to different frequencies. The static magnets only offer one frequency, so an individualized treatment is not possible.

Horses react very individually to magnets. Some horses won't tolerate them: they get twitchy and nervous. It's possible the wrong frequency has been selected. So, try again with a different program/frequency. If problems persist, you need to stop the treatment. However, most horses respond with beautiful muscular relaxation, which also has a positive effect on your horse's psyche.

My Tip

Try out how your horse reacts to magnetic therapy. If you have a nervous, forward horse and you would like him to be calmer during work, it is worth a try to treat him with magnetic therapy before you ride. If your horse is a little too quiet and you are looking for a little more activity, there are frequencies that help with that, too. Ask the manufacturer which frequencies would be appropriate. I personally always put a magnetic blanket on my horse after intense work to support the recovery phase.

Areas of Application

- Preventive measures
- Fractures and fissures, ganglia
- Arthrosis
- All forms of soft tissue injury (ligaments, tendons, muscles)
- Muscle tightness

When You *Shouldn't* Use Magnetic Therapy

Magnetic therapy has the advantage that it can be applied almost everywhere.

Contraindications are:

- Sepsis
- Kidney disease
- Pregnant mares
- Existing tumors

Laser Therapy

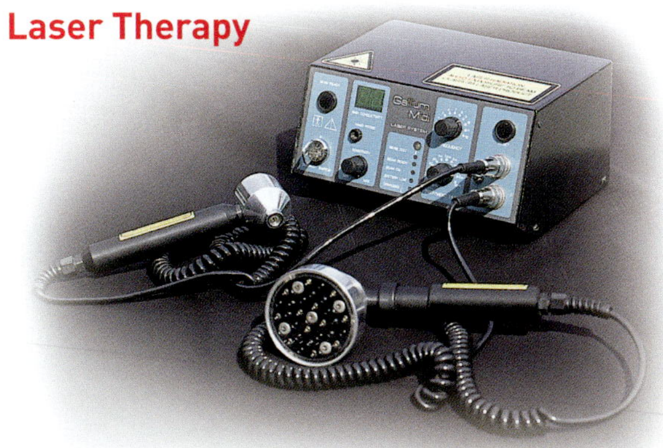

The application of laser can work wonders for poorly healing wounds.

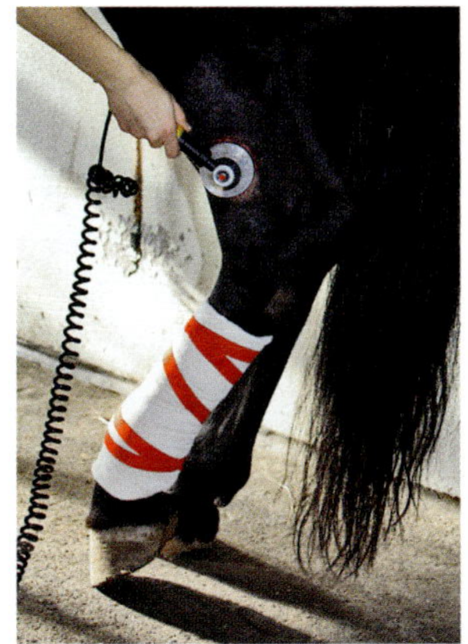

Laser stands for "Light Amplification by Stimulated Emission of Radiation." This means generating an intense or focused beam of light through stimulated emission of radiation. Laser therapy is used in diverse areas of medicine. High Intensity Laser Therapy is used for surgical procedures. It is, among other applications, used in eye care. Low level laser is therapeutic light that finds its application in physical therapy. It is also known as "cold laser" or "soft laser" since it does not lead to a warming of tissue.

Effects

I will explain the effects of low level laser therapy. This laser only has a stimulating effect on the treatment area and does not injure the area. The effect of soft laser light on the organism happens on different levels. On the one hand, it has a positive impact on the force center of the cell, which leads to an increased metabolism. On the other hand, the cell can be influenced by specific oscillatory information of the low level laser. It has been proven that regulatory processes in the brain and spinal cord as well as hormonal reactions respond to treatment by soft laser light. Regulatory processes in the brain and spinal cord and hormonal reactions have been observed after laser treatment. More recent studies have shown that a laser only penetrates between .5 and 4 centimeters (an inch and a half or less) deep, but this initiates a chain reaction in the cells that goes much deeper. How deep the laser penetrates depends on the thickness of the horse's coat and skin. Therefore, there are special laser devices used in veterinary medicine.

It has also been demonstrated that laser therapy offers great support for poorly healing wounds. With such wounds, daily progress can be observed. In addition, when treating scar tissue, the laser has turned out to be a "miracle worker." Many acupuncture practitioners use laser light instead of needles with great success. In addition, laser light has been used successfully in the treatment of ligament, tendon, and joint injuries of the lower limbs.

Application

The laser is applied directly (touching) to the treatment area. The length and frequency of treatment is dependent on the specifications of the device. Please make sure to familiarize yourself with the manufacturer's instructions. If your horse has a thick coat, you may want to clear and clean the laser points, which reduces resistance to the laser beam. There are big laser boxes available, which perform well, but even small laser pens can successfully be used by the layperson to treat superficial injuries.

When You *Shouldn't* Use Laser Therapy

There are basically no contraindications to the use of laser therapy. It is completely pain-free since it "only" uses light beams. Don't treat areas close to the eye of the horse, as light can injure the eye.

Important Hint!
Never look directly into the laser light and always wear the protective glasses that come with the device during treatments.

Ultrasound Therapy

Ultrasound therapy is being used widely in the medical field for examination, diagnostics, and treatment. When not used correctly, ultrasound can also be the most "dangerous" of the physical therapy devices. Irreparable injury can occur quickly. Damages can include death of tissue or burning, and injuries to cartilage and bones. Therefore, I advise you, let experts give this treatment. Do so yourself only if you have received a 100-percent-correct introduction and you feel confident handling the device.

Effects

Ultrasound uses sound waves. All cells that are hit by these waves receive a "micro-massage." This activates the cell membrane, so metabolism is positively influenced by the massage. The tissue is slightly warmed by the waves. As a result, the elasticity of the soft tissue increases. One advantage of ultrasound is that it can reach the deeper structures of the body.

Ultrasound has a positive impact on tissue where tension has accumulated. The waves can dissolve adhesions and scar tissue. Positive results can be observed from treating tendon and ligament injuries. Even bursitis and arthritis are being treated with ultrasound therapy. In addition, poorly healing fractures can be improved with ultrasound treatment. The micro-massage also helps with pain reduction.

Application

In order to transmit the waves from the head of the device, as little as possible resistance is necessary. Hair in the treatment area needs to be shaved. A gel is applied to transmit the sound waves into the tissue. The head of the device should always be in motion during treatment, either in small circles or in straight lines. There is another option for treating the lower limbs. You can stand the horse's leg in a bucket of water. Water is a fantastic sound-wave transmitter. For the sound waves to transmit optimally, there should not be any air in between the hairs (so run your hand down the leg in water to press out the air bubbles). You put the head of the device into the water, 1 to 2 centimeters (about half an inch) away from the treatment area. Here, too, you need to constantly move the head of the device. You will be able to see how the waves are being transmitted in the water.

When You *Shouldn't* Use Ultrasound Therapy
- Sepsis
- Vascular disease
- Tumors
- Thrombosis

The treatment with ultrasound should not exceed four weeks. If the injury is not completely healed, please take a two-week break in the treatment before you start another round. You can cause harm to your horse if you treat for a prolonged period.

Electric Muscle Stimulation

When a nerve is injured within a single muscle or muscle group, the muscle/muscle group will immediately become inactive and atrophy will occur within just a few days. Atrophy means that the body has less strength at its disposal. It is often believed that the body can correct this muscular imbalance itself during the recovery phase, but unfortunately, this is not actually the case. For example, if your horse injures his right hind leg, it will be his weak leg for a very long time to come. The body is not capable of targeted development of just the affected muscle. In these cases, electric muscle stimulation can help your horse tremendously.

Effects

The muscle stimulator externally stimulates the nerve that controls the muscle through electricity/current. This causes a muscle contraction in the specific muscle. In this way, it is possible to stimulate the metabolism in the affected muscle or muscle group and counteract muscular atrophy and adhesions of the tissue as a result of injury and tension. The muscle is being rehabilitated and strengthened "from the outside."

Application

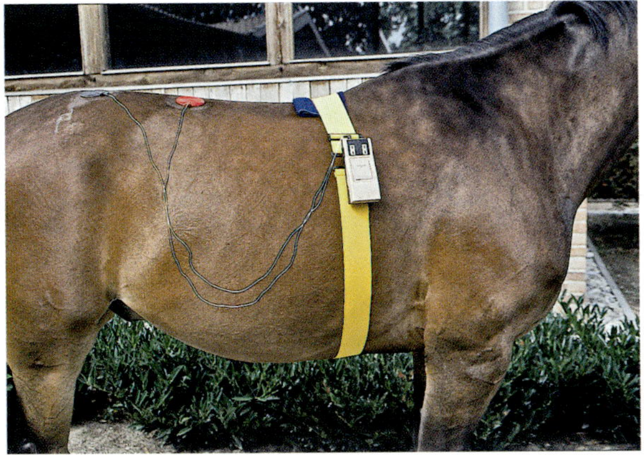

Electric muscle stimulation to build up the back and croup muscles.

The energy that is needed is being produced by a small device that is run by batteries. During a therapy session, electrodes are attached to the nerve of the affected muscle. The muscle function is stimulated by a low-level electrical current. The muscle is supposed to show a small contraction, just a small flicker, not a strong muscle pump. The electrodes are attached directly to a wet skin area. If resistance is too high, go ahead and wash the area with soap. It is best to also use gel that's specifically intended for electrodes. If you don't want to use gel, you need to keep the area wet throughout the treatment session. Self-adhesive electrodes are available, and I think they work well for treating the limbs. I would advise you to start with a low frequency and observe your horse's reaction. However, it has also been my experience that some horses react negatively to low frequencies but react well to high frequencies. Note: It is important to clean off the gel thoroughly after treatment because it can cause a skin reaction.

My Tip

You should use the electric muscle stimulator daily. The duration of the treatment should be between 30 minutes and one hour. If the horse can be worked, the muscle stimulation should happen before work. This way the muscle can best regain its elasticity, coordination, and strength.

Areas of Application

- Muscular atrophy
- Peripheral nerve damage
- Muscle tension
- Soft tissue injury (treatment should begin three to five days after injury)

When You *Shouldn't* Use Electric Muscle Stimulation

- Fever
- Thrombosis
- Sepsis
- Immediately after an injury

TENS (Transcutaneous Electrical Nerve Stimulation)

With the help of a TENS device, electric impulses are created and transmitted via the skin to the horse's nervous system. These impulses stimulate the body's own pain-relief system and influence the overstimulated nervous system. To put it simply: when using this, you are blocking the spinal cord's transmission system. The pain signal is blocked and stopped from being transmitted to the brain. In addition, hormones (endorphins) are released that have a pain-relieving effect.

TENS can be used in the case of an acute injury as well as for chronic pain, such as arthritis or muscular tension. In the case of acute injury, it is a good measure for preventing muscular tension from developing. As you know, tension results from pain and it causes circulation to decrease and hinders the healing process. As with an electric muscle stimulator, treatment with a TENS device triggers muscular contraction, which, over time, leads to the relaxation of muscle tissue.

Application

The application of the TENS device is similar to the muscle stimulator. For humans, the recommended treatment time is between 20 to 50 minutes, but with horses, I have the best results when treating between 20 and 30 minutes. With acute pain, a higher impulse is needed, and with chronic pain, a lower impulse is needed. Although this device causes a slight tingle on the skin, most horses react positively to it.

Hint: If the injury is very old, it can take a few weeks before the treatment is successful.

When You *Shouldn't* Use TENS

There is no specific pain that cannot be treated with the TENS device. But you should not attach the electrodes to open wounds or areas of skin disease.

In addition, do not use with:

- Tumors
- Thrombosis
- Fever
- Heart problems
- Acute inflammation/infection

Fact: It is very important that the cause of the pain has been diagnosed before you start treatment with the TENS device. Otherwise, you could suppress important information regarding the source of the pain.

My Tip

If you want to use this device on a limb for arthritis, first try it on the *longissimus dorsi* in order to test your horse's reaction. If he reacts negatively and doesn't like the treatment, keep the device in the same place until your horse gets used to the "tickling." Only then should you apply the device to the treatment area/the joint.

Medium-Frequency Electrotherapy

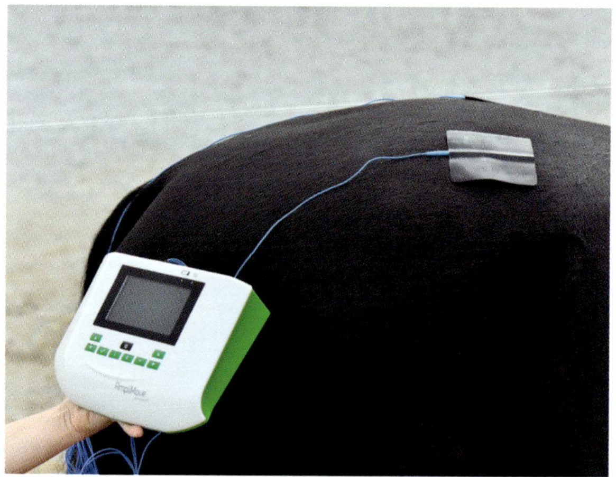

Medium-frequency electrotherapy uses medium frequency (1000–100,000 Hz) voltage. Just like electric muscle stimulation and TENS (which only work with low electrical frequencies, 1–100 Hz), medium-frequency electrotherapy is applied to build muscle and treat pain, among other uses. The advantage of medium-frequency electrotherapy is the option to treat larger muscle areas than you can when using electric muscle stimulation or TENS. In

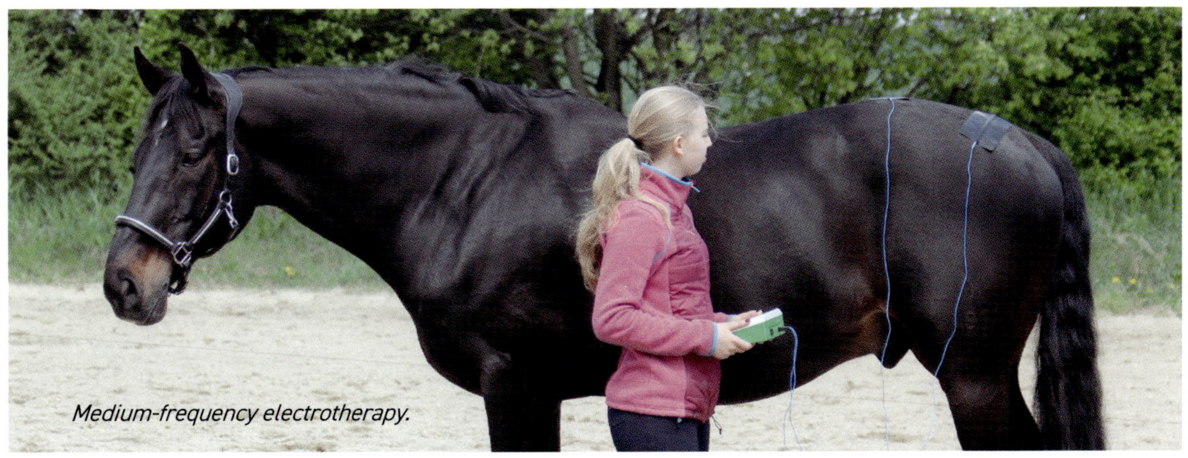

Medium-frequency electrotherapy.

addition, there is a better flow of current through the tissue when using higher frequencies. Scientific studies have shown that this therapy is able to activate muscle fibers over their complete length and muscle contraction reaches almost the physiological stage of activated muscle tone.

Frequencies:
Low frequency:
Pain management and building of muscle (frequency range: 1–100 Hz).

Medium frequency:
Pain management and building of muscle (frequency range: 1000–100,000 Hz).

High frequency:
Specific heat therapy (frequencies higher than 100,000 Hz).

Application

Just like TENS and electric muscle stimulation, the skin needs to be cleaned and moistened before you begin. You should work with a contact gel to guarantee good transmission of the current. With medium-frequency electrotherapy, you can use larger electrodes, and therefore, you can treat larger areas. The most commonly used devices have preset programs that choose the appropriate frequencies and treatment duration automatically, depending on the desired therapy results, like pain management, muscle activation, or returning lymphatic circulation support.

Hint: In my experience, horses perceive the medium-frequency electrotherapy as pleasurable.

When You *Shouldn't* Use Medium-Frequency Electrotherapy

You should not apply medium-frequency electrotherapy when inflammatory disease of vessels and arteries is present. In addition, it is contraindicated with all forms of skin injury. If you want to apply this form of therapy on yourself, please be aware that it cannot be applied to patients with metal implants or pacemakers.

Kinesiology Tape

Kinesiology tape was developed for human use by Dr. Kenzo Kase, a Japanese chiropractor. The underlying idea was to develop a bandage that could be worn over a longer period and that would not restrict the mobility of the patient. Kinesiology tape is a breathable, elastic, self-adhesive tape that can be applied directly to the horse's skin or coat. This technique became popular after the Olympic games in 2008, where many human athletes were seen wearing kinesiology tape.

Application

We've now discovered the benefits of kinesiology tape for prevention and rehabilitation for our equine athletes. Especially after illness or injury, it can be applied to remedy the following: muscular symptoms (tension and weakness), lack of stability, poor lymph drainage, and fasciae immobility. Beyond these applications, it has an outstanding healing effect in the case of ligament and tendon injuries. As a preventive measure, it can accelerate recovery after a training session, among other things.

For people, the effect of these tapes is based on how they raise the skin and stimulate the fascia; therefore, they also stimulate the body's ability to self-heal. In horses, the tape is applied directly to the coat (no shaving/clipping). The root of the hair is being stimulated and the connected fasciae as well as nerves and blood vessels are activated. The great thing about the tape is that it works particularly well for horses, thanks to the abundance of receptors in their skin. A tape bandage can influence all levels/layers of the body, since they are all connected through fasciae. This means that the tape influences the deeper structures such as muscles, fasciae, tendons, and joints. Even the inner organs can benefit from the stimulating effect.

It looks very easy to apply the tape. You should know, however, that different ways of taping are used for different health problems. In addition, different colored tape supports the healing process in various ways.

The goal of taping is to stimulate the body's self-healing processes. It can be applied before or after a treatment to support recovery. For the best possible outcome, it's important that a trained person applies the tape. It can stay on the horse for several hours up to a few days (three to five) and can be removed by pulling it off in the direction of hair growth.

Fact: Kinesiology taping can decrease pain, increase mobility, support the healing process in the body, and improve muscle activity and lymphatic flow.

When to Use Kinesiology Tape

- Muscle, tendon, and ligament injury
- Correction of incorrect movement patterns
- Lymphadenitis
- Neurological dysfunction
- Adhesions of the fascia
- Scar tissue
- Acute and chronic pain

When You *Shouldn't* Use Kinesiology Tape

- Open wounds
- Skin inflammation
- Kidney and heart disease
- Hormonal imbalance
- Tumors

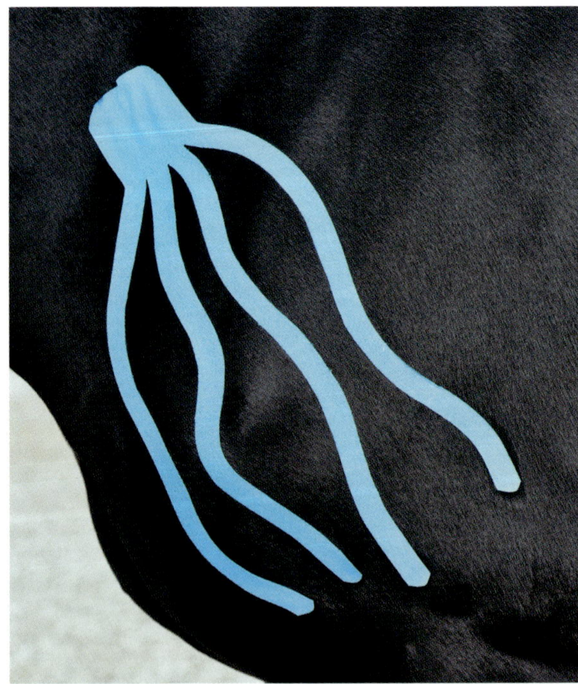

Kinesiology tape is applied to treat tension/tightness and injuries, as two examples. In addition, weak muscle areas can be deliberately stimulated to support building of muscle. In this picture, you see tape applied to improve lymphatic flow.

Physical Therapy for Horses

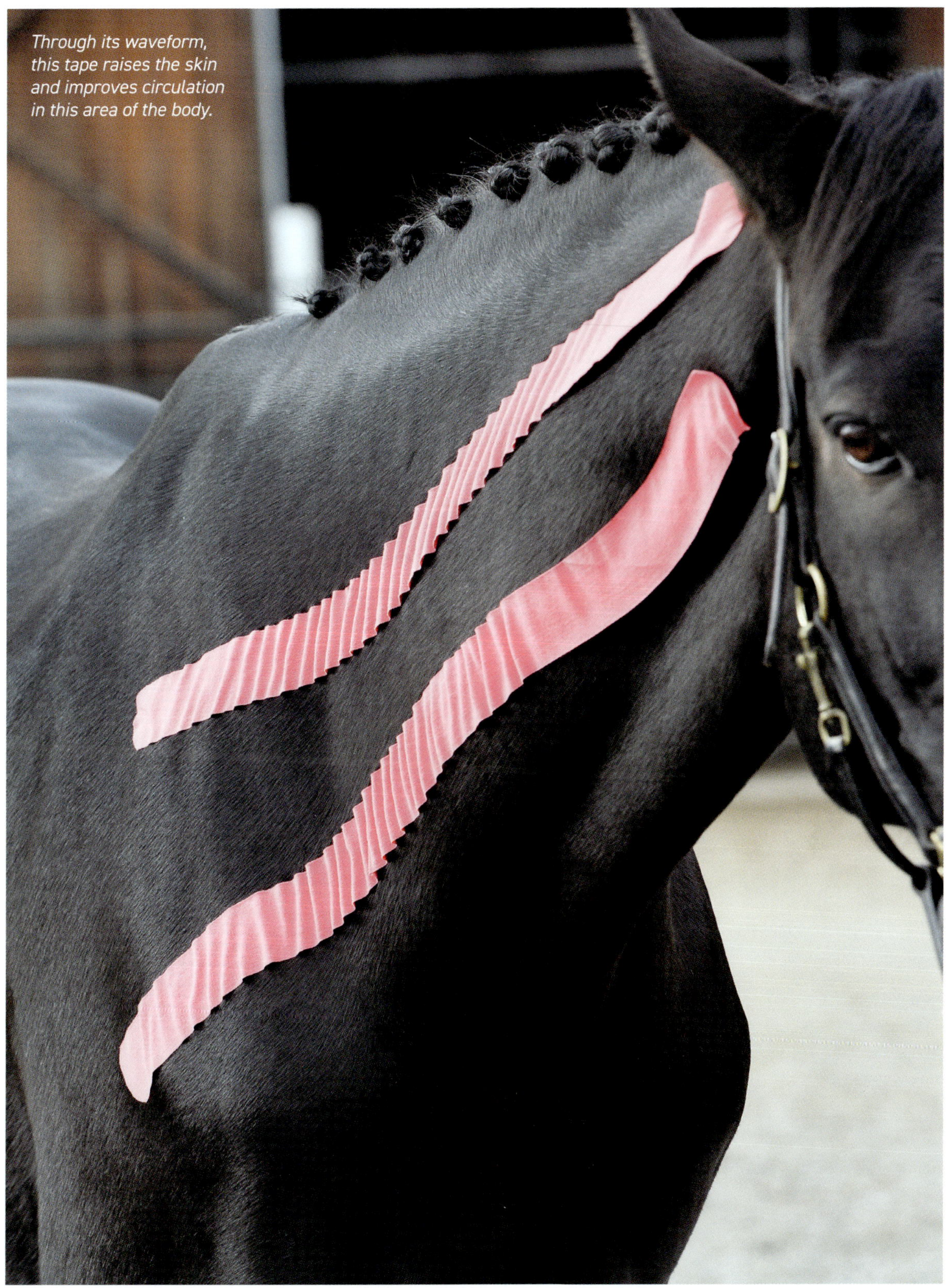
Through its waveform,
this tape raises the skin
and improves circulation
in this area of the body.

Rehabilitation

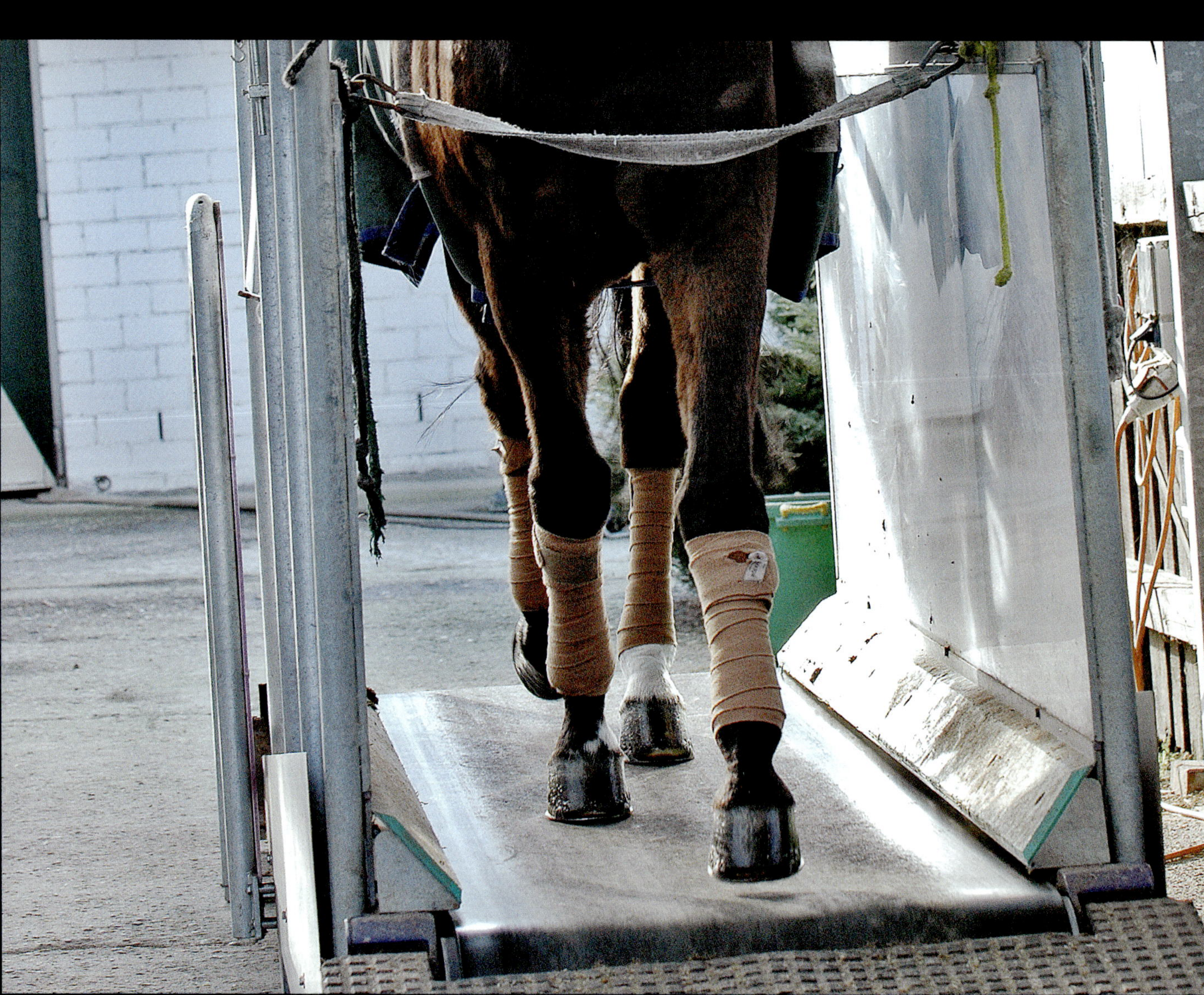

Rehabilitation means to restore and recover. This term describes the effort made by a person or animal to recover a former level of physical conditioning that existed prior to an illness/injury. In this phase, the body is being physically and/or mentally built back up.

Unfortunately, you often can't make an exact plan for rehabilitation and say, "In two weeks, all will be healed again." We, people and animals, are too individualized for that. Many influences come into play; for example, the degree of injury, the physical condition, and the emotional strength of the affected individual. There are some who have tissue that heals quickly and a good metabolism, while others don't. Other factors are also important, such as swelling, inflammation, secondary injuries. Our psyche also plays an important part in healing quickly and successfully.

Passive Rehabilitation

When your horse is injured or ill, it means that normal conditioning must be scaled back in order to allow the body to heal. In even a short time, your horse loses condition, and his whole body is affected by this.

You can already begin to counteract the muscular atrophy and limited movement that come about as a result (i.e. during stall rest) in the time directly after the injury. I've already described the implementation and effects of passive rehabilitation in chapter 10 (p. 176). To recap, important tools for rehabilitation include massage, mobilization, stretching, stabilization exercises, and physical therapy such as ice, water, heat, kinesiology tape, and electrotherapy.

When the body has recovered enough that it can sustain work again, the active rehabilitation phase begins.

Active Rehabilitation

When it comes to active rehabilitation, you're working with functional movement. At the beginning of treatment, passive measures will outnumber active measures of rehabilitation, but one by one, the passive measures will be replaced by active measures.

Active measures must be chosen based on what's appropriate for your horse's weakest body part, and that's most often the part affected by injury. For example, if your horse has suffered a tendon injury, he can only be worked so hard that the tendon is being rehabilitated positively as a result of the stress. If the stress on the tendon is too much or too little, you run the risk of the tendon having a negative response to the stimuli and that doesn't support the rehabilitation. Finding the exact stress level to implement is a challenge. Not too much and not too little!

During active rehabilitation, it comes down to the fact that you need to "reprogram" your horse's movement patterns. A horse is moving as a reflex, which means, he's not thinking about how he's moving. If he has an injury or compensatory posture, he will inevitably change his way of going. When the reason for his compensatory stance goes away, or the injury heals, the horse will not automatically go back to his healthy movement pattern—the altered gait has become normal for him!

Those among us who have ever worn a plaster cast will know exactly what I'm talking about. People who have worn a cast for six weeks or so will also continue to "limp" after the injury has healed and the cast has been removed. This condition can last weeks. But humans have the advantage that we recognize the unnatural movement pattern and are able to correct it with physical therapy and visual support.

In this chapter, I'll describe the options available to horse owners when their horse requires rehabilitation.

The Plan

Every horse that sustains an injury requires an individualized plan for rehabilitation. It's advisable to collaborate with a veterinarian and physical therapist to establish the plan. The plan should not be fixed, but should be adjusted over time based on the healing process.

When establishing a rehabilitation plan, it's important to keep in mind not only the type and degree of the injury, but also the horse's general circumstances and mental health. It doesn't make much sense to prescribe a horse to stall rest if he's going to constantly be circling around the stall and bucking because he's so bored and has too much energy. You also need to pay attention to the general condition of the places that the horse may use: it's a problem when the horse is only allowed to go on soft footing but the footing in all the riding areas at your facility are too hard.

Fact: Only a correct, purposeful and patient rehabilitation can bring about healing.

Purposeful Rehabilitation

- First, it's important to diagnose the injury and determine the seriousness and extent. Next, the veterinarian can prescribe a rehabilitation plan that's based on the diagnosis.
- The injury should be examined regularly so that the healing process is monitored. After any prescribed daily exercise or turnout, you should observe the injury to see if swelling, temperature changes, or pain sensitivity are present in the tissue. When you're uncertain, call your vet!
- You must never lose sight of the problem. Even when, let's say, the swelling goes down after a tendon injury, it doesn't mean that the tendon is fully repaired for use.
- Build both passive and active rehabilitative measures into the treatment plan. For example, this

includes massage, stretching exercises, physical therapy, work on the double lunge, treadmill, or walker.

Methods for Active Rehabilitation

Equibands®

The Equicore Concepts® system was developed over many years by physical therapists and veterinarians in the United States. It's well-suited for rehabilitative purposes as it effectively promotes muscle development. The Equiband® system consists of a specially designed saddle pad and two latex-free, rubber bands, which are fastened to the saddle pad during training. The advantage of the system is that you can ride as well as longe with it.

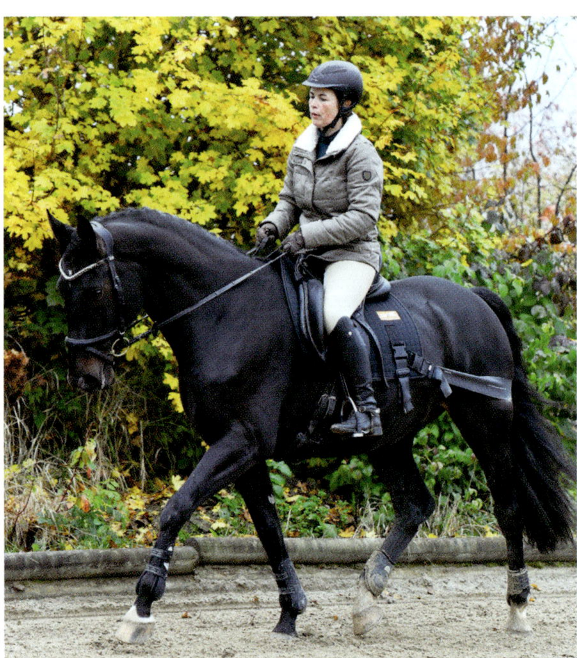

The Equiband system was specifically developed to stimulate receptors in the horse's skin and hair follicles. As a reaction to the stimulation, the trunk muscles (especially the abdominals and deep, stabilizing muscles) are activated. The abdominal muscles lift the back and bring the spine into a position where it can swing. In this way, the deep muscles of the back are activated. The band that runs around the hindquarters stimulates the hindquarters. They become more active and the hind limbs are brought more in the direction of the horse's center of gravity. Because the Equibands are relatively tight when fastened, they create resistance when the hind legs extend, which also serves to strengthen the extensor musculature. As you already know, well-trained trunk muscles prevent back pain and injury. With the Equicore Concepts system, you can improve strength, stability, and balance.

When Can Equibands Be Used?

- With young horses during in-hand training or on the longe line in order to strengthen and prepare the musculature for training under saddle.
- With older horses, to maintain the strength and stability of the spine.
- For rehabilitation after injury, illness, joint treatments, and surgery.
- To increase performance capability through optimal muscle training.

My Tip

When longeing, the Equiband works the horse from back to front. Therefore, don't use side reins. Because of the band, the horse must actively lift through the back, and over a longer period of time, carry the head and neck lower (about the height of the stirrups is desirable). In this way, you can check whether the horse is able to carry himself in this head/neck position. In my experience, most horses can't do this. They always lift the head and bring it to the outside. Over time, your horse will get stronger in the neck and trunk, and will be able to carry his neck in the lower position more consistently.

Longeing

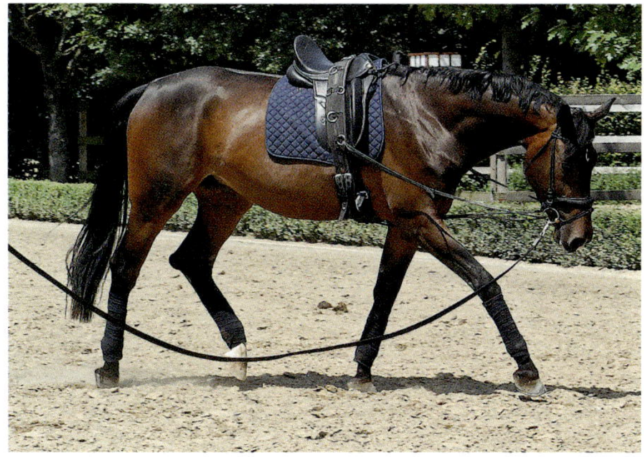

Longeing with the saddle provides the back muscle with an additional stimulus, resulting in muscles developing more quickly.

Longeing can be utilized with many disorders where the horse must start working again but is not yet able to be ridden; for example, with serious back pain. The work on the longe gives you the chance to purposefully prepare the horse for further work, without losing conditioning or strength. Longeing promotes suppleness, muscular development, and coordination. The horse can rediscover his balance without being disturbed by the rider.

The work on the longe can be set up to include lots of variety. For example, you can integrate ground poles or cavalletti work. A study has determined that when training with ground poles/cavalletti, there will be an increased bend in the joints, and the time the limbs take as they extend forward will be prolonged significantly. In addition, it was determined that this work positively affected visual coordination during schooling, and had a strengthening effect on the flexor muscles. This training is good for the development of the trunk musculature, which again, is so very important to the horse's physical stability and helps to correct abnormal movement patterns.

The disadvantage of longeing is that the horse is constantly on a circle, which places higher stress on the extremities.

My Tip

Before you begin longe work, remember to first lead your horse at a walk on a long rein for 15 minutes. Don't secure side reins immediately; instead, allow him to go a few rounds without them at trot and canter. Make side reins only so tight that the horse carries himself, not so he comes behind the vertical or leans on them. In addition, the horse must also move from back to front when being longed.

Double Longeing/Long-Lining

Generally speaking, and especially during a rehabilitation, I prefer double longeing or long-lining over longeing with a single line. Through the outside longe line or long line, you have additional options for influencing the horse: you can keep his hindquarters more under control and influence them more effectively. In addition, when double longeing, you can also work on a straight line (along the rail as in long-lining) and reduce the stress on the limbs (joints and soft tissue).

You see the horse's movement patterns (way of going) from "below" (on the ground). When there's progress and improvement in the way of going, you can more easily track this and value it. In addition, for young horses that don't yet have much strength, coordination, and stability, this work without a rider as a preparation for riding is especially useful.

My Tip

On the longe line, keep a slow tempo. The higher the tempo, the more stress on the lower legs.

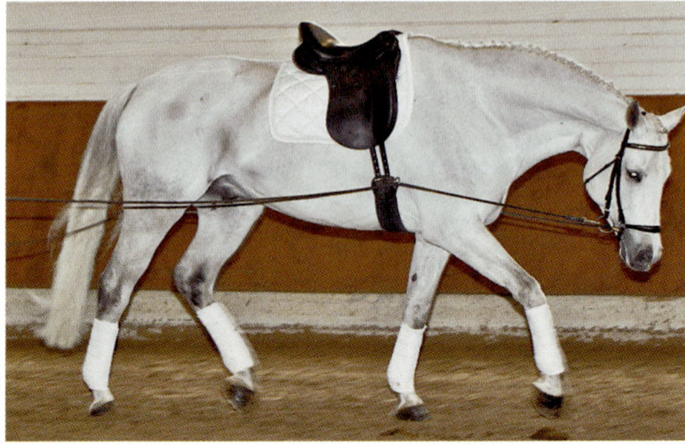

Double longeing or long-lining is ideal for improving coordination, stabilization, and building up strength.

Round-Penning

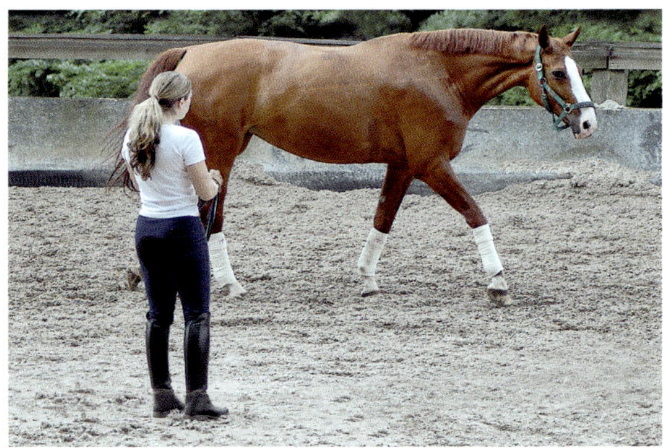

A walled or fenced round pen has the advantage that you can work without a longe line.

Round pens[8] are becoming more popular and can be useful in active rehabilitation.

The advantage of the round pen is that the horse can move freely. Because the area is limited by the fence, there's less danger that he can "get charged up" and

---

8 A round pen is a round, fenced area that has a circumference of about 18 meters (60 feet).

too out of control. It makes it easier for your horse to find his balance and this, in particular, applies to horses that have back issues or problems caused by rider error, such as being "rein lame," leaning on the bit, rooting the reins from the hand, and abnormal movement patterns. In a round pen, you only need one person to keep the horse moving in the desired direction, without him stopping in the corners, which isn't possible in a regular riding arena.

Through the unattached, free movement, you'll recognize that your horse seeks contact with you of his own accord, which can bring the two of you closer together. Groundwork can also be utilized to support rehabilitation, for which the round pen is ideally suited as your horse can move there without a lead or longe line.

But nothing advantageous is without its disadvantages. Through movement on a relatively tight circle, there's increased stress on the limbs. So in the round pen, as when longeing, please don't do the work for too long!

Horse Walker

Unfortunately, it's not always possible for us to meet the horse's needs in regards to movement. Horse walkers are a good compliment to training, including during rehabilitation. Studies have shown that after 10 days of stall rest, horses begin to lose their conditioning. Those that spent an hour a day on the horse walker were able to maintain the condition of their musculoskeletal systems. Only cardiovascular performance was slightly lowered. In addition, healthy horses were also tested and it was determined that the ones that were both ridden and worked on the walker were in distinctly better shape than those that were only ridden. It's totally clear that horses are animals meant for movement and that movement is what keeps them in shape.

Here are a couple of hints: With work on a horse walker, you still need to pay attention to the footing. This must be appropriate for your horse's injury. For example, if your horse has a tendon injury, he

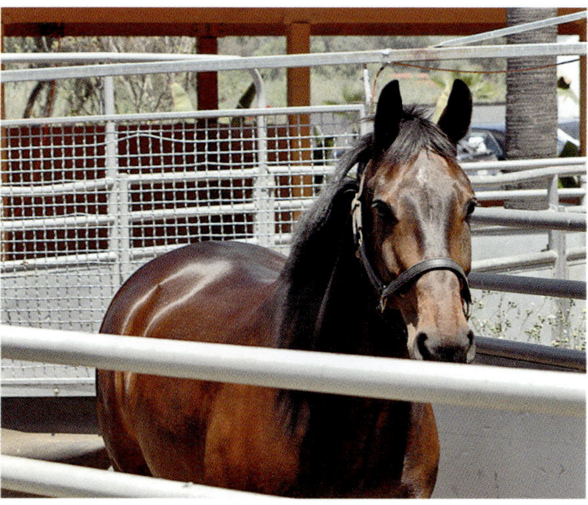

Movement is the best therapy. An automatic horse walker can improve your horse's conditioning.

shouldn't be worked using a walker where the footing is too soft. For horses with joint problems, a softer footing is preferred. You need to check this out before you allow your horse to be worked in a walker. Often, horses only walk along the inside wall (depending on the style of walker) and so, over time, deep tracks develop in the footing. Such worn-out footing is extremely damaging for a horse undergoing rehabilitation, just as it is for those that are healthy and sound. Further, you should make sure that your horse can move freely on the walker and is never tied. Tethered horses move differently, unnaturally, with more restriction.

Rehabilitation aside, the horse walker provides an additional option for movement, though it is no substitute for work under saddle, work at liberty, and daily turnout.

My Tip

Please keep in mind that horses are made for movement. If you have access to a horse walker at your facility, use it. It is definitely better to allow the horse to move in a walker than to just stand in a stall. His musculoskeletal system will thank you.

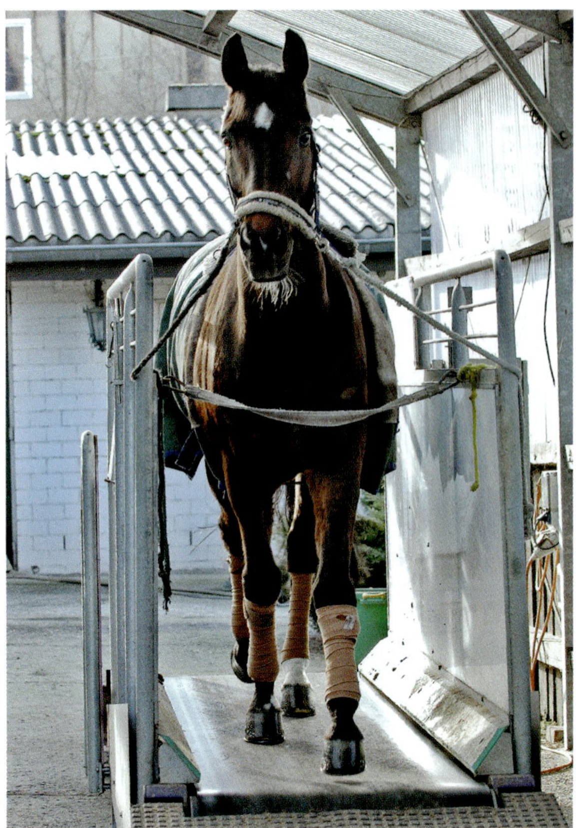

The treadmill can be used successfully as a supportive measure for building muscles and condition.

Treadmill

Some horse facilities have treadmills these days. Good treadmills have the advantage of providing the horse with a non-slip, shock-absorbing base on which to move, which in turn, improves the joints. The speed is adjustable from walk to gallop. Often, treadmills have an incline feature. This height/ incline adjustment leads to more demand on the heart and cardiovascular system, but also on the muscles. Consequently, the *longissimus* muscle in the back and the *extensors* of the hindquarters can be trained in a purposeful way, for example.

On a treadmill, the horse moves actively forward, as the legs are passively guided toward the back. The active push from back to front, the horse's "motor," is not optimally trained this way; it causes a movement pattern that is not physiologically based: the

treadmill cannot replace natural movement. But the treadmill does have many advantages anyway. Horses that have developed anomalies in their gaits due to compensatory posture or injury, must once again take even strides with all four limbs when they're on the treadmill. Because of the moving ground, the horse simply can't take the shortened step. This would cause him to lose his balance. At the same time, the small stabilizing muscles of the spine, which are often so weak, are more engaged and strengthened without the burden of rider and saddle. In addition, work on the treadmill is schooling balance, equilibrium, strength, and coordination.

> **My Tip**
>
> **Movement is the best therapy.**

I've observed that when horses are on the treadmill, their center of gravity shifts forward. This causes the horse to roll over his limbs not as quickly as on a normal surface when bringing his limbs backward. This has an advantage as well as a disadvantage. The advantage is that the muscles responsible for bringing the limb forward will get a light stretch every time the limbs come back on the treadmill. These muscles, such as the *brachiocephalicus* muscle and *hip flexor*, are often very tight. Frequently, this can have a relaxing effect on this muscular group. A disadvantage pertains to the joints of the lower leg and flexor tendons. Due to the slowed rollover, they are put under greater strain, which can lead to overstressing. The overstressing can also occur as a result of increasing the incline of the treadmill. Therefore, if your horse has an injury in these areas, you should be careful with the treadmill. And never let your horse go at a steep incline for a long time. When your horse is sound, multiple intervals at incline are recommended as they provide the musculoskeletal system with a significantly greater challenge.

Riding

The last stage in a rehabilitation plan is work under saddle. From here, you must newly "program" your

Physical Therapy for Horses

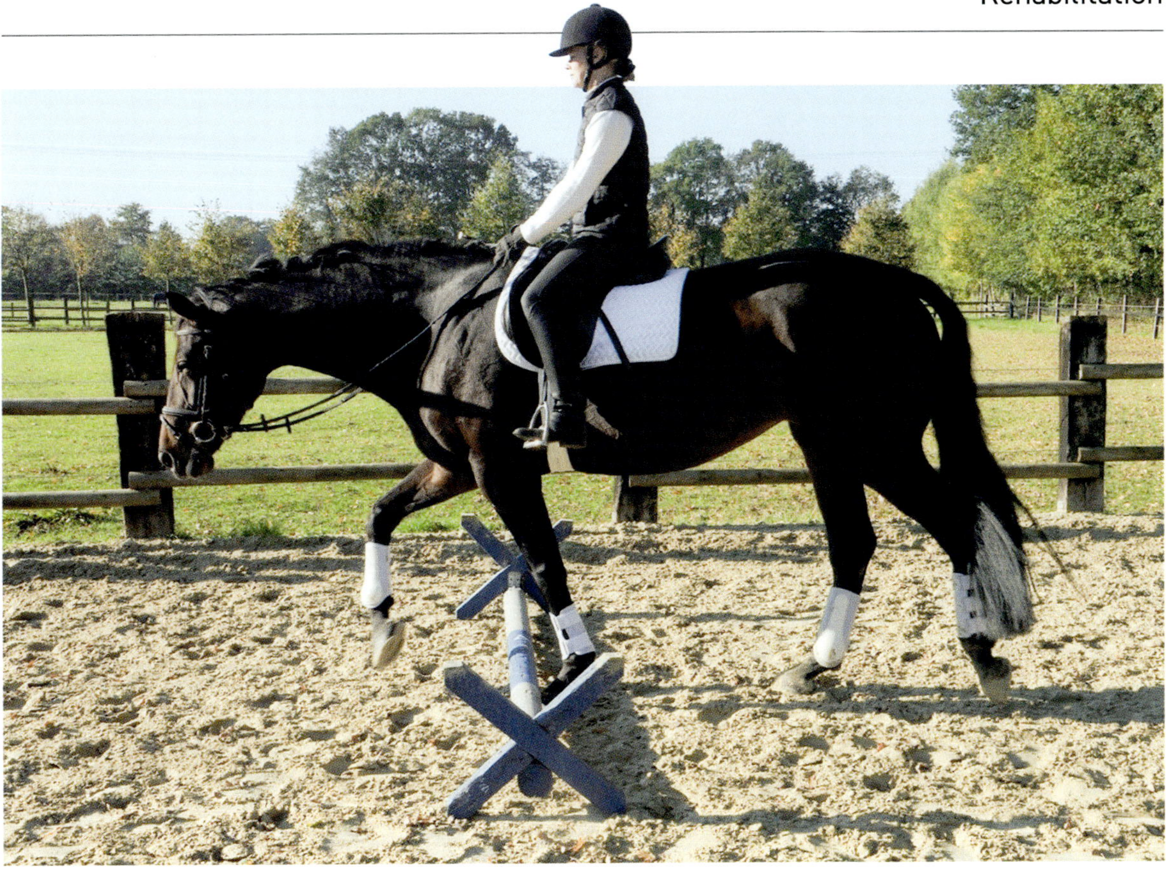

All other exercises and rehabilitative measures cannot replace riding.

horse to change back from his altered movement pattern to his natural one. This means: back to basics! Here, the classical Training Scale comes into effect: rhythm, *losgelassenheit*, and contact are called for. In the beginning, riding of specific movements is once again taboo.

It's important for the horse to be gradually reintroduced to work under saddle. The danger of overdoing it is great. If the injury had its origins in an incorrect movement pattern and/or rider error, you must be careful that both you and the horse avoid falling back into the incorrect way of going.

No matter what the cause of the injury, it's important to pay attention to footing when you start riding again. Work on diverse types of ground in order to stimulate the horse's nervous system and musculoskeletal system. You'll find the best opportunities for this by going trail riding (see chapter 4, "The Nervous System," p. 86).

Of course, you could incorporate all the above suggestions into your normal training program.

Hint:
After an injury the goals are:
· *Build muscle strength*
· *Increase endurance*
· *Expand flexibility*
· *Restore coordination*

My Tip

To correct riding errors, you must have a riding instructor who can identify the riding errors you tend to make. This is the only way you can possibly correct these mistakes and, in the end, prevent further/recurring injury to your horse.

Preventive Measures

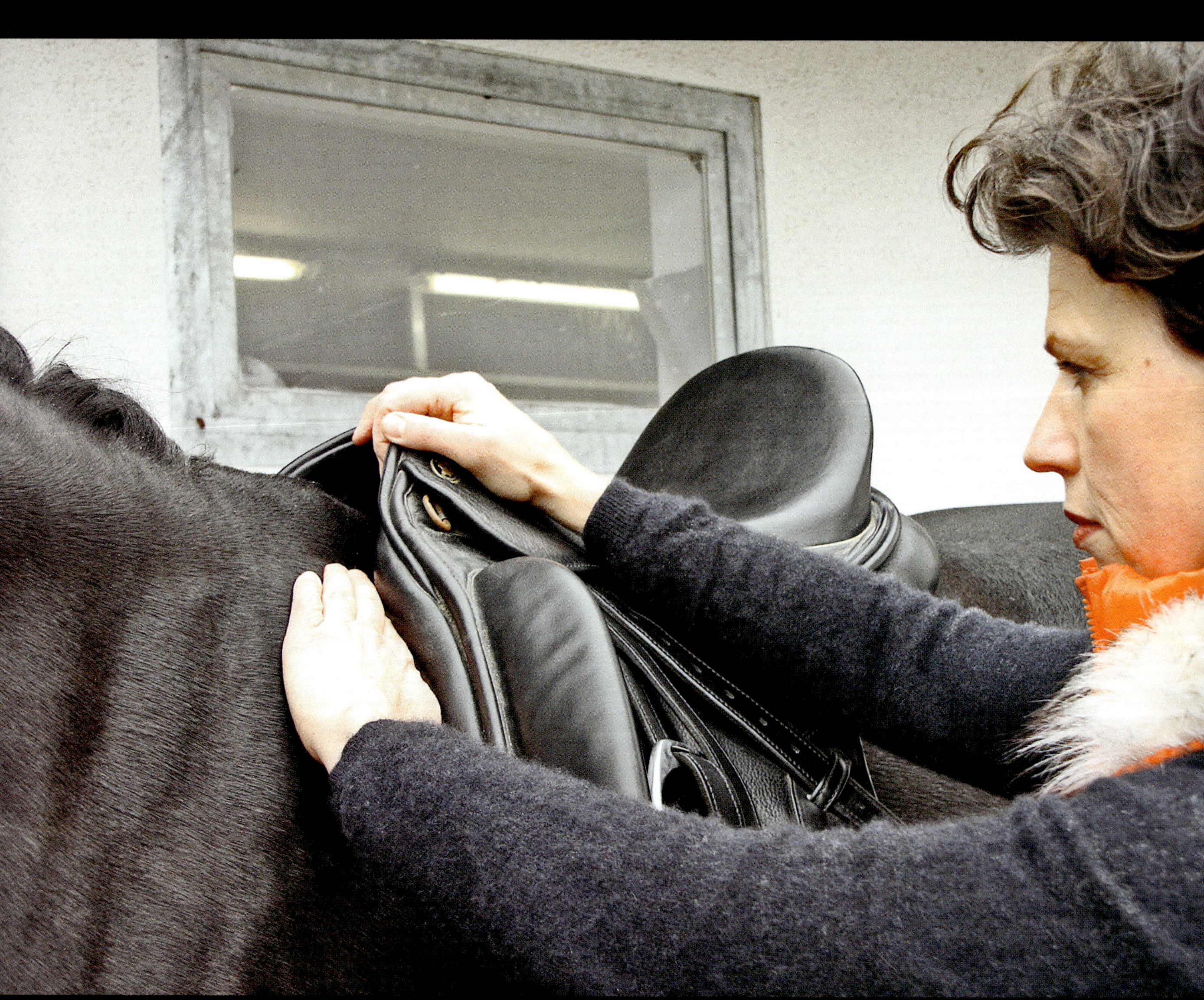

At the beginning of this book, I described the many different sources that can lead to tension and injury of your horse's musculoskeletal system. Some of these, unfortunately, are "homemade," so in this chapter, I want to make you aware of a few such sources of danger.

Tying

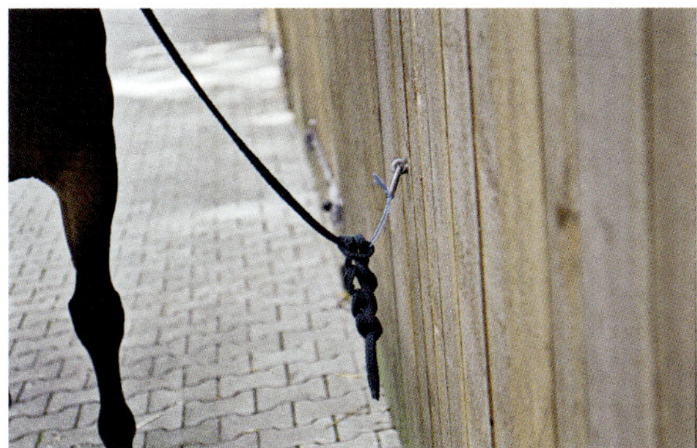

A thin piece of baling twine prevents injury should the horse panic and need to break free.

Picture this: Your horse is standing tied in the barn aisle and gets spooked. Using lots of strength, he pulls back, realizes that he's tied, panics even more, and pulls harder.

This panicked situation leads to an enormous transmission of pressure from the halter onto the poll, and you already know how sensitive and important the poll is. The health consequences that follow this situation can be grave. I unfortunately treat many horses that have developed a serious blockage or instability in the neck region as a result. And if the panic snap, halter, or lead rope falls apart, the horse can also be hit with it. As a result of tying accidents, I've seen horses with cranial damage and fractured withers, to name just a couple of examples.

In order to avoid this, we can all learn something from the British, who are more careful with tying than the rest of us. When they have a horse that doesn't like to stay tied, they connect the lead rope to the tying hook with a small ring made from a thin piece of baling twine. This a simple, but effective, "defined breaking point." If the horse pulls hard against this, the baling twine will quickly rip and the horse will avoid the serious injury that might otherwise follow. Therefore, I recommend that you use this method of tying when executing the exercises presented in this book and especially when you don't have an assistant.

Saddle Fit

When you consider the diverse saddle areas horses have as well as their diverse ways of going, it's clear that it's no easy task to find a saddle that fits. Have you already experienced firsthand how frustrating the search for a saddle that fits both you and your horse can be? And, if you're lucky enough to find that saddle that fits you both, the whole picture can look completely different just six months later. Horses, saddles, and riders are all changing, all the time.

Unfortunately, the importance of a well-fitting saddle is still greatly underestimated. Often, saddles are mainly fit to the rider and it's forgotten that the saddle must also fit the horse's back. When you don't check to see if the saddle fits the horse, you can be confronted with serious problems. Many of my "back patients" have been ridden in saddles that didn't fit them. One thing is for sure: a saddle that doesn't fit leads to trouble, whether that is back pain, muscular atrophy, a decline in performance, lameness, and—worst case scenario—irreparable damage to the musculoskeletal system.

There are two basic criteria for a saddle. A saddle must:

- **Help the rider achieve an elastic, correct seat.**
- **Comply with the form of the horse's back in both length and width and ensure an even distribution of pressure in the saddle area. This makes it possible for the horse to achieve optimal freedom of movement.**

Saddle Test

At least twice a year, you should check the panels and fit of your saddle, in regard to the following:

Panel Design and Flocking

1 Check the panels, allowing your hands to glide over them. This should feel smooth and evenly flocked. Unfortunately, I often find unevenly flocked saddles, which are only padded at the front and/or the back but are soft and weak in the middle. This causes too much pressure at the front and back of the saddle.

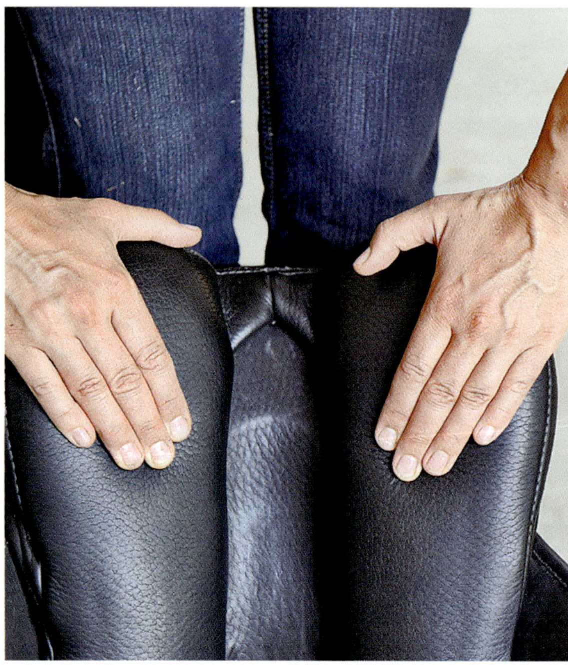

The saddle's flocking should be checked regularly.

2 The flocking should not be too hard, which poses the risk that the panels get too round, decreasing the contact area on the horse's back.

3 Between the panels (the gullet), you should be able to fit two to three fingers width-wise, in order to avoid limiting movement of the horse's spine and causing pressure on the spinous processes. The spine should also move freely during lateral movements and bending lines.

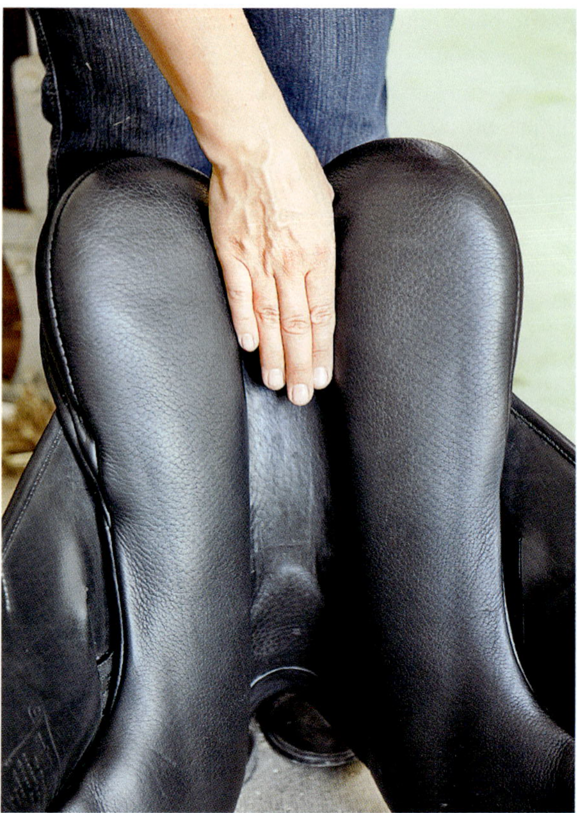

A broad gullet is important in order to avoid limiting the movement of the horse's spine.

■ Saddle Fit on the Horse's Back

You should also check this at least twice a year and especially after illness or breaks from riding. Place the saddle on the horse's back without a saddle pad.

Pay attention to the following:

1 The saddle must lie behind the shoulder blade.
2 The middle of the saddle should be the deepest point.
3 The panels must lie evenly on the horse's back.
4 The saddle should sit in a balanced position.
5 Check for freedom through the gullet, around and above the withers.
6 Consider the shape of the tree.
7 Check the length of the saddle.
8 Consider the positioning of the billets and girth.
9 Check that the horse's spine moves freely in the gullet.

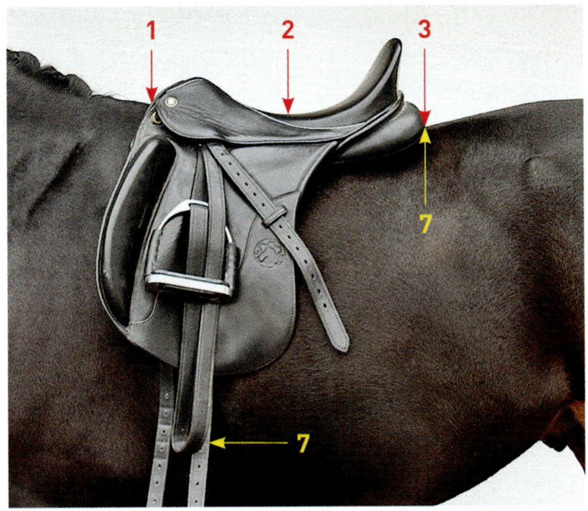

1 The saddle must sit behind the horse's shoulder blade. Many riders have their saddle too far forward over the shoulder blade, which can lead to an injury in the cartilage of the shoulder blade. When the saddle sits on the shoulder blade, you have also automatically changed the saddle's center of gravity; it is now too far back. This is especially prevalent among jumper riders who fix their saddles in this incorrect position with foregirth billets.

2 The middle of the saddle must be the deepest point of the seat. If you have a saddle that doesn't sit have this center of gravity, it's not only bad for the horse but also for the rider. When the center of the saddle is too far back, the horse will have a pressure point at the back of the saddle. As there are reflex points here, the horse must push away with his back to avoid too much pressure on these points. What follows is that his head goes up and it's impossible for the hindquarters to step up fully and accept weight. Moving into the bit is now impossible, too. In the worst case, these horses suffer from terrible back pain, which can cause them to panic under saddle, buck, rear, or refuse to move altogether.
This displaced center of gravity is also not doing you as the rider any good. As your pelvis tips backward (chair seat), you must engage too many muscles in your trunk and pelvic area in order to just be able to sit up. It will, therefore, be impossible to achieve the following seat you desire. In addition, your backward-tilting pelvis will cause your thighs to slide forward. Where will the driving leg aids land when you're positioned this way? That's right—too far forward to have a driving influence.

3 To check the evenness of the panels, place one hand against the saddle and apply a light pressure. Place your other hand beneath the saddle and glide it from front to back underneath the saddle and along the horse's back. Here, you should be able to feel an even pressure. If the pressure varies, there's an uneven distribution of the pressure that comes from the rider's weight.

4 When you apply pressure to the pommel of the saddle or tighten your girth, the back of the saddle should not lift upward and lose contact with the horse's back.

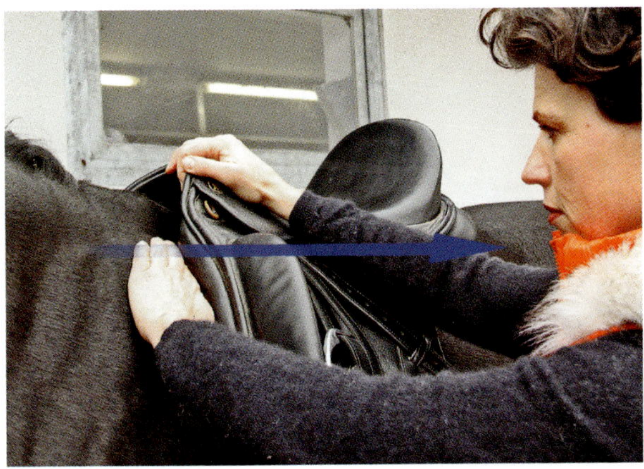

To test the saddle panels, place one hand under the saddle and stroke along the horse's back from front to back.

5 Check for freedom of the withers in the gullet. You should be able to fit three fingers there. Also check this when you're seated in the saddle. Pressure on the withers is painful and your horse will try to avoid the pain by pushing away with his back or shaking his head.

6 Check the fit of the gullet plate. You can test this by positioning your hand parallel to the gullet plate. It should form a parallel line to the shoulder blade. This fit can change quickly as muscle develops. If the gullet is too wide, the saddle will either sit on the withers and/or just put pressure on certain points along the upper edge of the withers.

Fact: The saddle pad should not lie tightly against the withers.

When the gullet is too narrow, it will press directly on the *trapezius* and *latissimus dorsi* (broad muscle of the back). This can cause a limited range of motion for the front limbs, or even trigger lameness.

7 The panels/contact area of the saddle must never sit farther back than the end of the thoracic vertebrae. This goes for all types of saddles: English, Western, endurance, dressage, cross-country,

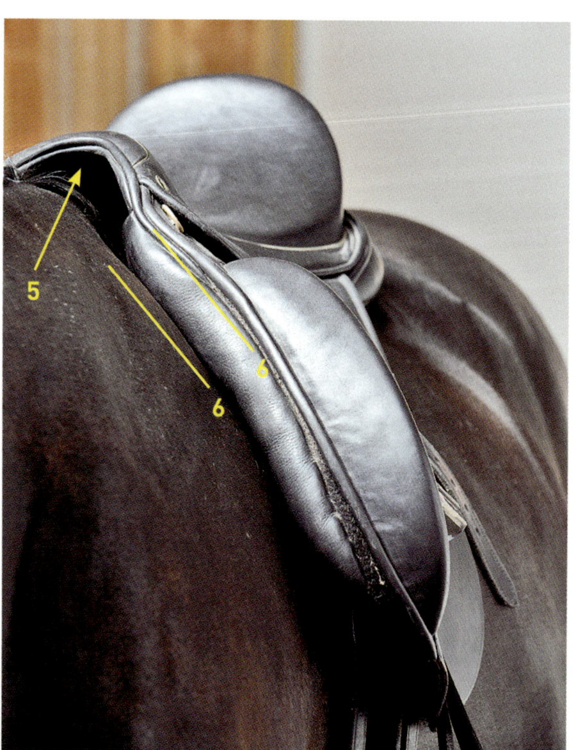

The gullet plate should run parallel to the shoulder blade.

and so on. The reason is that after the 18th rib, the spinal column no longer has support for carrying weight, as the ribs aren't there. The lumbar vertebrae "swing in the air" and should never be asked to carry weight. But, how do you find the end of the thoracic vertebrae? It's really easy to find, as long as your horse isn't too fat. Coming from the back, stroke sideways and forward along your horse's side. You'll automatically "bump into" the 18th rib. Follow the rib up toward the spine. When you reach the point where you can no longer feel the rib, go straight up to the spinous processes and you will have reached the last thoracic vertebrae. This is absolutely as far back as the panel of the saddle is allowed to go.

8 Check the billet straps on your saddle; they should fall to the height of the girth area. When dealing with a saddle that tends to slide out of place, I've often found that the billet straps are way too far back or too far forward in comparison to the horse's natural girth area. This girth area is different from horse to horse and must be taken into consideration when shopping for a saddle. Note that the position of the billets can be corrected by a saddler.

9 Check the saddle from the back to be sure that the spinous processes are completely free. To do so, you need to stand on a stool and look through the gullet from the back of the saddle.

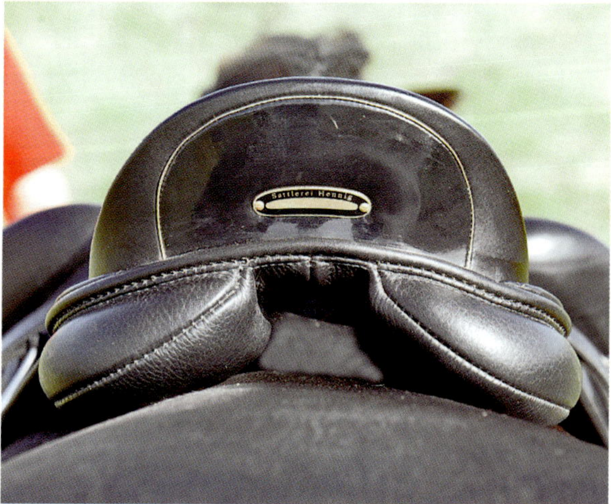

Physical Therapy for Horses

■ Saddle Test in Movement

I've seen how many saddles that seem to fit when the horse is standing in the barn aisle, no longer fit once the horse starts moving. The reason is that when the horse steps, he slightly lifts his back. This mechanism is different for every horse and must be monitored. You do want a saddle that fits when the horse is moving, right? Therefore, this is an important test.

During saddle testing, I like to tighten the girth just lightly and lead the horse about 20 meters (65 feet). The horse's head should stay at medium height, not too low or too high, as the height of the head influences the line of the back.

Pay Attention to the Following Important Points

1 Does the entire paneling of the saddle have contact with the horse's back or does it move up and down from back to front like a seesaw?

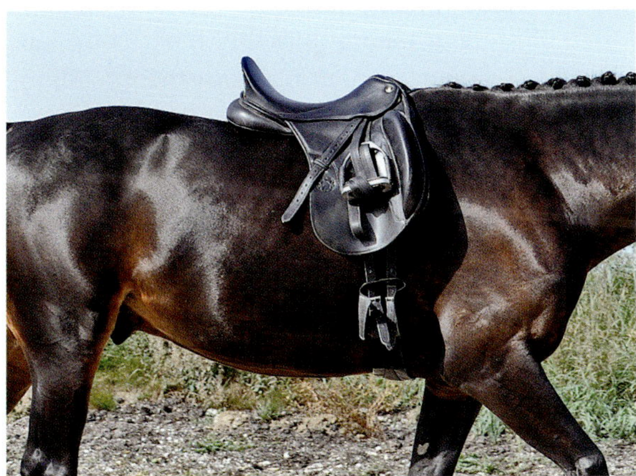

When in movement, the saddle should not seesaw...

2 Does the saddle, when viewed from behind, stay in the middle? It's not acceptable for the saddle to suddenly sit crookedly on the horse's back when he starts to move.

You also need to check the position of the saddle after you ride. Feel the saddle area for swellings or pain points and take note of how the horse's hair lies. Hair moving means there is too much pressure and movement from the saddle.

My Tip

If possible, try to find a saddler who can flock your saddle on site. The saddler needs to see how the saddle fits and observe your horse's biomechanics.

Regardless of your riding discipline, you should pay attention to these hints. Of course, there are some differences: unflocked saddles, like Western saddles, have bars, which are hard panels covered by woolskin.

Fact: The horse's back changes over time. Through good training, more muscle develops and when there's a break, they diminish. This can also affect saddle fit.

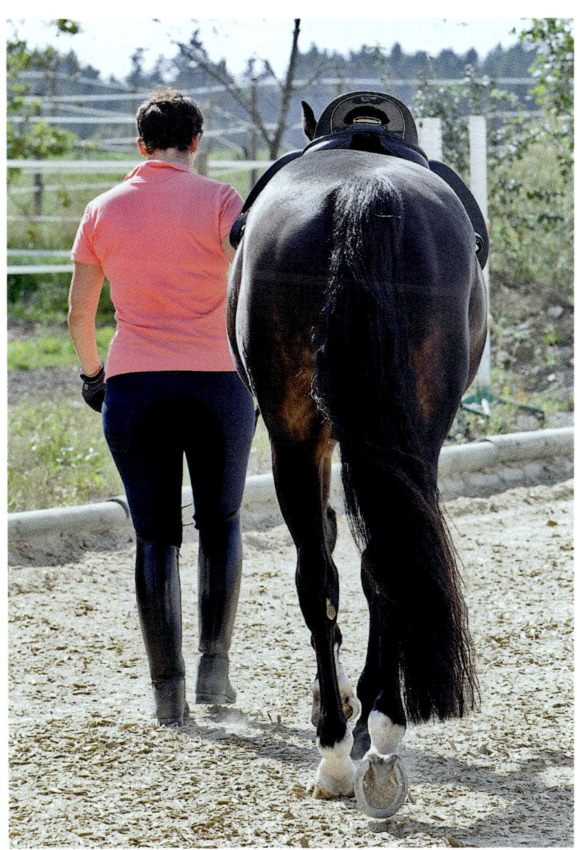

...or sit crookedly on the horse's back.

The advantage of Western saddles is that they have larger panels, which distribute the rider's weight more evenly over the horse's back. The disadvantage: since the bars are often very long, it can increase the likelihood of bridging, which means that the saddle is only sitting on the shoulder and/or lumbar area and forming a hollow "bridged" space over the thoracic vertebrae. In addition, Western saddles often reach all the way back to the lumbar region, which is not good from a biomechanical perspective. Originally, they were developed to provide a comfortable seat for the rider for long distances. But remember, since that time, a lot has also changed with Western horses. Today, Western riders often ride with much more bending and positioning than in earlier times. Therefore, these long bars (and big saddles) can restrict movement in the thoracic and lumbar regions.

Hint: When you've bought a new saddle, you might notice after three or four weeks that it does not fit your horse optimally and/or he's developing pressure points.

Saddle Pads

The English saddle should fit so well that it really doesn't require anything underneath. The saddle pad simply protects the saddle and not, as many believe, the horse's back! For Western saddles, the pad does the job the flocking does in an English saddle.

There are countless saddle pads on the market. Pay attention to their position: they can never be allowed to fold or wrinkle under the saddle, as this can lead to pain and eventually pressure points. It's also important to have a saddle pad of the right length. It must cover the entire length of the panels.

Many riders use a saddle pad to improve the fit of their saddle. My advice is that this should only be done as a temporary solution. For example, this might work when a horse has lost muscle mass after an illness, but which he'll quickly build back

up when he starts to work again. In every case, you must take into account that everything you put between the saddle and the horse's back makes the saddle narrower/tighter. This situation changes the deepest point of the saddle and, therefore, can cause more compression on the withers. Most of the time, the communication from the rider's seat is no longer optimal.

Certainly, there are horses who will work with a looser back when they are provided with a thicker saddle pad. Then, it's important to ensure that the gullet is wide enough so that it's not restricting the musculature of the withers.

Fact: The saddle must fit the horse 100 percent; anything less is a makeshift solution.

The Girth

Many horses don't like being girthed up at all. They show their displeasure through their body language, by pinning their ears, tossing their heads, or even biting or kicking. You need to take these behaviors seriously as your horse is telling you clearly that he's in pain and uncomfortable. Look for the reason. Here are a few common causes:

1 The girth is too tight.
2 The girth is too narrow.
3 The girth is too short.
4 There's only elastic on one side.
5 The billet straps are creating pressure.

1 A girth that's too tight places negative compression on the ribs and soft tissue in the girth area. Over and over again, I find many horses have a high degree of pain sensitivity and swelling in this area. The muscles that are especially affected include the *ventral serratus* and the *pectorals*. When horses have too much tension in these muscles, they lose their important ability to absorb shock when the forelegs touch down. From a mechanical point of view, the mobility of the withers can also become compromised. These horses are no longer able to shift

Physical Therapy for Horses

the spinous processes forward and, thereby, to lift the back. As a result, the biomechanics of the entire body are negatively affected.

Australian researchers conducted a study on race-horses where they tightened their girths with 5, 10, 15, and 20 kilograms (10–40 pounds) of pressure. They were attempting to test whether the girth influenced performance. As a frame of reference for the weight specifications, you can imagine the following: with 5 kilograms (about 10 pounds) of pressure, the girth is loosely around the trunk, but the saddle is not secured and can slide. With 10 kilograms (around 20 pounds) of pressure, the girth is tight around the trunk and the saddle is stable. With 15 kilograms (close to 30 pounds) of girth pressure or more, it's very tight. And, at 20 kilograms (over 40 pounds), you can no longer shove your hand in between the girth and the horse and the girth leaves a print on the horse's side.

Here's the result of the study: Even with the lowest amount of pressure, the researchers discovered a considerable reduction in performance. In addition, the horses tired more quickly. When the girth was tightened even more, performance declined even more. Why is that? It is possible that the girth and the saddle put too much pressure on the shoulder-girdle muscles, restricting them in their contraction and extension. Likewise, the compression in the horse's heart and lung area limits both organs in their function and therefore, performance is affected.

My takeaway from this study: always keep your girth as loose as possible, but, of course, tight enough to be safe.

Hint: When the girth is tightened optimally, you should still be able to gently slide your hand between the horse and the girth.

2 There are many girths that appear to have a broad surface area, but in reality, there's just a small strip that's holding it on the horse. Less width means a more concentrated pressure.

3 A dressage girth that is too short means the buckles are at elbow-height. This causes irritation at every step and over time leads to pain around the elbow.

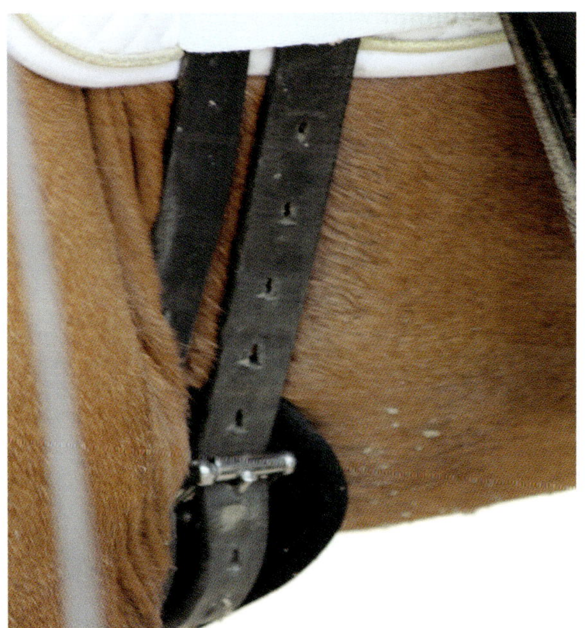

This girth is too short. With each step, every time the limb comes back, this horse's elbow bumps against the buckles. In addition, there's too much concentrated pressure on the trunk because of the long billet straps.

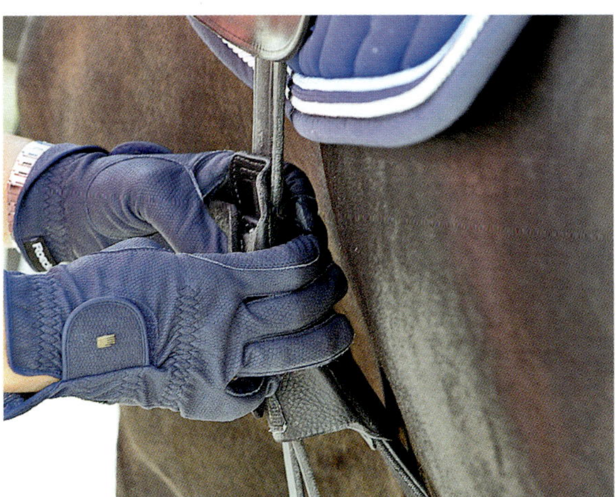

In order to avoid obstructing the muscles in the saddle and girth area, the right girth is important.

4 I advise my customers to choose a curved girth that has elastic on both sides and is broader at the sternum (breastbone) and more narrowly formed around the elbows. Thanks to the elastic, the mobility of the sternum is maintained, and breathing is impacted less. But, be careful with the elastic attachments: there's a risk of over-tightening the girth.

When it comes to girths, please be careful that you never have elastic on just one side. That's extremely bad for the mechanics of the rib cage. Just by putting this girth on, you have automatically caused uneven muscular engagement/tension in the rib cage as it becomes fixed on the side where there's no elastic. The other side, with the elastic, allows a certain degree of mobility.

My Tip

If you have a horse that's very sensitive when being girthed, gradually make the girth tighter, hole by hole. Lead your horse a few steps in between tightenings. Stretch the forelegs forward (see photo on p. 150), as this measure often brings a positive result. In addition, there's the option of a sheepskin cover for the girth. This can bring the horse relief, but be sure there's still enough wiggle room in the elbow area.

---

5 Many billet-strap buckles are not padded sufficiently and they put pressure on the horse's ribs. After you tighten the girth, see if you can still feel where the buckles are located and, after your ride, check to see if the horse is sensitive in just that spot. If so, buy a new girth—there's just too much at stake here.

A further study done in England has proven that the girth places the most pressure directly behind the elbow and on the sternum. Scientists used this knowledge as the basis to develop a new girth: they've cut back the section directly behind the elbow and also added padding and width to the sternum area. The result was impressive: the amount of concentrated pressure in the elbow region and on the sternum was significantly reduced (from 76 to 98 percent). In addition, the horses were better able to extend their forelegs toward the front (from 6 to 11 percent), bring the hind limbs farther forward under the belly (from 10 to 20 percent), and flex more deeply with their knee and hock joints (about 3 percent). To me, these numbers make totally clear that the girth has an influence on the horse's body mechanics and not only in the trunk area. In addition, this study has proven that a well-fit girth will greatly improve a horse's well-being. The new girths were tested by 22 members of the British team at the London 2012 Games. The results were so spectacular that all the British horses wore them to the 2016 Olympics. This scientific study was first made public *after* the Olympics were over!

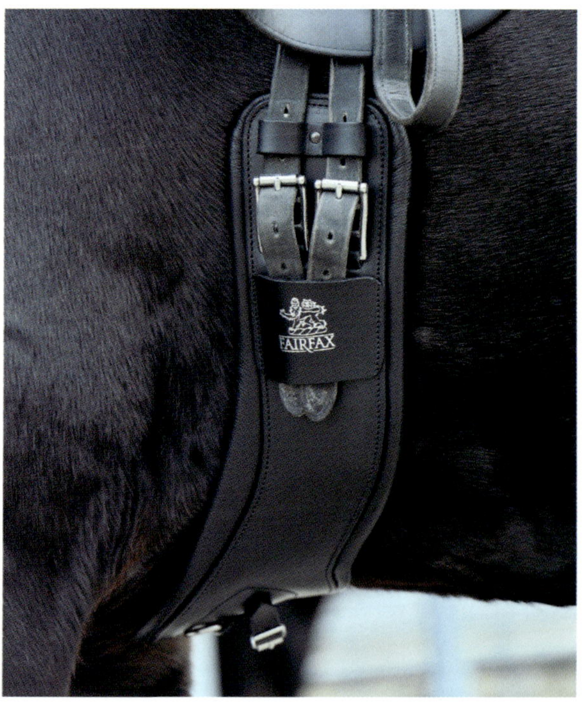

Studies have shown that when a girth is tightened, the highest pressure is on the sternum and just behind the elbows. Therefore, it's important to protect these areas—the sternum area should be well-padded and the sensitive area behind the elbow cut back.

Bridle Fit

As I described in the introduction to physical therapy, a horse's bridle—especially the cavesson, noseband, and flash—can be the source of injury or tension. Often, nosebands and curb chains are overtightened. In the following pages, you'll find a few hints about what to watch for and what effects a bridle that's been incorrectly fit or tightened can have.

Of special importance is the effect of the snaffle bit on many structures of the head. It applies pressure to the bars, the tongue, and the corners of the mouth, which leads to the yielding of the lower jaw. A gentle reminder: the yielding is important in order to release the muscles along the underside of the horse's neck and the jaw joint, which is what allows your horse to achieve and/or maintain *losgelassenheit*. Unfortunately, this all-important mobility of the jaw is often restricted due to an overtightened noseband. The result is tension in the temporo-mandibular joint, which, in turn, leads to heightened tension in the muscles that are responsible for bringing the forelegs forward.

> *Hint: Avoid over-tightening the noseband as you want to allow enough wiggle room for the jaw to move.*

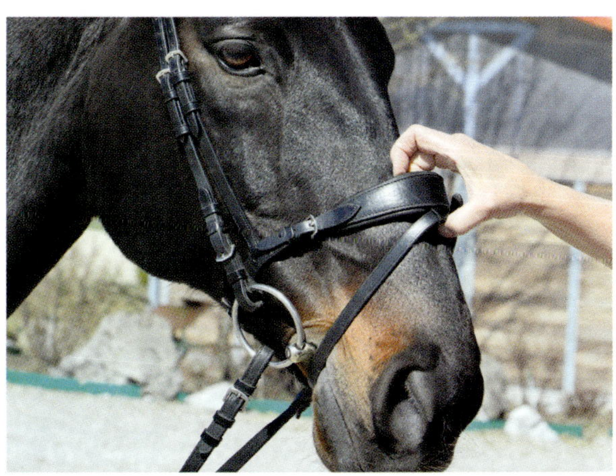

A correctly fastened cavesson has an enormous influence on your horse's losgelassenheit. *Above the nose, two fingers should fit easily between the noseband and your horse's face.*

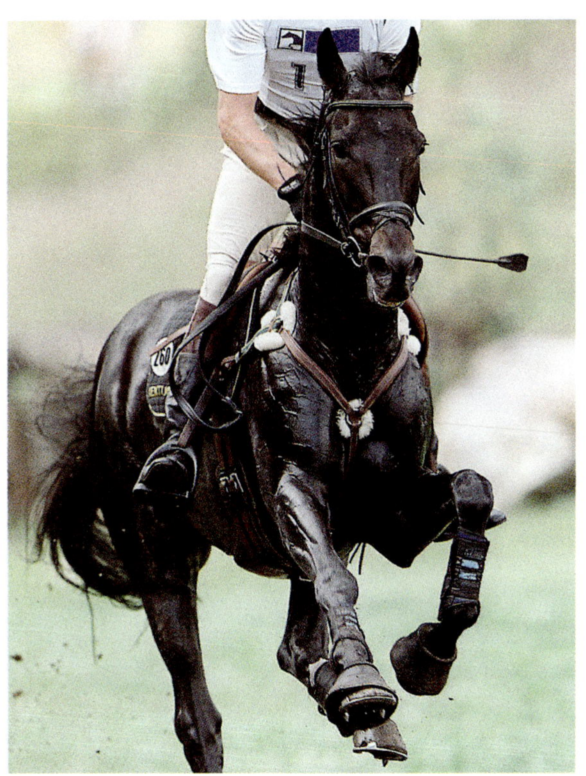

When the noseband is too tight, it can restrict the horse's breathing.

Let's not forget that an overly tightened noseband also triggers pain. Look inside your horse's mouth and you'll see that the teeth of the upper jaw are positioned farther out than the teeth of the lower jaw. So, the teeth don't lie against each other as they do for people. If you tighten the noseband too much, the cheeks and gums will be tightly pressed against the upper teeth and this can cause injury to the gums. It's very painful when the teeth have developed hooks. You try it—press your teeth hard against your cheeks. You'll notice it doesn't really take much pressure before it becomes uncomfortable.

In addition, there's the danger with all bridles that if you overtighten the noseband or curb chain, you will compromise the nerves that run along the upper cheek bone and lower jaw area (see photo). The result will be pain and sensory disorders in the mouth and nostril area.

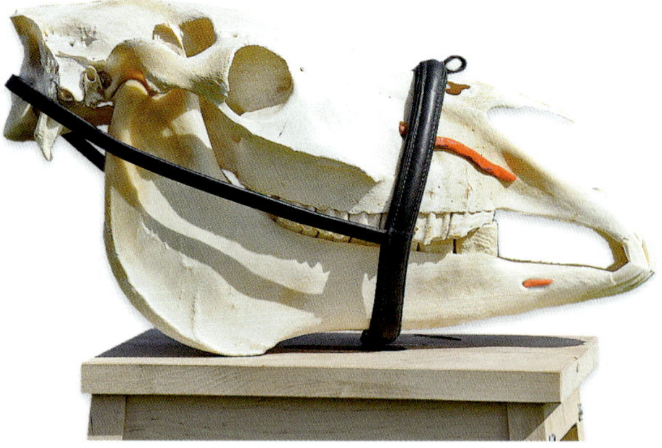

When you overtighten the noseband, you're compromising the important nerves in the horse's nose and mouth area. This goes for flash and figure-8 nosebands as well.

There's yet another problem that occurs when the bridle cavesson is overtightened; it comes about because of the strap that runs behind the horse's ears, under the crown piece, which is usually very narrow. If you make the noseband too tight, you'll cause heightened, concentrated pressure at the poll. This comes about because of the horse's cone-shaped head. The noseband constantly pulls down, with the result that the small area of the poll is under a whole lot of pressure. This permanent pressure at the poll can lead to immense pain. Because many nerves run through this area and this is also the attachment point for many muscles, a variety of symptoms will be triggered; for example, problems with contact, playing with the tongue, and/or headshaking—just to name a few.

My Tip

To test the amount of pressure that the bridle is putting on the poll, place one finger under the bridle at the poll after you have fastened the bridle overall. It should be easy to lift the bridle with one finger and possible to place two fingers between the bridle and the horse's head. A bridle with a poll piece is also advantageous, in that the bridle will be wider at the poll (to better distribute pressure) and it will also be padded.

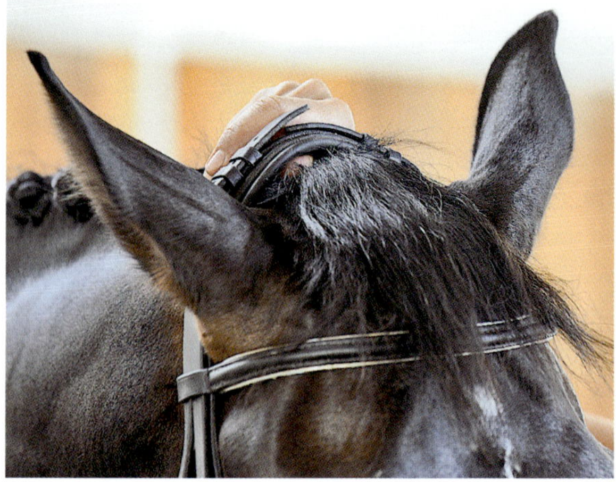

When the noseband is tightened correctly, there will also be less compression at the poll.

The same British research team that studied girths has also put bridles under the microscope. Horses were first examined in their normal bridles. Then, they were outfitted with the newly developed bridles and the results were compared. Here, too, the results were astounding.

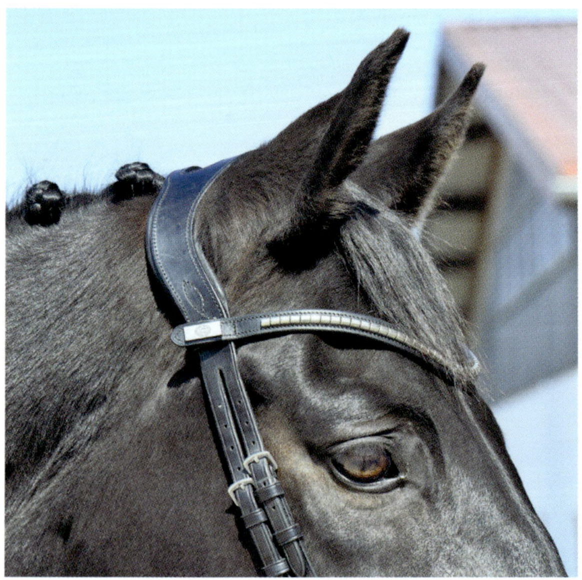

A well-fit bridle improves a horse's well-being and performance. Because of the anatomically shaped poll piece, the pressure on the poll and ears is greatly reduced.

A traditional bridle put 106 percent more pressure on the horse's poll than the newly developed bridle. On the noseband alone, there was a 47 percent difference. Interestingly, the researchers have also measured the influence of the bridle on the horse's biomechanics. They determined that when there was less pressure at the poll and on the bridge of the nose, the scope of the horse's ability to bring his forelegs forward and to flex his knee and hock joints increased by 3.5 to 4.2 percent. The data shows that there's a likely connection between less pressure on the poll and better movement. This can be attributed to the horse's improved well-being.

Auxiliary Reins

In tack shops, you'll find many types of auxiliary reins that are designed to bring the horses into a correct frame when they're being ridden or longed. Some are useful, others not so much, and some are "highly dangerous" for your horse's health.

Now, I'm going to write about a type of auxiliary reins that is very popular and explain why you should be very careful about using it, or better yet, not use it at all. I'm talking about *draw reins*. And now, I'll explain why I personally advise you to never use them.

What Happens When You Ride with Draw Reins?

Draw reins are frequently used when a rider is having problems with contact or collection. Here, it often comes down to finding a "quick solution," without "getting to the root of the problem" by resolving the rider's problems that lie beneath. In addition, draw reins are often attached much too short, which leads to increased stress throughout the horse's entire body.

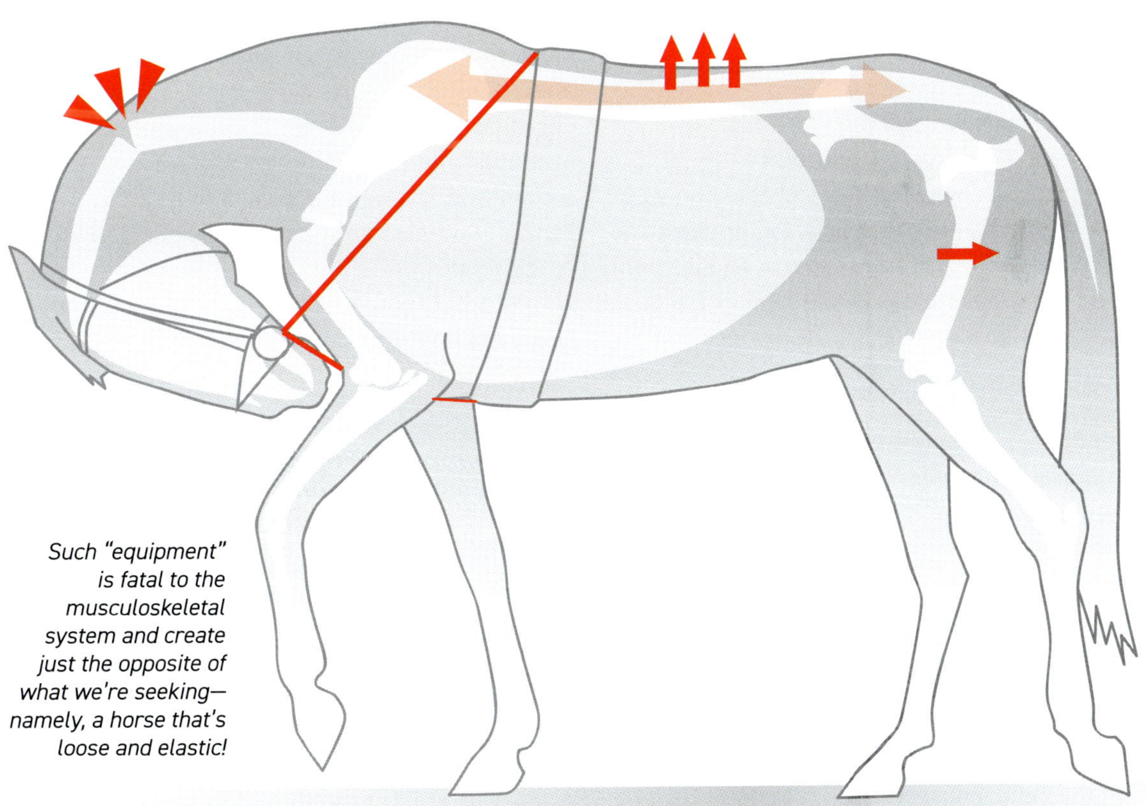

Such "equipment" is fatal to the musculoskeletal system and create just the opposite of what we're seeking— namely, a horse that's loose and elastic!

Let's begin at the head. Through the pull on the draw reins, the head comes into an incorrect frame. We also must acknowledge that all horses that are ridden with draw reins go too deep and are behind the vertical. The forward-downward stretch and the ability of the back to actively swing are, therefore, being limited more than promoted.

The nuchal ligament is being pulled upon. This pull goes farther over the supraspinal ligament. The back lifts, yes, but the sacrum is being pulled too much toward the front. The pelvis tips and goes flat. What happens to the hind legs? Because of the tipped pelvis, there's a negative stretch stimulus on the strong flexor muscles of the hindquarters, and the hind legs are, therefore, pulled toward the back. This causes accumulated tension in the *ischium* muscle, the *longissimus* muscle of the back, and the *gluteus medius* (trunk extensor muscles). As a result, the loin and abdominal muscles (*trunk flexors*) are no longer able to raise the pelvis, and the hind legs cannot step up and under. Both correct collection and flexion of the joints of the hindquarters are now impossible.

For this reason, the horse falls onto the forehand. The *pectorals* and *ventral serratus* muscles of the forehand are overstressed and tense up, so the forelegs lose the ability to absorb shock. The muscles of the forehand responsible for bringing the legs forward no longer have natural engagement and can't bring the forelegs forward much. Because of the lack of shock absorption, the tendons and ligaments of the lower forelimbs are strained.

The cervical spine becomes kinked in way that is physiologically unnatural, which causes tension and blockages in the small, deep muscles. This can cause irritation where the nerves leave the spinal column, as the incorrect positioning of the spine causes the spinal canal to become too narrow. Over time, this can lead to instability of the spine and/or calcifications on the ligaments as these are constantly overstretched. In addition, inflammation that eventually becomes calcification on the nuchal ligament can result.

When the horse is ridden with the line from his forehead to his nose behind the vertical, the rider is automatically locking the first cervical vertebra opposite the head. Therefore, a sideways longitudinal bend is no longer possible. The horse makes a compensatory movement, in that he turns his whole head between the 1st and 2nd cervical vertebrae when asked to turn.

The more the rider pulls/positions her horse's neck in hyperflexion, the more vertebrae become locked. This means, the mobility of the spine is greatly reduced.

Fact: A horse that is ridden behind the vertical can never demonstrate a true longitudinal bend in the neck.

Now I'm going to present an exercise to help you understand something close to what the horse feels: bend forward and try to touch your toes with your fingertips. But, with your current level of flexibility, you only reach your knees. And then I come along (I'm acting like draw reins) and push your neck and upper body down. I hold you in this position over a long period of time, without a break, without a chance to recover. My goal is to make you more flexible. Can you just imagine how painful this is?

With this background information in mind, can you justify the improper use of draw reins?

Fact: The painful hyperflexion can also take place without using draw reins. But, the resulting symptoms and injuries are just the same.

Auxiliary Reins for Support

The word "auxiliary" means "providing help or support." And, there are auxiliary reins that can actually be "helpful." These may include side reins and sliding side reins like Vienna reins and Lauffer reins. They help correct the horse, improving contact and trust in the rider's hands. In addition, these reins can be helpful for inexperienced riders. They can achieve better control and/or concentrate more fully on their seat. As your horse's rider and trainer, you must be clear what purpose you are trying to achieve by using these reins. And, of course, you should also know how to attach these reins correctly, otherwise your "helping" reins will become "forcing" reins.

It's important that the auxiliary reins are attached correctly in order to avoid cramming the horse together and forcing him to work statically. The horse must not be restricted in his natural movement. Only then can the rider experience and maintain the feeling of *losgelassenheit*.

> *Fact: Incorrectly applied auxiliary reins can cause many problems from tension and strain all the way to doing enormous damage to the musculoskeletal system.*

Teeth

Dental problems can cause injury to the gums. In addition, they cause digestive problems, neck and back pain to the point of lameness, behavioral changes, problems under saddle, and drop in performance. I recommend you have your horse's teeth checked by a vet or equine dentist at least once a year in order to avoid the problems listed here.

Shoeing

A shoeing that is no longer suitable will inevitably lead to incorrect stress on the body and it can also cause a change in the horse's way of going: stumbling, shortened strides, or uneven rhythm. It can even get to the point of causing accumulated tension in the neck and back areas. Later, there will also be injuries and changes to ligaments, tendons, joint capsules, and joint surfaces of the affected limbs.

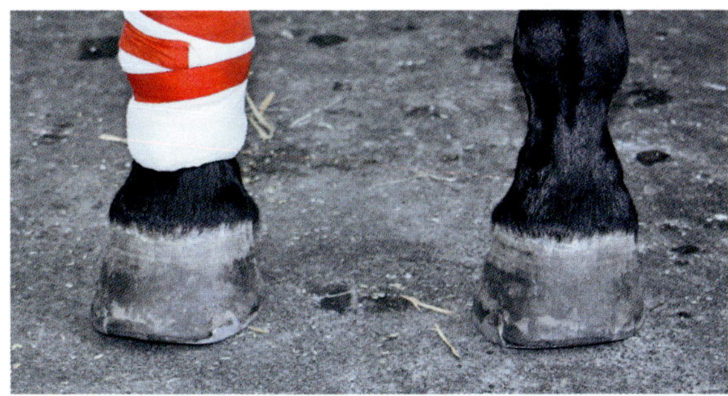

To avoid injury and tension of the musculoskeletal system, good farrier care is indispensable. This horse's inside walls are somewhat too long so the horse has to roll over the outer edges.

The horse should be shod every 6 to 8 weeks. To check the shoeing, you should observe how the horse sets down and weights his hooves, both when he's standing still and walking. In between farrier visits, you should monitor the shoes for correct position and size. The hoof should never be larger than the shoe.

Many horse owners prefer their horses go barefoot. This is definitely better for the mechanics of the hoof, but then not every surface is made for a horse to walk barefoot, and not every horse has the right hoof quality for this. Again and again, I treat horses that are suffering from back problems, and that have lost their looseness and impulsion because their feet hurt. Try for yourself to walk barefoot down a gravel path—you certainly won't walk very quickly, and your movement definitely won't be very relaxed. Horses' feet are sensitive, despite their walled hooves, and some footing will cause them to tense and stiffen.

Mounting

The mounting block: in England, you would be scolded for trying to mount a horse without one, and in Germany, you will get laughed at for using one. How come?

The English have caught on!

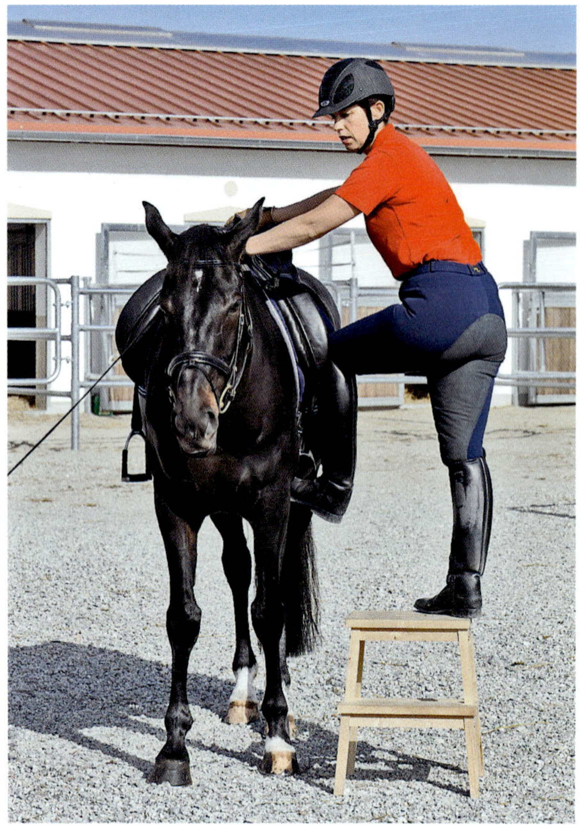

To avoid strain on the horse's withers and on the saddle itself, the best policy for every riding facility is that riders mount from a block.

If you once again consider the anatomy of the saddle area, it will be clear to why we need help when we mount up.

In the anatomy section, I described how long the spinous processes at the withers can be and that the vertebral joints that belong to them tend to be really small. When you mount up from the ground, the effect is that the long levers of the spinous processes put an uncomfortable stretch and immense pressure on the small joints. In addition, nerves run in between every vertebra, which control a section of the horse's body: through the uncomfortable pressure and stretch, these can be compromised. Pain is transmitted outward.

You're not only damaging the joints and nerve pathways, but also the soft tissue (the *trapezius* muscle). You're causing more pressure on the right side (opposite from where you get on). Here, I often also feel swelling or old scar tissue. It's no wonder that so many horses suffer from immobility and muscular pain around their withers!

What Can You Change?

When you sit down, it's important to make sure the horse gets only a vertical pressure near his withers. You can only achieve this by getting on from a mounting block and/or having a person on the other side who applies pressure to the off-side stirrup to counterweight the saddle as you mount. Getting on from a block is not only beneficial to the horse, it's also easier for you and a relief to your entire body.

Of course, this applies in reverse when you are dismounting—don't put your whole weight in just one stirrup iron. Your horse, your sciatic nerve, and your saddle will thank you for it. Let others laugh at you!

Hint: Don't forget that the saddle tree can also become altered or twisted due to mounting.

Warming Up

Take time to warm up and relax your horse. These are easy tasks that prevent injury and tension in the musculoskeletal system. As described in chapter 1 (p. 1), you must prepare the musculoskeletal system for the stress of work. There are no true athletes who train or compete without warming up first. I recommend walking your horse for the first 15 minutes of your warm-up. That's a long time, but it pays off! This also applies to horses that are being lunged, worked at liberty in the arena, or being free jumped.

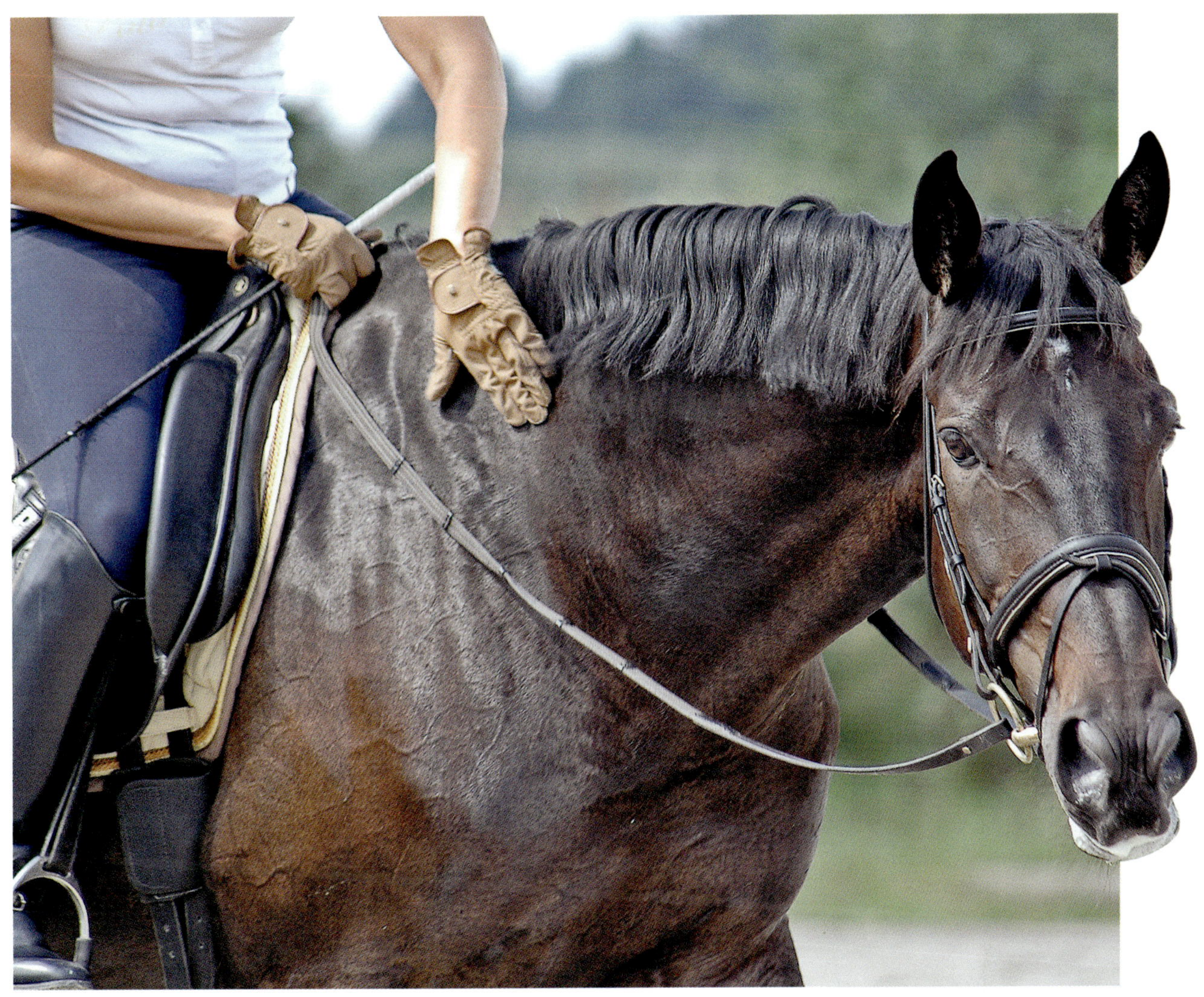

Cooling Down

In order to relax the musculoskeletal system and calm the horse's mind after work, you need to walk for about 10 minutes. Giving him this time to walk on a loose rein is a wonderful stretching exercise for the entire musculoskeletal system. There are riders and trainers who just stand still during the cool-down. It's certainly good for your horse's mind to leave him alone for a moment, but it's no gift to his musculoskeletal system. The effective muscle pump (the tensing and relaxing of the muscles that take place during movement) will be shut down this way, so that metabolism is no longer optimal and the musculature becomes cool and stiff. When you've watched high-level athletes perform, you've certainly observed that they never just stand still after they're done performing. They constantly stay moving so that they don't cool down too fast and get stiff.

The Skeleton

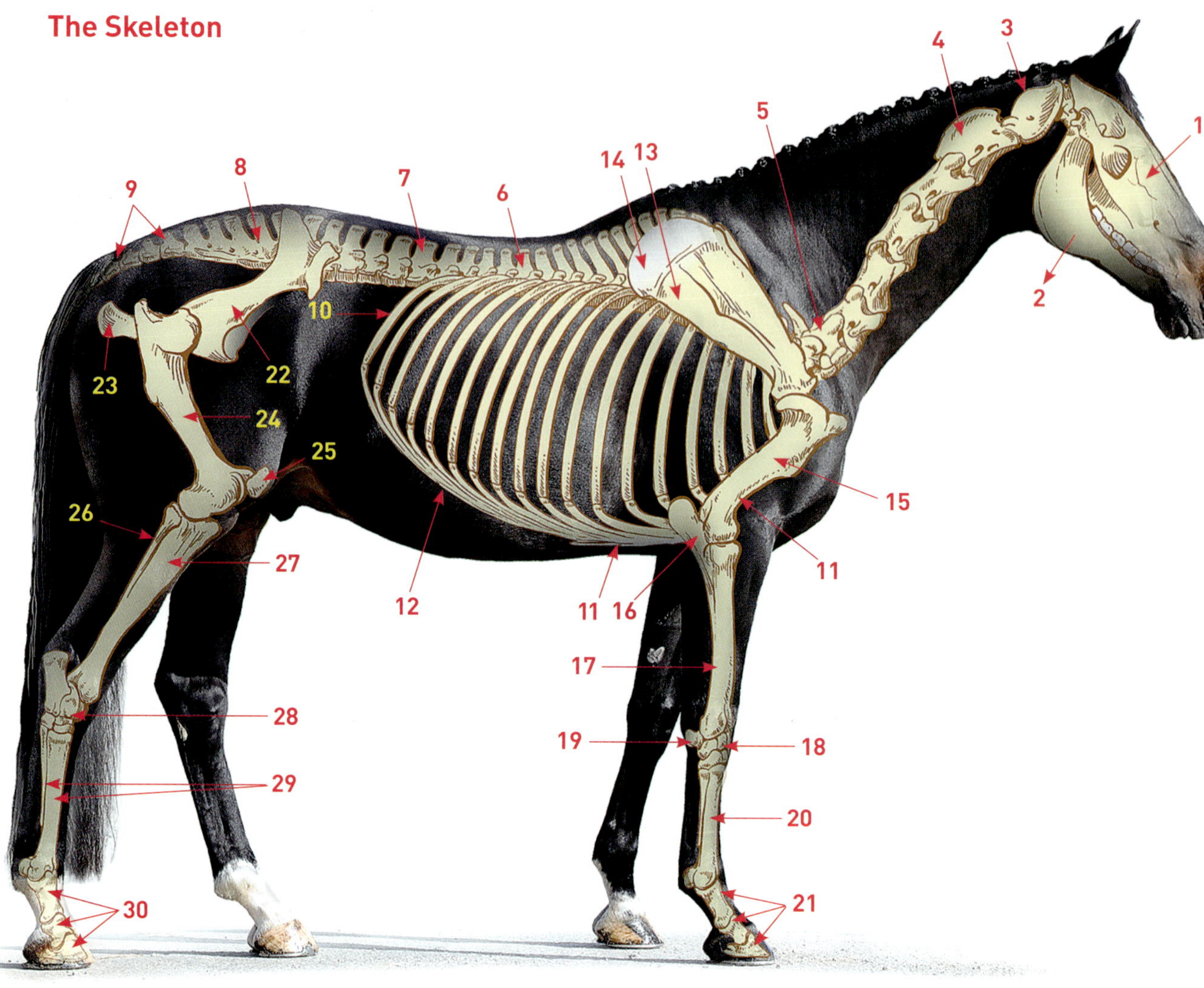

1	Upper Jaw	*Maxilla*
2	Lower Jaw	*Mandibula*
3	First Cervical Vertebra (C1)	*Atlas*
4	Second Cervical Vertebra (C2)	*Axis*
5	Seventh Cervical Vertebra (C7)	*Vertebra cervicalis*
6	Fourteenth Thoracic Vertebra (T14)	*Vertebra thoracica*
7	First Lumbar Vertebra (L1)	*Vertebra lumbalis*
8	Sacrum	
9	Coccygeal Vertebra	*Vertebrae cuadales*
10	Eighteenth Rib	*Costa*
11	Breastbone	*Sternum*
12	Bottom edge of rib cage	*Costal arch*
13	Shoulder blade	*Scapula*
14	Scapular cartilage	*Cartilago scapulae*
15	Upper arm	*Humerus*

16	Ulna	
17	Radius	
18	Knee joint (carpus)	*Ossa carpi*
19	Accessory carpal	*Os Pisiforme*
20	Cannon bone (front)	*Ossa metacarpalia*
21	Bones of the foot	*Ossa digiti manus*
22	Hip bone (ilium)	*Os coxae*
23	Seat bone (ischium)	*Os ischiadicum*
24	Thigh bone (femur)	*Os femoris*
25	Patella	
26	Fibula	
27	Tibia	
28	Hock	*Ossa tarsi*
29	Rear cannon and splint bone	*Ossa metatarsalia*
30	Phalanx bones	*Ossa digiti pedis*

Deep Musculature

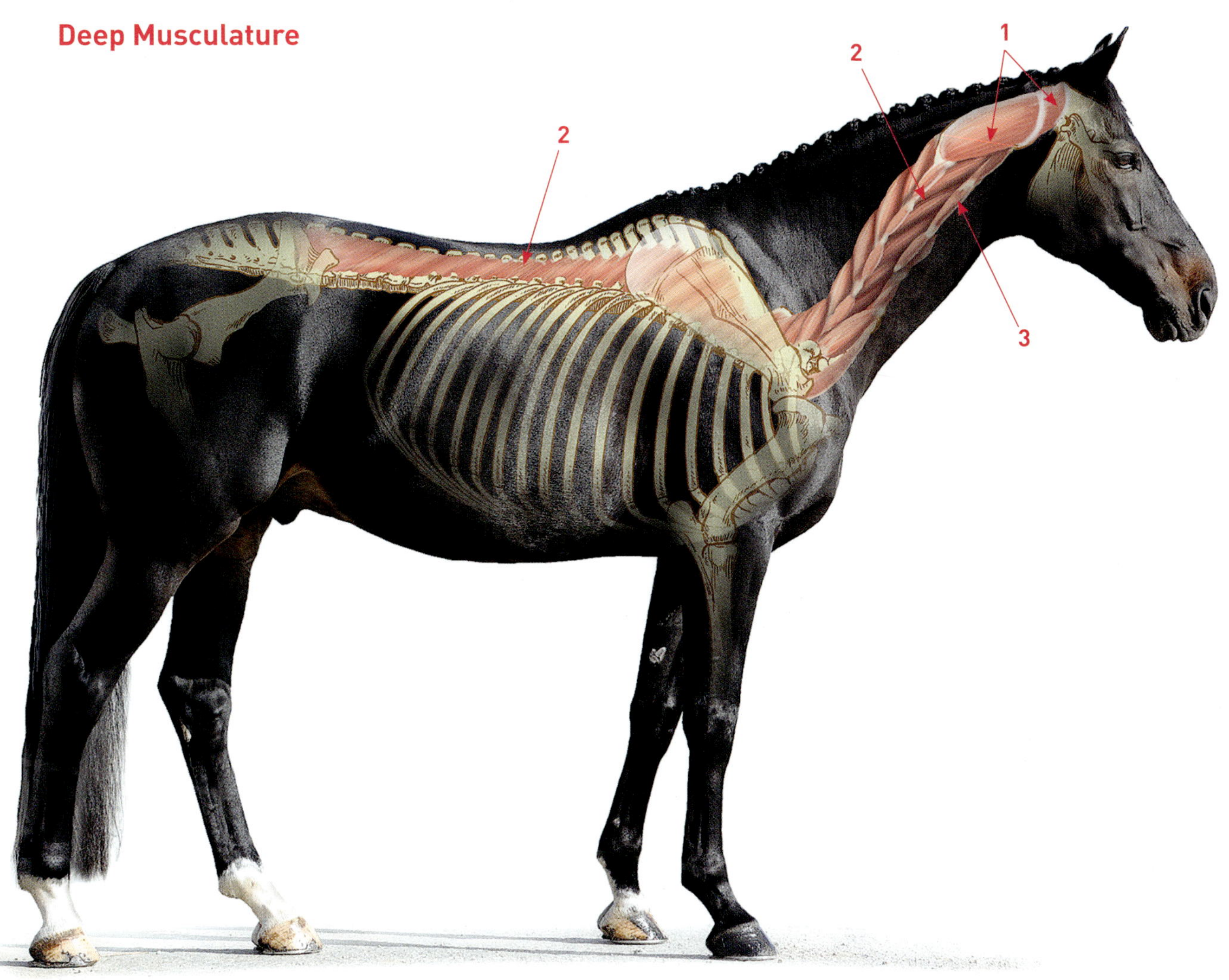

1 Deep muscles of the poll   *M. obliquus capitis cranialis*
                                         M. obliquus capitis caudalis

2 Multi-part spine musculature   *Mm. multifidi*

3 Cervical intertransverse muscles   *Mm. intertransversarii*

Middle Muscle Layer

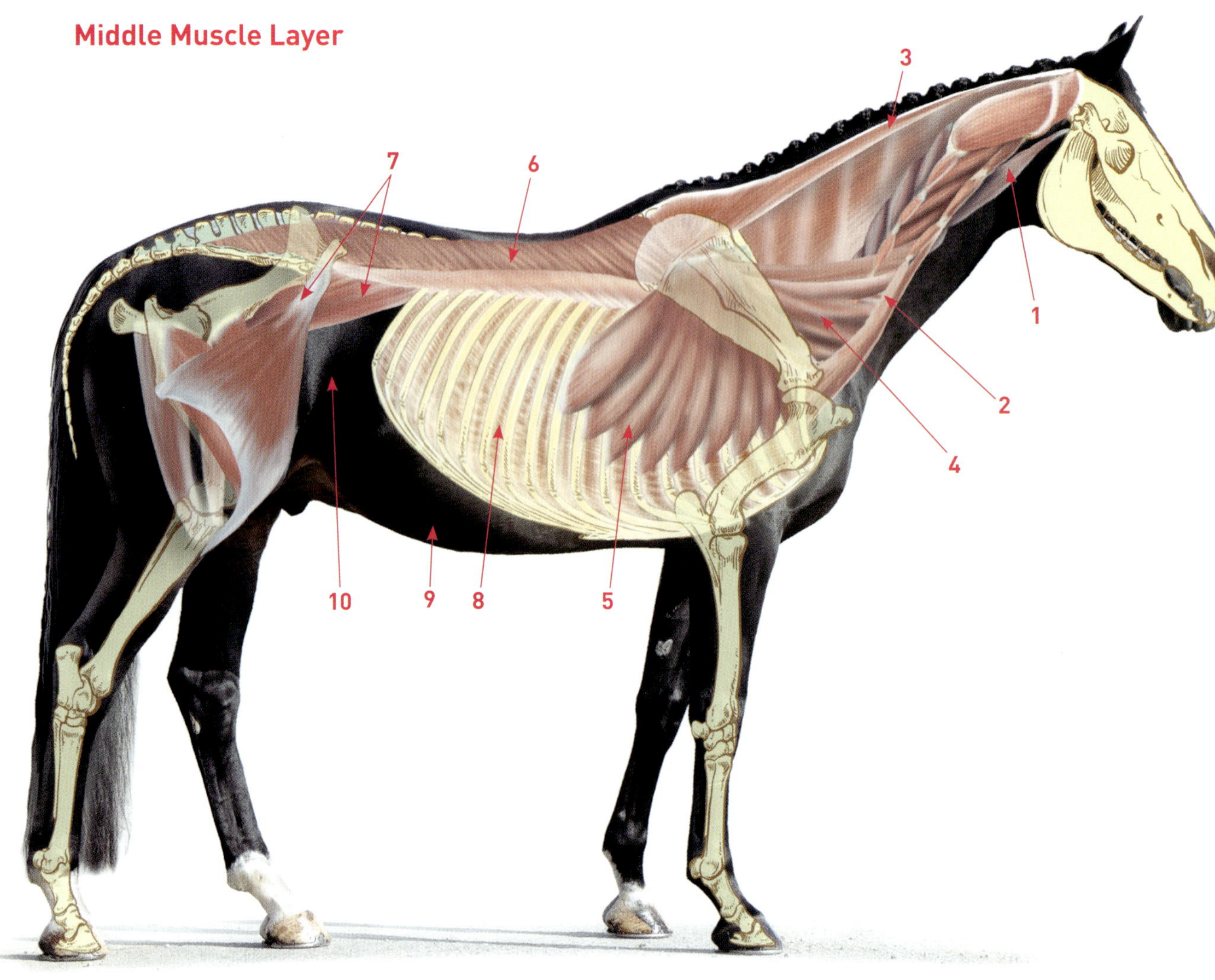

1	Long muscle of the head	*M. longus capitis*
2	Scalene muscles	*Mm. scalenii*
3	Rhomboid	*M. rhomboideus*
4	Ventral Serratus (neck portion)	*M. serrates ventralis cervicis*
5	Ventral Serratus (thoracic portion)	*M. serrates ventralis thoracis*
6	Longissimus Dorsi (long back muscle)	*M. longissimus dorsi*
7	Lumbar/loin muscle	*M. iliopsoas*
8	Intercostal muscles	*M. intercostales externi*
9	Rectus abdominis	*M. rectus abdominis*
10	Transversus abdominis	*M. transversus abdominis*

Superficial Muscle Layer

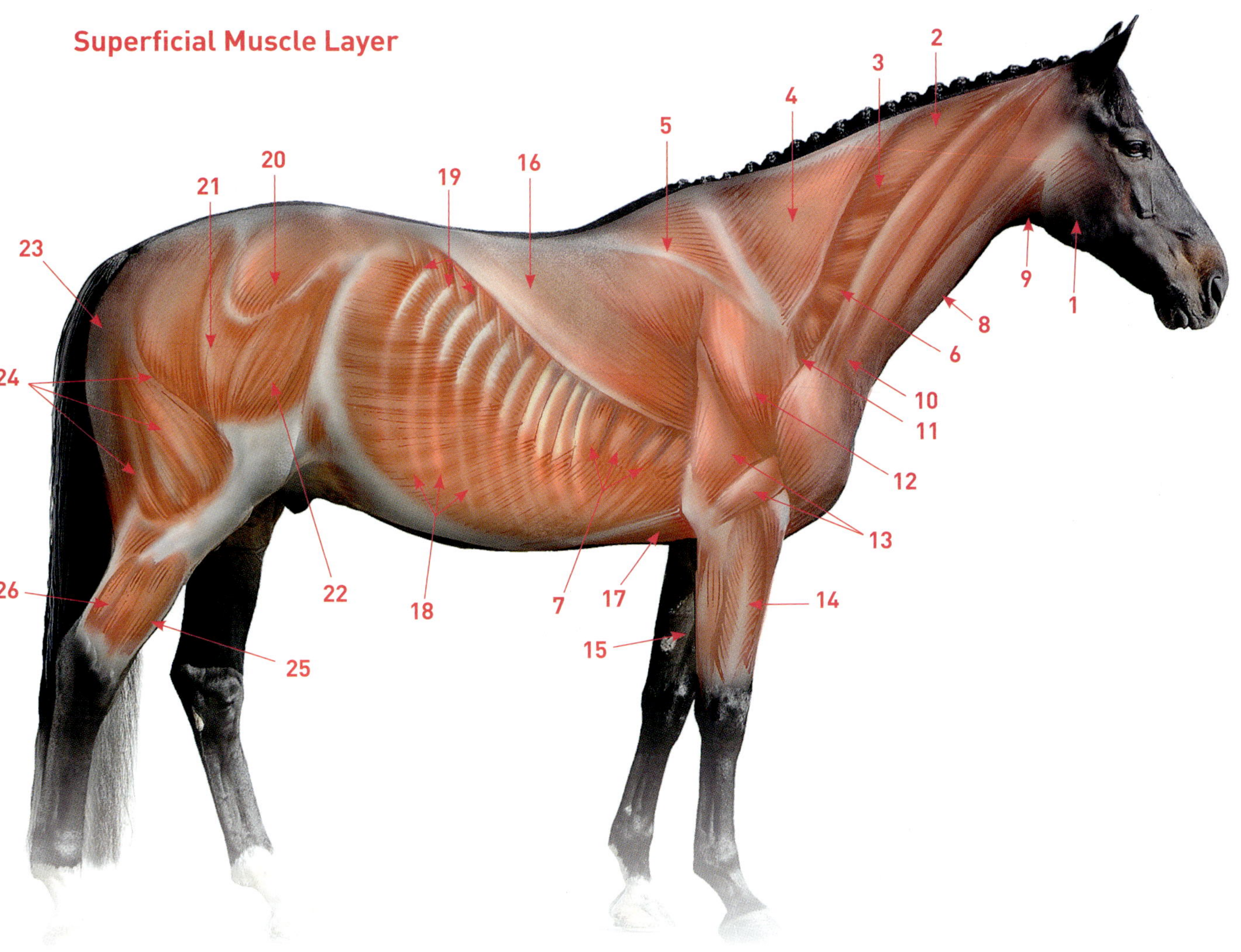

1	Masseter	*M. masseter*	**14**	Common digital extensor	*Mm. extensorii*
2	Rhomboid	*M. rhomboideus*	**15**	Superficial flexor	*Mm. flexorii*
3	Splenius	*M. splenius*	**16**	Latissimus dorsi	*M. latissimus dorsi*
4	Trapezoid (neck portion)	*M. trapezius cervicis*	**17**	Pectoral	*M. pectoralis profondus*
5	Trapezoid (thoracic portion)	*M. trapezius thoracis*	**18**	Oblique Abdominal	*M. obliquus externus abdominis*
6	Ventral serratus (neck)	*M. serratus ventralis cervicis*			
7	Ventral serratus (thoracic)	*M. serratus ventralis thoracis*	**19**	Dorsal Serratus	*M. serratus dorsalis caudalis*
			20	Gluteus medius	*M. gluteus medius*
8	Sternomandibular	*M. sternomandibularis*	**21**	Superficial gluteal muscles	*M. gluteus superficialis*
9	Sternohyoideus	*M. sternohyoideus*	**22**	Tensor Fascia Lata	*M. tensor fasciae latae*
10	Brachiocephalicus	*M. brachiocephalicus*	**23**	Semitendinosus (hamstring)	*M. semitendinosus*
11	Supraspinatus	*M. supraspinatus*	**24**	Biceps Femoris	*M. biceps femoris*
12	Deltoid	*M. deltoideus*	**25**	Long digital extensor	*Extensoren*
13	Triceps	*M. triceps*	**26**	Deep digital flexor	*Flexoren*

Fascia

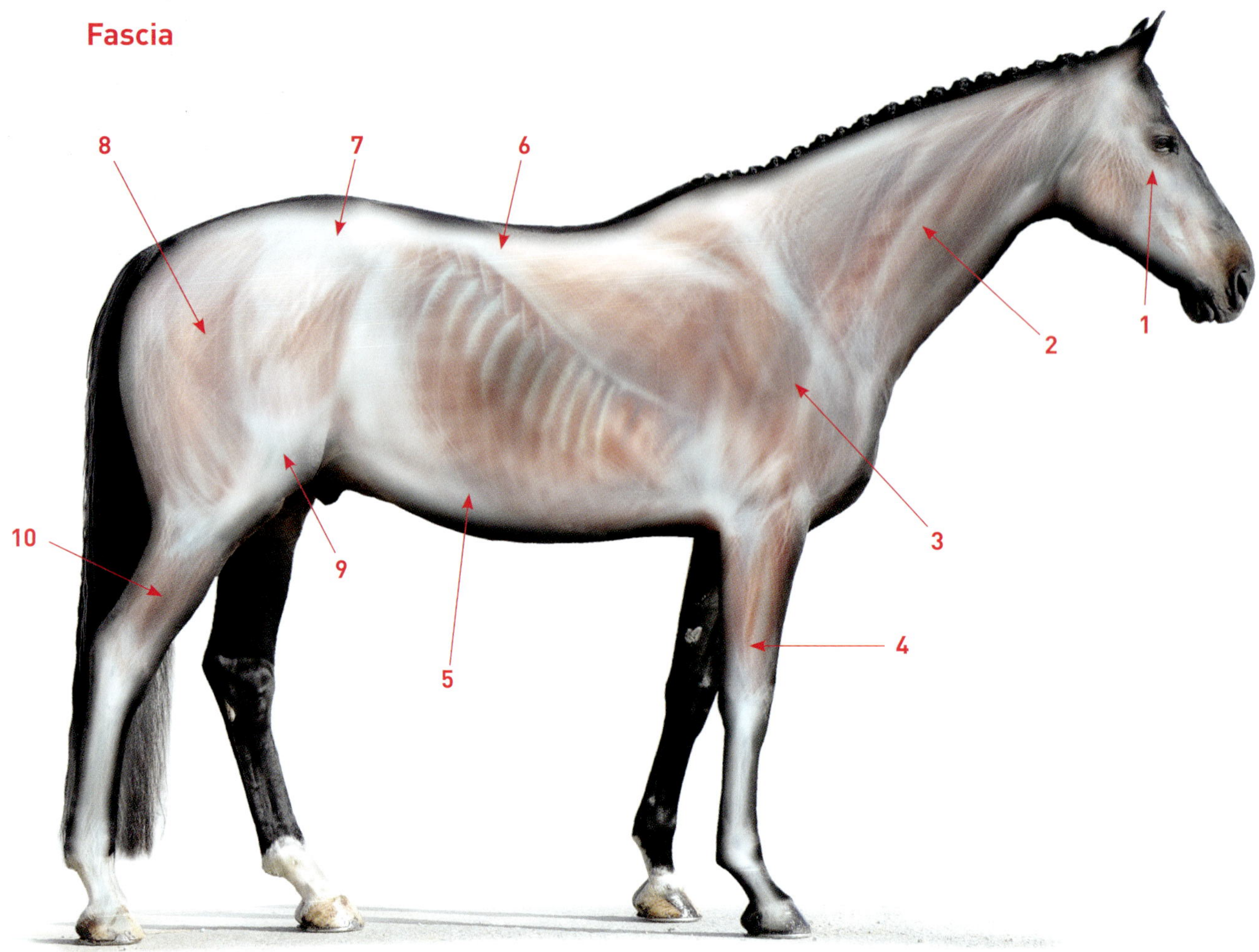

1 Superficial fascia of the head
2 Superficial fascia of the neck
3 Superficial fascia of the shoulder
4 Superficial fascia of the arm
5 Superficial fascia of the abdomen
6 Superficial fascia of the back
7 Superficial fascia of the croup
8 Superficial fascia of the hip
9 Superficial fascia of the stifle
10 Superficial fascia of the lower leg

Glossary

Abduction .... A movement of a limb or other part of the body away from the body and/or the axis of a limb.

Acetabulum .... Hip socket.

Adduction .... A movement of a limb or other part of the body toward the body and/or axis of a limb.

Adhesion .... Fasciae sticking together closely in a certain area; causes loss of movement.

Agonist .... A muscle that interplays with its counterpart (antagonist) to execute a specific movement.

Antagonist .... The counterpart of an agonist muscle.

Arthritis .... Degenerative joint disease.

Ataxia .... A coordination disorder.

Atrophy .... Muscle "wasting"/ decrease in muscle mass.

Axis .... The second cervical vertebra (C2).

Biomechanics .... Study of the musculoskeletal system.

Blockage .... A restriction/limitation of movement.

Bursa .... Synovial sac.

Bursitis .... An acute or chronic inflammation of the synovial bursa.

Capillaries .... Small blood vessels.

Cartilage .... Firm but flexible connective tissue.

Caudal .... At or near the tail or toward the hindquarters.

Cervical .... Belonging to the neck region.

CNS .... Central Nervous System.

Cranial .... At or near the skull, toward the head of the horse.

Diaphragm .... A major respiratory muscle.

Dorsal .... The back of a body part.

Edema .... Swelling.

Extremities .... Limbs.

Extension .... Stretching.

Fascia .... A thin layer of tissue that covers a muscle .

Flexion .... Contracting.

Golgi Apparatus .... Muscle spindle (sensory receptor).

Hematoma .... When injured blood vessels bleed into body tissues, otherwise known as a bruise or "black and blue" mark.

Iliosacral Joint .... Sacroiliac joint.

Knee joint .... Carpal joint of the front leg.

Lactate .... Lactic acid, produced in muscles during strenuous exercise.

Lateral .... Away from the center of the body, sideways, positioned to the side.

Lateral flexion .... Turning to the side.

Ligaments .... Dand of connective tissue.

Ligamentum funiculus nuchae .... Nuchal ligament/laminar portion of nuchal ligament.

Lumbalis .... Lumbar.

Luxation .... A dislocation/separation of the joint surfaces.

M. (musculus) biceps femoris .... *Biceps femoris.*

M. brachiocephalicus .... *Brachiocephalicus.*

M. iliopsoas .... Loin muscles/*iliopsoas.*

M. gluteus medius .... Superficial gluteal muscles.

M. obliquus capitis caudalis .... An oblique muscle of the head that lies between C1 and C2 (caudal).

M. obliquus capitis cranialis .... An oblique muscle of the head that lies between the head and C1 (cranial).

M. obliquus externus abdominis .... Outer oblique abdominal muscle.

Glossary

M. obliquus internus abdominis	Inner oblique abdominal muscle.
M. latissimus dorsi	A broad muscle of the back.
M. longissimus cervicis	The neck segment of the body's longest muscle.
M. longissimus dorsi	The longest muscle of the body (the back muscle).
M. quadriceps	Quadriceps.
M. rectus abdominis	Rectus abdominis.
M. rhomboideus	Rhomboid.
M. semimembranosus	Semimembranosus muscle.
M. semispinalis cervicis	Semispinalis muscle, neck segment.
M. semitendinosus	Semitendinosus muscle (hamstring).
M. serratus ventralis cervicis	Ventral serratus (neck).
M. serratus ventralis thoracis	Ventral serratus (thoracic).
M. splenius	Splenius muscle.
M. transversus abdominis	Transversus abdominis.
M. trapezius	Trapezius.
M. triceps brachii	Triceps.
Medial	Positioned toward the center of the body.
Membrana synovialis	Specialized tissue that lines joint surfaces.
Meniscus	A cartilage disc in a joint, for example in the stifle.
Mm. (Musculi) abdominales	Abdominals.
Mm. adductores	Inner adductors.
Mm. extensores	Muscles that stretch/extend.
Mm. flexores	Muscles that bend/contract.
Mm. glutaei	Croup muscles.
Mm. intercostales	Intercostal muscles (between the ribs).
Mm. intertransversarii	Cervical intertransverse muscles.
Mm. pectorales	Pectorals.
Mm. scalenii	Scalene muscles.
Muscular Insertion	The point where a muscle attaches to the body, oriented away from the middle of the body.
Muscle Origin	The point where a muscle attaches to the body, oriented toward the middle of the body.
Myo	Of or relating to muscles.
Myogelosis	Muscular knots/hardenings.
Palpate	Examine by touch.
PNS	Peripheral Nervous System.
Prevention	Avoiding injury or disorder.
Proximal	Oriented toward the center of the body.
Rotation	Turning.
Scapula	Shoulder blade.
Subluxation	A slight misalignment of the joint surfaces.
Synergist Muscles	Muscles that work together to generate movement in the same direction.
Synovial	Joint fluid.
Tendinitis	Tendon inflammation.
Tendo	Of or relating to the tendons.
TENS Therapy	Transcutaneous Electrical Nerve Stimulation therapy.
Therapy	Treatment.
Thoracic	Area of the breastbone and rib cage.
Thrombosis	A blood clot in the circulatory system.
Ventral	Positioned toward or on the abdomen, on the abdominal side.

Acknowledgments

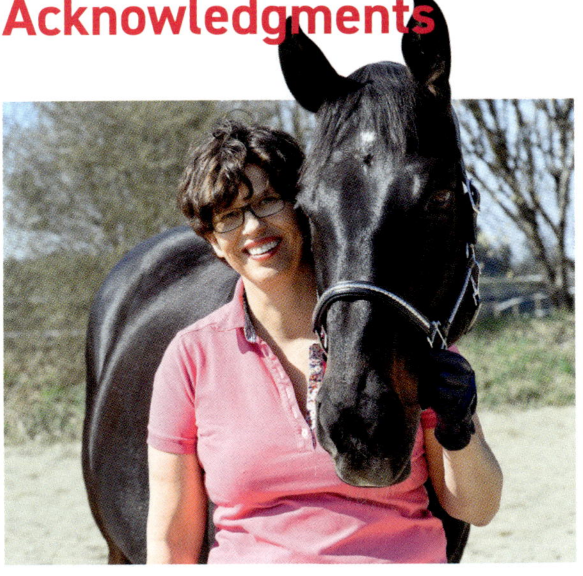

I would like to thank...

Gaby Pfleiderer-Ehrl, above all. You did such a super job "translating" my "Norwegian-German" into German (and I know that was hard work!). You also kept me motivated to keep writing. Without your enormous help, this book would never have come to be. MANY THANKS, GABY! Starting with the fourth edition my thanks go to Karin Ottemann, Hannover. You supported me exceptionally well with the writing. Thanks to your horse knowledge and curiosity, you "discovered" many places where the text wasn't clear and the collaboration with you was just so much fun!

I also must thank all the horse owners who have allowed me to handle their horses. Thank you for your trust in physical therapy. Even after many years of practicing physical therapy, I'm still fascinated by how to help horses and riders. Each individual horse responds differently and with every treatment, there's a new challenge. I'm so happy to get lots of positive feedback, which is truly motivating to me.

Thanks to those who have helped me along the way and support me today in the development of my own riding knowledge—above all Lars Kjörsvik (Norway), and Isle Leeb and Johannes Grupen (both from Munich). You've managed to tie my knowledge of biomechanics together with riding instruction in a more intense way. And theory doesn't work unless applied to practice. A huge thank you to my friend and trainer, Petra Huml, from Herbrontshausen. Every riding lesson with you is an "aha moment." From you, I've come to understand how much influence a rider has on the movement of the horse.

My colleague Anna Großler from Hamburg. When faced with problems, I count on your clear vision to help me sleep at night.

Thanks, too, to Michaela Grau, from Baldham, and Eleni Junkernheinrich, from Poing, for the daily support in our practice and shop. Because of your support, I was able to concentrate on this book.

To the Tristl Family from Ingelsberg, near Munich, thank you for allowing the photo shoot to take place at your beautiful equestrian facility.

The whole Pferdeklinik Parsdorf team near Munich, with whom I've been working together for so many years now. This teamwork has made it possible to provide first-class care and treatment.

To my sister, Anne Gry. You have guided me in the right direction.

To Nadieh Abayan-Stoef, for your help with structuring the section on biomechanics.

Thanks to those whose hard work led to this book's successful design: Dr. Carla Mattis, from FN*verlag*; Jeanne Kloepfer, from Lindenfels; Maximillian Schreiner, from Unterstall; Ute Schmoll, from Bad Schwalbach; Dr. Petra Smital, from Munich and Dr. Beatrice Dülffer-Schneitzer, from Steinbach.

Thank you to my "two- and four-legged friends," and especially to my horse, Sir Colin, who is always so patient when it comes to photos.

Index

Page numbers in *italics* indicate illustrations.